T0224678

Key Themes in Health and Social Care

This revised and expanded second edition of *Key Themes in Health and Social Care* is a learning resource for students in health and social care. It provides an overview of foundational issues and core themes in the field and introduces key areas of debate, moving from an introductory level to in-depth discussion as the book progresses. Divided into three parts:

- the first part sets the scene, addressing introductory psychology and sociology, social policy, equality and diversity, skills for practice, and working with people
- the second part considers key themes such as mental health and wellbeing; management of services; the relationship between place and wellbeing; research in health and social care; and person-centred interventions
- the third part looks at discrete areas of practice such as mental health; ageing, leading and managing health and social care; working with vulnerable populations; and health promotion

Each chapter begins with an outline of the content and learning outcomes and includes reflective exercises to allow students to reflect on what they have read, review their learning and consolidate their understanding. Time-pressed readers wanting to 'dip into' the book for relevant areas can do so but, read from cover to cover, the book provides a comprehensive introduction to the key areas of contemporary health and social care practice. It will be particularly helpful for students undertaking health and social care undergraduate and foundation degrees.

Adam Barnard (PhD) has worked in Higher Education for over twenty years. During this time, he has worked with a variety of students and learners across educational contexts. He is programme leader for Professional Doctorates in Social Practice at Nottingham Trent University. His latest works are *Developing Professional Practice in Health and Social Care* (2019), *Key Themes in Health and Social Care* published by Routledge in 2011, and *Value Base of Social Work and Social Care* with Open University Press (2008). He is involved in the leadership and management of research in social science including ethics, governance, supervision and development. He is working on a book on developing reflective practice in Health and Social Care. He is committed to challenging policy, research and practice that does not contribute to ethical and value-based professionalism of frontline workers.

Verusca Calabria (PhD) is a Senior Lecturer in Health and Social Care in the Department of Social Work, Care and Community, School of Social Sciences, Nottingham Trent University, Nottingham (UK). Verusca is an interdisciplinary qualitative researcher working across the Social Sciences and Humanities. Her PhD research combined participatory-action-research with oral history to explore the transition from institutional to community care practices. Her research interests include the history of mental health care in the UK, patient and public involvement in health and social care, oral history, participatory action research, researcher vulnerability. She has presented her research at several international conferences and co-convenes the NTU cross-faculty Oral History Network.

Louise Griffiths is a Senior Lecturer in Social Work, Care and Community at Nottingham Trent University. Louise's research interests include prison peer support with particular attention paid to the Prison Listener Scheme and the self-harm behaviour of prisoners. Louise's PhD thesis explored the Prison Listener Scheme's contribution to the reduction in self-harm within the female prison estate. Louise has a multi-disciplinary background as she completed her MSc in Psychology and PhD in Criminology at Nottingham Trent University.

Bailey Foster is a Research Assistant in the Social Work, Care and Community department at Nottingham Trent University. Before entering academia, Bailey worked as a Teaching Assistant across schools in Nottinghamshire, whilst also completing an MSc in Forensic Psychology. This has led Bailey to be interested in inequalities within the justice system for people with additional needs. As Bailey is a researcher across the Social Work, Care and Community department, she has also worked on projects relating to child sexual exploitation and transitional support, consent education and mental health.

Key Themes in Health and Social Care

A Companion to Learning

Second Edition

Edited by Adam Barnard, Verusca Calabria, and Louise Griffiths

Editorial Assistant Bailey Foster

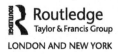

Routledge
Taylor & Francis Group

LONDON AND NEW YORK

Cover image: 'Teach kids how far a little care can go'.
Credit: PeopleImages © Getty Images

Second edition published 2023
by Routledge
4 Park Square, Milton Park, Abingdon, Oxon, OX14 4RN

and by Routledge
605 Third Avenue, New York, NY 10158

Routledge is an imprint of the Taylor & Francis Group, an informa business

First edition published by Routledge, 2010

British Library Cataloguing-in-Publication Data
A catalogue record for this book is available from the British Library

Library of Congress Cataloguing-in-Publication Data
Names: Barnard, Adam, editor.
Title: Key themes in health and social care : a companion to learning / edited by Adam Barnard, Verusca Calabria and Louise Griffiths ; editorial assistant Bailey Foster.
Description: 2nd edition. | Abingdon, Oxon ; New York, NY : Routledge, 2023. | Includes bibliographical references and index.
Identifiers: LCCN 2022044707 (print) | LCCN 2022044708 (ebook) | (ebk)
Subjects: LCSH: Medical care. | Medical policy. | Social service.
Classification: LCC RA393 .K49 2023 (print) | LCC RA393 (ebook) |
DDC 362.1--dc23/eng/20221007
LC record available at https://lccn.loc.gov/2022044707
LC ebook record available at https://lccn.loc.gov/2022044708

ISBN: 978-0-367-52934-5 (hbk)
ISBN: 978-0-367-52932-1 (pbk)
ISBN: 978-1-003-07987-3 (ebk)

DOI: 10.4324/9781003079873

Typeset in Sabon
by MPS Limited, Dehradun

Contents

Figures

Tables

Contributors

Amy Allen has 10 years of experience in teaching and course coordination. She has delivered a wide range of health and social care courses in colleges, schools and higher education settings. Amy is the Course Leader for the FdSc Assistant Practitioner in Health Apprenticeship and module leader for Managing Health and Social Care.

Jessica Arnold is a registered Mental health Nurse and holds a Masters of Science (MSc) in the specialism of Mental Health Nursing. She was chosen to be a Scholar with the Royal College of Nursing for her graduate nurse training and undertook this at the University of Nottingham. Jessica has a wealth of experience being a clinical supervisor, mentor and practice assessor to student nurses (mental health and learning disability) in clinical practice throughout her nursing career.

Melanie Bailey has worked in a range of Health and Care settings over the last 10 years which included Primary care, Mental Health and Secondary care. After gaining practical experience in her specialised field of public Health and Alcohol misuse Melanie moved in to full time Academia in January 2021. She has taught on a variety of health related courses including Undergraduate and Postgraduate at a variety of institutions across England including the Health and Social Care Degree at Nottingham Trent University.

Monique Duncan has recently graduated from Nottingham Trent University with a BA (Hons) Health and Social Care degree and currently works as a Support Worker within the speciality of Acquired Brain injury. Prior to this, Monique worked within the speciality of Mental Health. Monique is an Alumni Fellow at Nottingham Trent University and shall be returning to study MSc in Paramedic Science.

Dolores Ellidge (MA, RGN, RHV) currently works as a senior lecturer in nursing at the University of Lincoln and Associate Lecturer with The Open University working on both nursing and health and social care programmes. She is a Fellow of the Higher Education Academy. Dolores qualified as an adult nurse in 1986, as a Specialist Community Public Health Practitioner (Health Visiting) in 1997 and gained a Masters in Online and Distance Learning in 2018.

Alice Lee completed her BA (Hons) Health and Social Care at Nottingham Trent University. The degree is for people wanting to work in a helping, restorative and supportive capacity to a range of people and service users. Alice is starting her journey in health and social care.

Richard Machin is a Senior Lecturer in Social Work and Health at Nottingham Trent University. He teaches social policy across a range of undergraduate and postgraduate courses including Health and Social Care, Social Work, Public Health and Public Policy. His research focuses on the impact of policy on marginalised groups in society, and he has published in a wide range of academic and professional journals.

Aslihan Nisanci is an Assistant Professor at Marmara University. She received her Master of Social Work degree from Jane Addams College of Social Work, where her area of concentration was mental health. During her PhD studies at Jane Addams College of Social Work, her dissertation research focused on parenting and adolescent wellbeing relationship in Turkish immigrant families in the United States.

James Pike is a Lecturer in for Health and Social Care and a PhD candidate at Nottingham Trent University. He is researching **'Caring for Capital: Capital accumulation and the crisis in the English care sector'**.

Lee Reynolds is an Academic Developer. During her previous work of seven years tutoring study skills for undergraduate and postgraduate students in Social Sciences, she completed an MA in Education in 2020. Lee is currently undertaking a PhD in Education, investigating barriers to participation in doctoral study.

Jennifer Sanders is a Senior Lecturer in Health and Social Care. Following completion of her MSc Forensic Psychology she worked in adult social care, in a residential home for Autistic young adults, before moving into higher education in 2013. Combining her interest in forensic psychology and Autism, Jenny is undertaking a PhD in Psychology, to understand why Autistic individuals exhibit inappropriate sexual behaviour.

Dani Shepherd completed her BA (Hons) Health and Social Care at Nottingham Trent University, continuing education to complete a PGCE, recently becoming a Newly Qualified Teacher.

Penny Siebert (PhD) is a Lecturer in Health and Social Care who is interested in how theory is used in practice to support the design, implementation and evaluation of interventions aimed at improving health outcomes and reducing inequalities. Before entering academia she worked as Midwife, then as a Public Health professional in primary care settings in the East midlands region.

Martin Smith is a Senior Lecturer and Course Leader specialising in counselling and psychotherapy within various courses taught in the School of Social Sciences at Nottingham Trent University. Martin is a Psychotherapist in a Private Practice and Private training consultancy specialising in personality issues and extreme difficult behaviours in the workplace. He has been in clinical practice for the past 14 years.

Walters Tanifum is a qualified senior therapeutic social worker with 14 years experience including experience as a CAMHS lead professional and co-ordinating a regional service.

Chris Towers (PhD) has been a Lecturer for many years and has taught across all levels of the BA Health and Social Care Degree. He has also taught at master's level and across disciplines from social policy to public health, social work, and criminology. His passion for teaching helped him to be awarded the Vice-Chancellor's Award for Excellence in Teaching in 2018. He is a specialist in social gerontology.

Acknowledgements

Thanks for the acumen from Routledge with the expert guidance of Claire Jarvis who has steered this project through the process.

A thank you to Louise Griffiths, Verusca Calabria and Bailey Foster for their steady stewardship and congratulations to Louise for her new addition.

To all staff and students that we've had the pleasure and privilege to work with and for the inspiration and humbling experience of committed, invested and imaginative individuals working in solidarity.

A Note on Terminology

Terminology is a generalised terms for different specilised words and meanings relating to particular fields, and the study of such terms and their use. Terminology often involves acronymns and can result in jargon. Different practitioners in different professions use different language and terminology. For example, clients, patients, service users, people who use sevices, people who are eligible for services, people are all used and admissable terms. Similarly, terms are contested, change over time, are different in different socieites and cultures. Dual heritage is the prefered term for people with different heritages to draw from. BAME as Black, Asian, Minority Ethnicity is widely used but hotley contested and not agree upon. Given these challenges this book uses terms that fit within the context of the chapter whilst recognising that they are contested and not universaly agreed upon. The historical charting of changes of meaning are fascinating areas that provide an insight into social, pooitical and economic and cultural arrangements at a participalr time and place.

List of Abbreviations

HL	House of Lords
HC	House of Commons
BME	Black and Minority Ethnic
CPS	Crown Prosecution Service
CSEW	Crime Survey for England and Wales
HC	House of Commons
HL	House of Lords
HMPPS	Her Majesty's Prison and Probation Services
NHS	National Health Service
ONS	Office for National Statistics
PHE	Public Health England
WHO	World Health Organisation
ASD	Autism Spectrum Disorder
SOTP	Sex Offender Treatment Programme
MBTI	Myers-Briggs Type Indicator
ICS	Integrated care systems

Mapping the Chapters

This is the second edition of Key Themes

Part I

In **Foundations in Health & Social Care,** *Dolores Ellidge* suggests people's access to health and social care services is influenced by their lifestyle, needs, knowledge and experiences. The resources available in their community and the support people have to access those resources also contribute to individual health and well-being. This chapter explores the concepts of community and inequality to support the development of understanding of factors which influence individual health and well-being. Key factors which will be discussed including health, housing, crime, employment, education, ethnicity and support networks with a focus on how these factors may interlink. Accountability for health and well-being in relation to the individual and the state will be discussed alongside accessibility and equality of service provision in communities including statutory, private and voluntary sector services.

Human Growth and Development, *Martin Smith* examines development through the lifespan. Psychological, biological and physical changes people experience and key developmental theories are considered. Physical, cognitive, personal, social well-being are explored, assumptions challenged and life cycle and lifespan perspectives examines active vs passive, critical vs sensitive periods of development, continuity and discontinuity in change, stability and change, nature vs nurture are discussed before psychodynamic, behavioural and humanistic theory are considered.

In **Current Issues in Health and Social Care,** *Jenny Sanders, Lee Reynolds and James Pike* advise Health and social care issues are often emotive and divisive, making newspaper headlines and trending on social media platforms. This media information is often what forms people's opinions on such issues, whereas academic literature such as peer reviewed journals *informs* us. Assisted dying, mandatory childhood vaccinations, and loneliness and isolation are the topics explored, drawing on a range of sources of information to develop an understanding of these key issues, as well as cultivating information literacy through evaluation of the different kinds of writing. To facilitate this, essential academic skills necessary for studying at degree level will be introduced. These include: searching and evaluating literature, reading and note-taking, academic writing, critical thinking, citing and referencing using Harvard. The chapter aims are to: develop an understanding of key issues in health and social care; develop research and academic skills required to explore these issues and succeed at University; and encourage a critical approach to the use of information discussing the key issues.

In **Working with People,** *Amy Allen's* chapter explores the complexities of working with people in health and social care environments. Effective communication is vital to ensuring the provision of high-quality care to all. The first section of this chapter will examine the concept of equality and encourages an empathetic understanding of the needs of a wide range of service users. The second section aims to develop the interpersonal skills employed by practitioners to engage with service users in a range of settings. Throughout the chapter, the reader is encouraged to reflect on the effectiveness of their own interpersonal skills and explore how these could affect care quality.

In **Social Policy,** *Chris Towers and Richard Machin's* chapter identifies some critical issues in the teaching of social policy from the perspective of two lectures who have taught on the programme. *Chris Towers* explores how the use of film supports teaching. He focuses on the work of film maker Ken Loach and he has frequently used film in the classroom, bringing some key issues of social policy and conditionality to prominence and illustrating wider issues of pedagogy. With frequent reference to Loach's work, the chapter raises questions concerning how people learn from a visual perspective (Rose 1991) and in doing so gives focus to the place of the emotions in this learning and how emotive as well as intellectual responses can be part of that wider learning.

In **Professional Practice,** *Dolores Ellidge, Jessica Arnold, Monique Duncan and Dani Shepherd* argue the definition of professional is influenced by the context of their practice (Barnard 2017) and across the sphere of health and social care the roles and responsibilities of practitioners vary greatly. However, all practice within health and social care should be underpinned by reliable evidence. The World Health Organisation (2017) identify that evidence-based practice is beneficial to service users and practitioners and may improve the quality of care provided.

This chapter will discuss the evidence base which supports effective practice as well as the qualities required to build respectful relationships with service users and colleagues. Development of key graduate skills through participation in work experience is explored as an opportunity to develop understanding of theory in practice and promote lifelong learning. This focus will support students to progress towards graduate employment through development of reflective practice and knowledge and understanding of the context of practice in health and social care settings. Alongside practice the chapter has two underpinning themes: safeguarding and equality and diversity. These themes will be linked to concepts such as quality and professional standards, accountability, communication, team working and workplace well-being.

Part II

In **Health, Social Care and Crime,** *Jenny Sanders* proposes definitions, roles and the purpose of police, prosecution, courts, probation and prison service will provide an introduction to the criminal justice system of England and Wales. Critical discussion will explore demographics such as gender, age and race in relation to these criminal justice agencies. Individuals interacting with these structures will have committed, or be suspected of committing, a criminal offence. Therefore, an exploration of criminal behaviour and the links to wider health and social care provision and services is required. With a focus on gangs, sexual offences and burglary biopsychosocial theories explaining criminal behaviour will be critiqued, responses to criminal behaviour will be evaluated, and the impact of crime analysed. The chapter aims to: provide a detailed understanding of the criminal justice system; examine the explanation for, and impact of, criminal behaviour; challenge contemporary approaches of responding to criminal behaviour.

In **Person-Centred Interventions**, *Richard Machin, Dolores Ellidge and Dr Verusca Calabria* argue service users are at the centre of the delivery of health and social care services and developing a critical knowledge and understanding of the person-centred approach is essential for health and social care practitioners. This chapter discusses the principles and theory of person-centred care and its link to humanistic and existential philosophy. The legislation and policy which underpins person-centred care is set out and analysed. The chapter introduces the paramount importance of working with service users as equal partners in the planning and delivery of services, valuing them as experts in their own right and central to the decision-making process. The benefits and challenges of using the person-centred approach in a multi-disciplinary and multi-cultural setting are discussed, emphasising the intersectional nature of discrimination in the context of health and social care. A case study is presented which ask the reader to reflect on the ways in which they can develop their person-centred skills and apply them in a wide range of health and social care roles. These include coaching and guidance roles, professional supervision, negotiation and advocacy and care planning.

In **Valuing Research in Health and Social Care**, *Louise Griffiths, Dr Verusca Calabria and Melanie Bailey* say in recent years, an understanding of research paradigms has become increasingly important in Health and Social Care, not only for students during their University studies but even more so for practitioners and the Government to make welfare decisions within UK, due to the rising levels of inequality. This chapter introduces the significance of research within the Health and Social Care sector by developing an understanding of the different research approaches and identifying the key role of research in supporting evidence-based practice. The chapter draws on current research priorities, such as conducting remote qualitative research and quantitative research in relation to COVID-19. The key research concepts in the field are introduced whilst distinguishing between the producers and consumers within Health and Social Care research.

In **Managing Health and Social Care**, *Amy Allen's* chapter focuses on the wider context in which health and social care services operate. Managers of services face constant challenges and changes which they need to adapt to whilst ensuring care quality remains high. Changes in political aims, legislation, funding and policy can have a significant impact on the way a service operates day-to-day. Social factors such as consumer expectations, demographic changes, the use of technology and media coverage can put pressure on a service which needs to be managed effectively. Major events such as public enquiries and pandemics can add further uncertainty. The first section of this chapter explores how 'good practice' in the management of services can ensure high quality of care even in times of uncertainty. The second section examines specific challenges faced by managers within the industry in recent years.

Part III

In **Young People and Social Care** *Aslihan Nisanci* suggests young people may need assistance and care for reasons including, but not limited to, abuse or neglect, health and mental health issues, drug use, disabilities, sexual exploitation, immigration status, anti-social behaviours, harmful sexual behaviours, and being young carers. Service and intervention models are offered to young people and their families within the existing policies, legislation, and service delivery systems. Numerous complex, dynamic and interrelated structural issues like poverty, unemployment, racism, discrimination surround these service systems and social care experiences of young people and their families. In this chapter, social care provided to young people with different needs and conditions are discussed with reference to relevant legislation and surrounding social forces. As commonly used and overarching frameworks, ecological perspective and youth-centred approach are proposed for work with young people in social care. Examples of best practices from national and international contexts are also presented.

In **Engaging with vulnerable groups**, *Christopher Towers'* chapter discusses vulnerability and its importance. The double-edged process, social construction and structural aspects of vulnerable populations influences how decisions are made and safeguarding and personalisation are explored. The chapter reflects on how different groups and individuals in receipt of services experience vulnerability. The practice issues working with vulnerable service users is considered.

In **Children's and Young People's Mental Health**, *Jessica Arnold, Amy Allen, Dolores Ellidge and Richard Machin's* chapter reflects a growing concern about the state of services for children and young people with mental health problems and the need to develop strategies for promoting and sustaining mental wellbeing. The first section explores four mental health conditions which commonly appear in childhood or adolescence. Current understanding about the causes and effects of these conditions is discussed. The role of biological, psychological, developmental and social factors in the formation of mental illness are examined. The second section explores current policy and practice in the management of the mental wellbeing of young people in the UK. A range of therapeutic interventions are presented, and their efficacy is examined. The value of commonly used and alternative therapeutic interventions is explored. Throughout the chapter, the reader is encouraged to consider the wider context within which our mental health and sense of self develops.

In **Ageing in the 21st century**, *Chris Towers* examines changing demographics that mean that ageing is an increasingly critical issue facing policy makers, practitioners, people and governments as people continue to live longer, work and care for each other. The Co-vid 19 pandemic exposed issues of risk and vulnerability to people and this chapter considers issues of health, housing, care, employment, income and pensions. The chapter looks at issues of retirement and the so called 'dependency ratio, the ratio of people engaged in paid work to those not working and looks at issues of dependency and independence, caring and being cared for. The issues are reflected through the experiences of a fictional character, Donald Major and take a life course perspective focusing on Issues of sociology, social policy, health and social care. The reader is asked to consider his choices and the constraints he faces through a life into older age and takes this experience and considers it in relation to wider evidence. Each chapter takes a particular theme and follows the story of his life, inviting the reader to consider issues from 'the cradle to the grave' and from early beginnings through to issues of dementia, death and dying and how society could respond to various twenty first century challenges. The chapter asks question of the reader as to their response and attitudes towards the elderly in the light of the pandemic and other national and global issues.

In **Transcultural issues,** *Aslihan Nisanci, Adam Barnard and Walters Tanifum* suggest transcultural issues are necessary in the increasing multicultural and diverse world. Oppressive and discriminatory thoughts, beliefs, actions and behaviours operate on personal, cultural and structural levels. Understanding factors and issues in transcultural thought, belief, communication, action and practice enables a transnational cultural competence to be developed. Drawing understanding from anti-oppressive views challenges the interests of social groups who have power and devalues characteristics of individuals and groups in different positions such as being female in a patriarchal society, being black in a white world, being a personal with a disability in an able-bodied world. Multicultural sensitivity relates to issues of cultural competence and cultural awareness to understand and value devalued characteristics. Language is a central concern and is easily dismissed by 'political correctness' and a backlash against progressive moves towards of more progressive services, thoughts, beliefs and action. This chapter reviewing theoretical ideas to explore the issues and propose more inclusive, diverse and equal services. The chapter ends with reviewing the increased sophistication of oppressive views through 'dog whistle politics'.

In **Leadership in Health and Social Care,** *Jennifer Sanders* recommends in an environment of increasing and more complex need, and decreasing staff levels and funding, the call for inspirational leadership has never been stronger. A critical exploration of leadership models across time and culture, will introduce key concepts including motivation, coaching and managing change. Team development, role theory and the link between leaders and followers will be discussed, providing opportunity for reflection on own experience and expectations. The challenges of leading integrated health and social care services and working in partnership with organisations will involve a discussion of innovation, enterprise and thinking differently. Reflections on personal values and traits provide an opportunity to develop employability skills. The chapter aims to: develop a critical understanding of traditional and emerging leadership paradigms; explore the challenges of leading integrated health and social care services; aid reflection and preparation for graduate-level roles.

In **Conducting a Student Empirical Research Study in Health and Social Care,** *Louise Griffiths, Penny Siebert and Alice Lee's* chapter explores how to conduct a small-scale empirical research study in a stepped process. Discussing quantitative and qualitative research the building blocks for a research study on social networking sites and mental health is discussed.

1 Introduction

*Adam Barnard, Verusca Calabria, and
Louise Griffiths*

Welcome to the world of health and social care. It is a complex, fascinating and
challenging world. Everyone at some point in their life will have need to health and
social care services so to have an awareness of the high and lows of receiving, interpreting, understanding and working with services is a necessary set of understandings. Delivering these services and the way they are shaped, influenced, designed
and delivered is the remit for staff working in health and social care. This book is an
introduction to broad areas of service provision, the theory that informs services and
the experience of receiving services.

The landscape of health and social care has changed dramatically in the recent
years but the key themes and ideas that populate this book remain and are discussed
below. They are an interesting blend of theory and practice, policy and process, lived
experience and cultural issues, human growth and development, working with others.
The opening chapters establish a foundation to health and social care. The second
part of the book takes these themes and probes a little deeper of how services are
delivered, how we know in health and social care, and how we learn. The final part of
the book examines in breadth and depth particular groups such as young people,
older people. The key themes of leadership, community engagement, transcultural
issues, and engaging vulnerable people and developing a research project closes the
circle on learning in health and social care. The end of the book contains a glossary of
key themes and a time-line of significant events in health and social care. It is hoped
that readers will benefit from ideas contained within this book at they will ignite a fire
for further exploration.

There are many ways to cut a cake. Those wanting an introduction to health and
social care can pick and choose the most relevant chapters. Those wanting an in-
depth understanding of key themes in health and social care can read specific chapters, each page, line by line for depth and detail in the argument of the chapter.

There are many voices and experiences in health and social care of service users,
staff and students. To reflect this diversity, there is a deliberate attempt in this book to
utilise a range of voices and give voice to different experiences. As such, there are
different registers, tones, styles and expressions from the contributors.

DOI: 10.4324/9781003079873-1

Part I

2 Foundations in Health and Social Care

Dolores Ellidge

The chapter aims to:

- Explore what is meant by health and well-being and differentiate between factors which contribute to being healthy
- Consider communities and their influence on the health and well-being of individuals and groups
- Analyse health inequalities within the United Kingdom and illustrate the role of public health and policy in reducing inequality

Introduction

Understanding the concepts of health and well-being is a fundamental requirement for all practitioners in the sphere of health and social care, therefore this chapter explores the meaning of health and well-being and how perception of an individual's health is influenced by their experience and circumstances. Health cannot be considered in isolation as achieving optimal health is influenced by individual factors such as genetics and lifestyle as well as social factors including housing, education, employment, financial stability and access to resources and services to meet any identified needs. Underpinning these social factors are government policy, strategy priorities and allocation of resources including services, which promote public health – that is strategies and services which aim to improve quality of life by reducing preventable ill-health.

The chapter has three broad sections. The first focuses on health and well-being, which leads into consideration of community; what is a community and its influence on well-being of individuals and the community as a whole. This section will also consider community profiling as a method of identifying strengths and needs within communities making links to the social determinants of health. The final section considers health and the inequalities in health which have been reported on in Britain over recent decades.

As you work through, the chapter activities have been included for you to complete. These activities will support you to actively engage in your learning by reflecting on your existing knowledge and your own experiences in relation to the key themes of the chapter and developing your skills in finding and analysing information.

DOI: 10.4324/9781003079873-3

Health and Well-Being

Developing a clear understanding or definition of health is important as it underpins health and social care provision historically and currently. Although there are some established definitions of health, it is important to think about what they are and what they mean to us as individuals, communities and the world in which we live. Our expectations for health are dependent on the area of the world in which we live as the wealth and government of our country contributes to our health and our expectations and perception of our health and lifestyle. It is our perceptions and expectations of health which contribute to our experience of well-being.

Trainee health and social care practitioners were asked to share the words they associated with being healthy. As you can see in the Word Cloud below, students included factors related to both feeling physically and psychologically healthy, actions which can support health such as exercising and having a balanced diet and resources needed to be healthy such as food and water (Figure 2.1).

Activity 1

Think about what words you associate with being healthy – are they similar or do they contrast in the Word Cloud?

Write your own definition of health and compare that to the definitions in the discussion below. See activity below.

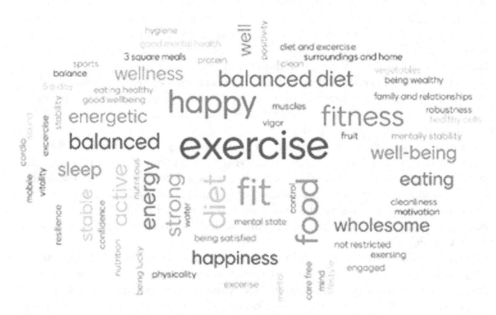

Figure 2.1 Words related to being healthy (NTU 2020).

Source: Hierarchy of Needs.

The trainee practitioners' perceptions of health are reflected in more formal definitions and emphasise the interconnections between physical, social and emotional well-being. The definition of health from the World Health Organisation (WHO) remains valid decades after its development: "Health is a state of complete physical, mental and social well-being and not merely the absence of disease or infirmity" (WHO 1946). For many people, however, this definition may not be completely true, for example people who have long-term conditions or disability may consider themselves to be healthy despite having an "infirmity". The Centres for Disease Control and Prevention (2020) report that most people with a disability feel that they are healthy, have a full life and feel that knowing that their condition can be effectively managed and treated is part of this. Huber et al. (2011) concur stating that a core component of being healthy is the ability to adapt and self-manage which links to the concept of well-being. Blatný and Šolvocá (2015) suggest that subjective well-being is an individual's response to their life experiences and the challenges they face. Well-being can be seen as dependent on personality factors such as resilience and positive outlook, therefore individuals with very similar life experiences and challenges may have opposing perceptions of well-being. Initially well-being was considered to be a static state; however, more recent research identifies that well-being fluctuates. Dodge et al. (2012) suggest that for stable well-being, individuals need the resources to meet the physical, social or psychological challenges they are experiencing; if the available resources are not sufficient to meet the needs generated by the challenges then the individuals' sense of well-being decreases.

It is important to remember that health is influenced by broader factors than an individual's capacity to be healthy. Health is influenced by personal health behaviours, but it is also influenced by structural factors such as the communities in which they live, resources available to them, genetic or inherited characteristics and political decision making. The Ottawa Charter states

> The fundamental conditions and resources for health are peace, shelter, education, food, income, a stable ecosystem, sustainable resources, social justice and equity. Improvement in health requires a secure foundation in these basic prerequisites.
>
> (WHO 1986)

Thus, similarly to well-being, being healthy is dependent on access to a range of resources and an individual's ability to manage or control them. In the document "Prevention is better than cure" the Department of Health and Social Care (2018) not only recognises the impact of the environment on individuals' health and well-being but the need for policy and strategies to improve factors such as housing, air pollution, work and social networks in order to prevent many of the common health conditions across England. The need to have access to certain resources relates to the broad definition of health; however, these needs and resources can be prioritised with some being essential for life.

Identifying Need

As a basic concept, need is something that can be identified as essential to life; however, we often use the word in different contexts, resulting in one person identifying something as essential but other people may not be view it in the same way.

This can be related to both fundamental requirements for life and everyday items. Most people in Britain have access to basic resources such as power and clean water, shelter, food and have access to a range of services all of which impacts on needs we may identify compared to people in less developed countries. However, access to resources and services does not fulfil needs for all people as access is impacted by income, for example, fuel poverty when people may have heating systems in their homes but not afford to use it to adequately heat their homes. Fuel poverty then can create a need which has a significant impact on health and well-being (Buck and Gregory 2018).

Activity 2   Needs analysis

First think about the last few days and the things you have felt you have needed. Allocate the things you have identified into three lists:

- Vital
- Important
- Helpful/nice

Then think about:

- Why you have categorised them in the way you have?
- Talk to someone you know well and ask them to do the activity. Do they have similar needs, and have they categorised them in the same way?

The activity and discussion above highlights that there are different types of need and prioritising of those needs. Bradshaw in 1972 developed a taxonomy of needs which focuses on assessing health in communities. He identified four key areas of need:

Normative; a standard which is defined by a specialist.

Felt; a need recognised by an individual which can be seen to be subjective.

Expressed; a need which is conveyed and leads to action.

Comparative; a need which occurs when services are provided unequally to different groups of people with the same condition.
(Bradshaw 1972, cited in Davidson, Iley and Ramsdale 2019)

Maslow (1987) identified fundamental desires of human beings, which he suggested could be expressed as a hierarchy. He stated that it was essential that basic needs were met and suggests that individuals were driven to meet lower order needs, which generates a desire to meet higher-order needs and achieve self-actualisation; that is, achieve their full potential. Although Maslow's ideas have been criticised as untestable, they have been the foundation for consideration of other models. Hale et al. (2019) identify that theorists have developed Maslow's ideas proposing that

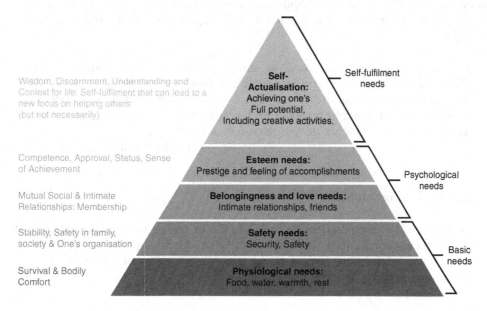

Figure 2.2 Hierarchy of needs.

Source: (Maslow 1987, see also Winston 2016).

needs can co-exist and that individuals can still meet higher-order needs even when lower-order needs are unmet. Hale et al.'s (2019) study focused on developing a model to support physician wellness; however, many of their findings are transferable to British society in general. Thus, the contemporary edition of Maslow's ideas builds on his perceptions but places them within the context of modern society. For example, broadening safety to encompass personal and financial safety alongside physical. Maslow's perception of esteem included both an individual's belief in their own worth and their desire for respect for others, whereas Hale et al.'s (2019) model suggests that individuals need respect and affirmation of their qualities and abilities through feedback, which becomes a cycle of building self-belief (Figure 2.2).

Needs are important in health and well-being as non-gratification of need can result in declining health and well-being and a lack of resources directly contributes to health inequalities, which we will consider later in this chapter. Doyal and Gough (1993, see also Marks, Murray and Vida Estacio 2018) suggest that health and autonomy are the two most significant needs which contribute to feelings of "need satisfaction". This sense of having needs satisfied is an important factor in people's perception of their quality of life – a subjective assessment of the positive and challenging aspects in a person's life (Marks, Murray and Vida Estacio 2018).

Community and Well-Being

Most people belong to one or more communities. Communities provide a sense of connection to others and can contribute to our social networks, which is an important factor in an individuals' well-being. As can be seen in the definition below, community is identified as a geographical area or a shared interest; however, it is the people within communities which generate a feeling of community and a sense of belonging.

> Community as a term is used as shorthand for the relationships, bonds, identities and interests that join people together or give them a shared stake in a place, service, culture or activity. Distinctions are often made between communities of place/geography and communities of interest or identity, as strategies for engaging people may vary accordingly.
>
> (Public Health England 2015)

Activity 3   Communities

Think about the communities you have lived in or belong to. Choose three or four of these communities and identify the characteristics of what you have liked, found helpful or is limited in the communities. How do you think the community could be developed?

  Discussion:

> My family moved to the village we lived in 20 years ago. It is relatively a big village with a lot of amenities, including a doctor's surgery, primary school, nurseries, small supermarket with a post office, newsagent, hairdressers, florist, takeaway shops, café, pub, community centre, village hall, and police and fire stations. The train and bus services provide regular access to the nearby city and towns. Having lived here so long we are accepted members of the village community and chat to other villagers regularly and engage in village social media groups for information and support however, when we first arrived, we were treated as "outsiders". Developing our sense of belonging and feeling accepted took years and initially we felt quite isolated within the community but being part of the school's parent teacher's association and attending village events helped us to make connections and be accepted into the community. The aspect of the community which is limited is activities for young people. The local groups and activities are more geared towards children with young people only being able to access specialist hobbies such as football or dance; however, other than a playing field there are no facilities for young people to hang out together.

Community Development and Participation

Community Development in Britain was founded in the 1960s with the development of organisations and strategies to reduce deprivation, and more recently this approach includes working towards social justice. It is defined as "a process where community members come together to take collective action and generate solutions to common problems". Adopting a community development approach means ensuring that the issues and priorities are identified and agreed by the communities themselves, and that people are encouraged to work together towards a collective solution to a shared concern (Gilchrist 2009). It promotes empowerment through a bottom-up approach and relies on people in the community, public services and government working in new ways.

One of the challenges with community development work is that it often happens informally or through local fundraising activities rather than statutory or grant funding, which means that initially there were few documented examples of the approach and its impact on health and well-being. Mtika and Kistlers (2017) suggest that the impact of community development is ongoing – like ripples from throwing a pebble into water – as a group develops a service, knowledge or skills, this is shared across the community and will support other people to develop services or resources. Examples of effective community development are seen in Saldana and Chamberlain's (2012) study, which included a project where foster carers came together to provide peer support on behaviour management, thus improving their parenting skills and a project which used peer support and community resources to support birth families for the successful transition of looked after children back to their care.

The concept of community participation is also significant when considering health and well-being in communities. Tudagbe-Obour (2022) suggests that "Community participation concerns the engagement of individuals and communities in decisions about things that affect their lives". The approach has the capacity to ensure access to health services and contribute to tackling the social inequalities in health (Marston et al. 2016). WHO (2002) identify that people engage more in projects in which they have contributed to the planning from the first stages rather than just being asked opinions of projects, which have already been planned. Community participation is fostered by projects and professionals having an understanding of the community dynamics and needs. Undertaking a community profile as discussed in the next section can support both the members of the community and health and social care practitioners to identify and understand the health and well-being needs within the area.

Community Profile

Undertaking a community profile is influenced by its purpose. In essence community profiling has developed as a social research method to create "... a picture of the nature, needs and resources of a locality or community" (Woodhouse 2010). In this chapter, the focus will be on community profiling as a mechanism to assess health and well-being needs within a community. Woodhouse (2010) suggests that this should involve active participation of the community members so that their views and priorities are incorporated into action plans which are developed.

Community profiles incorporate researching a range of factors related to the population of a community and the environment in which they reside. Information in Box 1 outlines the factors that should be considered when profiling a community to facilitate identification of strengths and needs within the community and gaps in services or resources which may reduce the needs within the community.

Box 1 Factors typically included in a community profile

Demographics of a population, including population size and breakdown, by gender, age, ethnicity.

Health, including life expectancy, incidence of diseases such as cancer, cardiovascular or respiratory, COVID-19, conditions such as mental health, long-term disability, obesity, teenage pregnancy, breastfeeding and unhealthy behaviours such as substance use, including smoking, alcohol and recreational drugs.

Educational attainment

Crime

Housing and homelessness

Employment and income

Any other factors which you identify have an impact on the health and well-being of the community's population.

Services in the community and key services in the wider geographical area which the community's population are recipients of.

To support identification of need within a community the statistical data can be compared to another community or to a nation. This enables the health and social care trainee to identify differences such as incidence of disease, condition or educational attainment may be higher or lower than the comparison area. This process is important both in identifying needs and inequalities but also in supporting appropriate allocation of resources and development of service provision. Comparison of data also facilitates the identification of factors which are interlinked. For example, van Zon et al. (2017) identified low educational attainment is a significant factor in unemployment as well as being an indicator of poorer health outcomes. Thus, considering statistical evidence in communities can support the researcher to identify needs and highlight inequalities in health and well-being, which will be explored further in the next section of this chapter. Residents within communities may be aware of the unmet need; however, despite changes in approach over recent years, many people feel powerless to make changes to support their individual needs or the needs within the community being met. This example highlights the role of social determinants in health. According to the World Health Organisation the social determinants of health:

> … are the non-medical factors that influence health outcomes. They are the conditions in which people are born, grow, work, live, and age, and the wider set of forces and systems shaping the conditions of daily life. These forces and

systems include economic policies and systems, development agendas, social norms, social policies and political systems.

(WHO n.d.)

These factors contribute to the unfair differences in health and well-being between countries and between populations in those countries. Many of these differences could be avoided and be more significant than access to health care services or the decisions people make around their lifestyle. These inequalities will be explored more in the next section of this chapter.

Health Inequalities

The earlier section focused on social inequality factors, which contribute to inequalities in well-being, but it is important to consider what is meant by health inequality. NHS England suggest:

Health inequalities are the preventable, unfair and unjust differences in health status between groups, populations or individuals that arise from the unequal distribution of social, environmental and economic conditions within societies, which determine the risk of people getting ill, their ability to prevent sickness, or opportunities to take action and access treatment when ill health occurs.

(NHS England n.d.)

Since 1980, several reports have been commissioned by the British Government to determine the extent of health inequalities within the country and to develop strategies to reduce inequality and improve the nations' health. The Black Report (1980) highlighted the inequalities in health outcomes within the population. Despite a key goal with the inception of the NHS in 1948 being to reduce inequality, the Black Report suggested that the gap between the poorest and wealthiest people in the country had increased since the introduction of the NHS in 1948 (McKintosh Grey 1982). The report identified key differences in life expectancy for adults and children between members of professional occupations and unskilled workers and their families; however, the report suggested that the inequalities in health identified were due to the "way members of the different social classes led their lives" (Marmot 2001).

The findings of the Acheson Report (1998) were similar in that they confirmed the widening gap in living standards with increasing income inequality, which was particularly impacting on families with children (Spencer 1999) and resultant poorer health outcomes being experienced by the population. However it also acknowledged the responsibility of the government and organisations in supporting the reduction of inequality. The paper made several recommendations related to improving financial well-being particularly for those in receipt of benefits as well as decreasing "… action to alleviate unemployment and the deprived condition of many ethnic minority groups, elderly and disabled people, and families with children; and increase benefit levels and real living standards." (Black et al. 1999). Increasing funding to develop societal infrastructure such as transport, schools the environment and housing was another aspect of the Acheson's recommendations which would contribute to reducing inequality.

Activity 4   Geography

Choose a geographical community that you are familiar with and look at the statistical data related to the factors in Box 1. If you live in a city or town, focus on a community which is the size of a council ward area such as the wards of St Ann's or Wollaton West in Nottingham City.

Compare the data you find with another ward in the same area of England to enable you to identify where health and well-being in your community is better or worse than the area you are comparing to.

Why do you think the differences occur?

In response to the Acheson report in 1999, the government publish the white paper "Saving Lives: Our Healthier Nation"; an action plan to support prevention of illness and premature death whilst improving the health of the whole population but particularly those with the worst health outcomes. The white paper included targets to reduce incidence in the areas determined to be priority including accidents, coronary heart disease and strokes, cancer and mental illness. In addition, the government committed to a review and change in policy, cross government focus and increased funding to support achievement of improved health with an emphasis on individuals needing to take responsibility for their own health and implement change to achieve good or improved health. The overall limited success of the interventions can be attributed to factors such as lack of evidence of the effectiveness of policy strategy prior to implementation, the slow pace of change and the unexpected complexity of health inequalities (Mackenbach 2011).

The existence of persistent health inequalities experienced in Britain are not explained purely by income and individual life choices. The ONS (2014, see also Dearden, Lloyd and Green 2020) suggest that it is a more complex gradient than "there being a straightforward divide between those who are deprived and those who are not", it is also about the place in which we live and consequently the deprivation experienced. Factors linked to deprivation have changed, including improvements related to overcrowding, access to a vehicle and unemployment; however, Dearden, Lloyd and Green's research (2020) identified that deprivation in urban areas has increased in the 20-year period up to 2011.

The Marmot Report commissioned by the Coalition Government strongly identified that health inequalities in England are associated with social justice and established a link between social gradient and health – that is that the lower a person's social position the worse their health is likely to be (Marmot 2010). The report clearly identified the majority of people in England spent a greater proportion of their life in ill health and did not live as long as those "best off" in society and proposed that addressing the social determinants of health such as the conditions in which people are born, grow, live, work and age is key to reducing inequality. Their recommendations focused on the principles that reducing inequality would benefit society as a whole and that a universal approach was needed but "with a scale and intensity that is proportionate to the level of disadvantage" (Marmot 2010). This was identified as proportionate universalism.

The report on health equity in England identified that over the decade since the publication of the Marmot report improvement in life expectancy has slowed dramatically, "almost grinding to a halt" (Marmot et al. 2010). Over the decade both health and society have stopped improving and links have been made between these findings and the austerity policy of the Conservative government.

Activity 5   Circumstances

Think about your family and own health and social circumstances. Can you identify any significant social determinants of health? Are there any factors which may suggest health inequalities? What contributes to this? What can you do to maximise your health and well-being?

Inequality and COVID-19

This chapter is being written during a global pandemic and therefore it is important to consider initial findings in relation to health inequality and the virus. Over the first year of the pandemic data has clearly shown that some people contracting the virus have a higher risk of mortality compared to others. Public Health England (2020a) identified that COVID-19 has not only followed the path of other health inequalities but in some case the inequalities have been heightened. The report identified that key areas of inequality included:

> Age: people under 40 years who contract COVID-19 are less likely to die than those over 80 years.

Males and people living in deprived communities are more likely to contract the virus.

The Black, Asian, Minority Ethnic (BAME) population have an increased risk of contracting the virus with higher rates of mortality. This is particularly significant as previously health inequalities in this population of the Britain were lower than in white British people (Public Health England 2020b).

Otu et al. (2020) report that mortality rates from COVID-19 for BAME individuals, irrespective of age, is 3.5 times higher than white British people. These differences in mortality are also seen in the health care workforce with a higher proportion of professional and support staff from BAME background dying from COVID-19 than their white peers. Otu et al. (2020) suggested that factors which contribute to differences in COVID outcomes related to ethnicity include that people of BAME background are more likely to live in cities were transmission rates where increased, to reside in areas of higher deprivation, high level of public facing roles for the BAME workforce increasing exposure and that cultural and language differences may create barriers to accessing essential services and advice.

The COVID-19 pandemic has had a broad impact on people's health and well-being that is not restricted to people who have contracted the disease. Lockdown measures although necessary have resulted in business closures, job losses and financial hardships despite government support through furlough payments. In addition, although important public health strategies to control the virus, the lock-down and social distancing measures of the last year have drastically reduced people's access to support networks and social activities which are key factors in resilience and psychological well-being, resulting in poorer mental health and greater demand on NHS and charitable services. Arslan et al.'s (2022) study identified that financial vulnerability due to COVID-19 was associated with stress and deterioration of mental health a concerning factor when the Child Poverty Action Groups survey (2020) identifies that people with the children in the lowest income groups where increasingly unable to afford basic essentials such as rent, food, utilities and child-related costs.

Working towards Health Equity

The pandemic has highlighted the inequalities experienced in Britain with the topic frequently hitting news headlines and raising society's awareness of inequality in a way which the reports by Black, Acheson and Marmot have failed to do. In the discussion above we identified that reports on inequalities have not resulted in policy and resources to support a move towards health equity. A broader approach is required. As Marmot (2010) suggests:

> Focusing solely on the most disadvantaged will not reduce health inequalities sufficiently. To reduce the steepness of the social gradient in health, actions must be universal, but with a scale and intensity that is proportionate to the level of disadvantage. We call this proportionate universalism. Action taken to reduce health inequalities will benefit society in many ways. It will have economic benefits in reducing losses from illness associated with health inequalities. These currently account for productivity losses, reduced tax revenue, higher welfare payments and increased treatment costs.

Recommendations from Marmot (2010) incorporate actions across the life span including:

> Increase spending for early years provision with proportionally higher allocation of resources in deprived areas to support the reduction of child poverty

> Improve equity of educational attainment with provision of services to reduce exclusions

> Increase the National Living Wage to reduce in-work poverty and ensure all have minimum income needed to support healthy lifestyle choices

> Develop work related training for the workforce and access to post-school apprenticeships

> Health equity to be at the centre of planning and strategy at all levels of government and health valued equally or above economic efficiency

> Decrease carbon footprint by achieving net zero emissions and carbon neutral new homes by 2030

Develop a national strategy and workforce to take action on the social determinants of health

Engage the public

These strategies to improve environment, housing and standards of living changes to health, care provision contribute to improving the health of the population across Britain; however, more than a decade later it is clear that health inequalities persist. A joint assessment of the NHS identified the service compares favourably to other health care systems but recognises that development is needed particularly focusing on preventable long-term health conditions (Dayan et al. 2018). The government has been criticised as needing to be more proactive in developing strategies and services, which focus on preventing ill-health and promoting healthier lifestyles (Buck et al. 2018). However, there have been some changes to improve the nation's health through the government taking a broad and inter-departmental approach. For example, plans to reduce obesity include increasing activity with the walking and cycling strategy (Department of Transport 2017), which outlines plans for financial investment to increase walking and cycling for short journeys by improving road safety, access to cycle routes, broadening options for commuters taking bikes on trains and investment in school bikeability programmes. Other obesity related strategies include The Soft Drinks Industry Levy Regulations (2018) which placed a levy on soft drink manufacturers which is titrated to the level of sugar in the drinks produced; drinks with a high sugar content incurring a higher levy. Increasing awareness of calorie content is another factor being tackled by the government. Calorie content is available for foods purchased through retail outlets and the government plans to build on this with legislation scheduled for implementation in 2022, which will require large businesses (more than 250 employees) to provide calorie information on foods which are not pre-packaged and are made for immediate consumption (UK Parliament 2021).

Access to services is another factor which contributes to health inequalities which the government is taking steps to improve. Access to mental health services is an example of this. No Health without Mental Health (Department of Health 2011) highlighted the need for parity of mental health and physical health services and recognised that access to mental health services should be as timely as access to other health services. Increased funding for mental health services since 2014–2015 focused on crisis support, effective hospital services, early intervention and targets for treatment waiting times, including self-referral as an element of the improving access to psychological therapies programme (Department of Health 2014). Undoubtedly, this investment in mental health services has made a difference; however, the increase in the prevalence of mental illness continues to impact on health inequalities and access to timely treatment.

Conclusion

This chapter identifies that definition and perception of health and well-being is multi-dimensional. It is influenced by individual circumstances and resources within themselves and within the communities in which they live and interact. Although a contributing factor, health is not focused on the physical as the capacity to manage physical health conditions is influenced by social and psychological factors, and psychological and social well-being are integral to a lifestyle, which support positive physical health. In addition, health and well-being are associated with identification of needs and the means to be able to have those needs met.

It has been established that despite having systems such as the NHS, Social Services and benefit system in place for the last eight decades, inequality continues to escalate in Britain. This inequity is impacting on opportunities for individuals to achieve their potential in key aspects of everyday life; health and well-being, financial and self-actualisation. The series of reports into health in Britain have painted a picture of health inequality between the most and least affluent in our society (Black et al. 1999; Marmot 2010) demonstrating that the lower a person's social position, the worse their health is likely to be, and despite multiple recommendations to support the reduction of these inequalities successive governments have either failed to act or not implemented successful policy strategies. Marmot (2010) states that "The fair distribution of health, well-being and sustainability are important social goals" and advocates that health and well-being is part of all government strategies. Health inequality is associated with social justice and government, organisations and individuals need to collaborate and cooperate and be motivated to strive for health equity.

References

Arslan, G., Yldrm, M., & Zangeneh, M. (2022). "Coronavirus anxiety and psychological adjustment in college students: Exploring the role of college belongingness and social media addiction". *International Journal of Mental Health and Addiction*, 20 (3), 1546–1559.

Black, D., Morris, J.N., Smith, C., and Townsend, P., 1999. Better benefits for health: plan to implement the central recommendation of the Acheson report. *BMJ* [online], 13(318), 724–727. [Accessed 5 February 2021].

Blatný, M. and Šolvocá, A., 2015. Well-being. In: Blatný M., ed. *Personality and well-being across the life-span*. London: Palgrave, 2015, 20–45. [Accessed 8 November 2020].

Buck, D., Baylis, A., Dougall, D., and Robertson, R., 2018. *A vision for population health Towards a healthier future* [online]. London: The Kings Fund. Available at: https://www.kingsfund.org.uk/sites/default/files/2018-11/A%20vision%20for%20population%20health%20online%20version.pdf [Accessed 15 February 2021].

Buck, D., and Gregory, S., 2018. *Housing and health opportunities for sustainability and transformation partnerships* [online]. London: The Kings Fund. Available at: https://www.kingsfund.org.uk/sites/default/files/2018-03/Housing_and_health_final.pdf [Accessed 29 October 2021].

Centers for Disease Control and Prevention, 2020. *Disability and health related conditions* [online]. United States of America: Department of Health and Social Sciences. Available at: https://www.cdc.gov/ncbddd/disabilityandhealth/relatedconditions.html#:~:text=Although%20a%20smaller%20percentage%20than,can%20lead%20full%2C%20active%20lives [Accessed 8 November 2020].

Davidson, H., Iley, K., and Ramsdale, S., 2019. Supporting and promoting health. In: Burns, D., ed. *Foundations of adult nursing*. 2nd ed. London: Sage, 245–274.

Dayan, M., Ward, D., Gardener, T., and Kelly, E., 2018. *How good is the NHS?* [online]. London: The Kings Fund. Available at: https://www.kingsfund.org.uk/sites/default/files/2018-06/NHS_at_70_how_good_is_the_NHS.pdf [Accessed 15 February 2021].

Dearden, E., Lloyd, C.D., and Green, M., 2020. Exploring the histories of health and deprivation in Britain, 1971–2011. *Health and Place* [online], 61, 1–11. https://doi-org.proxy.library.lincoln.ac.uk/10.1016/j.healthplace.2019.102255 [Accessed 29 January 2021].

Dodge, R., Daly, A.P., Huyton, J., and Sanders, L.D., 2012. The challenge of defining wellbeing. *International Journal of Wellbeing* [online], 2(3), 222–235. 10.5502/ijw.v2i3.4 [Accessed 25 September 2020].

Doyal, L., & Gough, I. (1993). Need satisfaction as a measure of human welfare. In *Mixed economies in Europe* (pp. 178–198). Edward Elgar Publishing.

Gilchrist, A., 2009. *The well-connected community (second edition): a networking approach to community development* [online]. 2nd ed. Bristol: Bristol University Press. https://doi.org/10.2307/j.ctt9qgrjc [Accessed 5 November 2021].

Great Britain. Department of Health, 2011. *No health without mental health: a cross-government mental health outcomes strategy for people of all ages* [online]. London: Department of Health. Available at: https://assets.publishing.service.gov.uk/government/uploads/system/uploads/attachment_data/file/138253/dh_124058.pdf [Accessed 5 November 2021].

Great Britain. Department of Health, 2014. *Achieving better access to mental health services by 2020* [online]. London: Department of Health. Available at: https://assets.publishing.service.gov.uk/government/uploads/system/uploads/attachment_data/file/361648/mental-health-access.pdf [Accessed 5 November 2021].

Great Britain. Department of Health and Social Care, 2018. *Prevention is better than cure: our vision to help you live well for longer* [online]. London: Department of Health and Social Care. Available at: https://assets.publishing.service.gov.uk/government/uploads/system/uploads/attachment_data/file/753688/Prevention_is_better_than_cure_5-11.pdf [Accessed 5 November 2021].

Great Britain. Department of Transport, 2017. *Cycling and walking investment strategy* [online]. London: Department of Transport. Available at: https://assets.publishing.service.gov.uk/government/uploads/system/uploads/attachment_data/file/918442/cycling-walking-investment-strategy.pdf [Accessed 5 November 2021].

Hale, A.J., Ricotta, N.D., Freed, J., Smith, C., and Huang, G.C., 2019. Adapting Maslow's hierarchy of needs as a framework for resident wellness. *Teaching and Learning in Medicine* [online], 31 (1), 109–118. 10.1080/10401334.2018.1456928 [Accessed 5 November 2021].

Huber, M., Knotterus, J.A., Green, H., Horst, J., and Anjelandro, R., 2011. How should we define health? *BMJ* [online], 346. 10.1136/bmj.d4163 [Accessed 27 September 2019].

Mackenbach, J., 2011. Can we reduce health inequalities? An analysis of the English strategy (1997–2010). *Journal of Epidemiological Community Health* [online], 65 (7), 568–575. 10.1136/jech.2010.128280 [Accessed 29 January 2021].

Marks, D.F., Murray, M., and Vida Estacio, E., 2018. *Health psychology*. 5th ed. London: Sage.

Marmot, M., 2001. From Black to Acheson: two decades of concern with inequalities in health. A celebration of the 90th birthday of Professor Jerry Morris. *International Journal of Epidemiology* [online], 30 (5), 1165–1171. 10.1093/ije/30.5.1165 [Accessed 29 January 2021].

Marmot, M., 2010. *Fair society, healthy lives: the Marmot Review: strategic review of health inequalities in England post-2010* [online]. London: Department for International Development. Available at: https://www.gov.uk/research-for-development-outputs/fair-society-healthy-lives-the-marmot-review-strategic-review-of-health-inequalities-in-england-post-2010 [Accessed 29 January 2021].

Marston, C., Hinton, R., Kean, S., Baral, S., Ahuja, A., Costello, A., and Portelaf, A., 2016. Community participation for transformative action on women's, children's and adolescents' health. *Bull World Health Organ* [online], 94 (5), 376–382. 10.2471/BLT.15.168492 [Accessed 4 December 2020].

Maslow, A.H., 1987. *Motivation and personality*. 3rd ed. New York: Harper & Row.

McKintosh Grey, A., 1982. Inequalities in health. The Black Report: summary and comment. *International Journal of Services* [online], 12 (3), 349–380. Available via: https://www.jstor.org/stable/45130747 [Accessed 29 January 2021].

Mitka, M., and Kistler, M., 2017. Contiguous community development. *Journal of Rural Studies* [online], 51, 83–92. 10.1016/j.jrurstud.2017.01.018 [Accessed 23 October 2019].

NHS England., n.d. *Reducing health inequalities resources* [online]. London: NHS England. Available at: https://www.england.nhs.uk/about/equality/equality-hub/resources/ [Accessed 30 January 2021].

NTU, 2020. *Word cloud; add the word you associate with being healthy*. Mentimeter [unpublished].

Office of National Statistics (2014). Annual Report. London: HMSO.

Otu, A., Ahinkorah, B.O., Ameyaw, E.K., Seidu, A., and Yaya, A., 2020. One country, two crises: what Covid-19 reveals about health inequalities among BAME communities in the United Kingdom and the sustainability of its health system? *International Journal for Equity in Health* [online], 19 (189), 1–6. 10.1186/s12939-020-01307-z [Accessed 15 February 2021].

Public Health England, 2020a. *Disparities in the risk and outcomes of COVID-19* [online]. London: Public Health England. Available at: https://assets.publishing.service.gov.uk/government/uploads/system/uploads/attachment_data/file/908434/Disparities_in_the_risk_and_outcomes_of_COVID_August_2020_update.pdf. [Accessed 15 February 2021]

Public Health England, 2020b. *Health equity assessment tool (HEAT)* [online]. London: Public Health England. Available at: https://www.gov.uk/government/publications/health-equity-assessment-tool-heat [Accessed 30 January 2020].

Saldana, L., and Chamberlain, P., 2012. Supporting Implementation: the role of community development teams to build infrastructure. *American Journal of Community Psychology* [online], 50 (3-4), 334–346. 10.1007/s10464-012-9503-0 [Accessed 4 December 2020].

Spencer, N.J., 1999. The Acheson report: challenges for the college. *Archives of Disease in Childhood* [online], 80 (6), 576–578. 10.1136/adc.80.6.576 [Accessed 5 February 2021].

The Soft Drinks Industry Levy Regulations, 2018. [online] Available at: https://www.legislation.gov.uk/uksi/2018/41/contents/made [Accessed 5 November 2018].

Tobin, J., 2021. *Eating out and takeaways: calorie labelling regulations* [online]. London: House of Lords Library. Available at: https://lordslibrary.parliament.uk/eating-out-and-takeaways-calorie-labelling-regulations/ [Accessed 5 November 2021].

Tudagbe-Obour, I., 2022. Appraisal of Challenges and Community Promotion in WASH Facilities in Senior High Schools in Ghana. *Universal Journal of Social Sciences and Humanities*, pp. 93–105.

van Zon, S.K.R., Reijneveld, S.A., Mendes de Leon, C.F., Bültmann, U., 2017. The impact of low education and poor health on unemployment varies by work life stage. *International Journal of Public Health* [online], 62 (9), 997–1006. 10.1007/s00038-017-0972-7 [Accessed 15 January 2020].

Winston, C.N., 2016. An existential-humanistic-positive theory of human motivation. *The Humanistic Psychologist* [online], 44 (2), 142–163. 10.1037/hum0000028 [Accessed 15 February 2021].

Woodhouse, D., 2010. Community profiling. In: Blackshaw, T., ed. *Key concepts in community studies*. London: Sage, 2010, 55–60. 10.4135/9781446279076 [Accessed 15 January 2021].

World Health Organisation, 1946. *Constitution* [online]. Geneva: WHO International. Available at: https://www.who.int/about/who-we-are/constitution [Accessed 27 October 2019].

World Health Organisation, 1986. *Ottawa charter for health promotion* [online]. Copenhagen: WHO Europe. Available at: http://www.euro.who.int/__data/assets/pdf_file/0004/129532/Ottawa_Charter.pdf [Accessed 27 September 2019].

World Health Organisation, 2002. *Environmental health in emergencies and disasters* [online]. Geneva: WHO International. Available at: https://apps.who.int/iris/bitstream/handle/10665/42561/9241545410_eng.pdf?sequence=1&isAllowed=y [Accessed 4 December 2020].

World Health Organisation, n.d. *Social determinants of health* [online]. Geneva: WHO International. Available at: https://www.who.int/health-topics/social-determinants-of-health#tab=tab_1 [Accessed 15 February 2020].

3 Human Growth and Development

Martin Smith

The chapter aims to consider a wide range of subjects related to our overall development across the lifespan of human growth and development including:

- Develop an understanding of key issues in health and social care
- Consider a range of psychosocial, biological and physical changes in human growth and development
- Key developmental theories and ideas central to human growth and development
- Develop understanding of the impact of life events on individuals and the effects of historical changes on the individual life course

Core Principles

As human beings we go through many stages in our overall development and are influenced by a range of different factors which ultimately shape who we are and how we evolve. There are many terms within the realm of human growth and development and we will consider and discuss a range of theories, concepts and ideas which go to make this area of study the interesting and fascinating subject it is.

The importance of understanding how we develop through our lifespan is vital to any aspect of work you may decide to undertake in the field of health and social care. Whether your focus is on children, adolescent or any stage of adult life, understanding key theories and ideas associated with human growth and development cannot be underestimated.

In this chapter, we will consider some of the psychosocial, biological and physical changes that people experience during their lifespan and the factors that affect and influence those changes. We will introduce you to key developmental theories and ideas and will consider and develop understanding of the impact of life events on individuals and the effects of historical changes on the individual life course.

The chapter will examine dimensions of human growth and development, lifespan development, key theories around human growth and development, human physical development, child development, adult development.

DOI: 10.4324/9781003079873-4

Dimensions of human growth and development (adapted from Rice, 1995) to be considered include:

Physical development

Includes the physical growth of the body and changes in motor development, the senses, and in bodily systems.

Cognitive development

Includes all changes in the intellectual processes of thinking, learning, remembering, problem solving and communicating.

Personal development

Includes the development of the concept of self; the development of attachment, trust, security, love and affection; and the development a variety of emotions, feelings and personality traits all of which go to make us who we are.

Social development

Includes the development of interpersonal relationships with family members, peers and other members of the community.

Defining well-being

When we consider the psychological literature on well-being, we find a range of authorities with over lapping ideas about how humans can live their lives to the full (Ryff and Singer 1998).

Examples of such terms/ideas we should consider include:

- Self-actualisation (Maslow 1968)
- Individuation (Jung 1933)
- The will to meaning (Frankl 1958)
- Personal development (Erickson 1963)
- The fully function person (Rogers 1962)
- Maturity (Allport 1961; Pilgrim 2017, p. 6)

All the ideas and theories we will discuss contain assumptions which can be challenged. Beckett and Taylor (2019, p. 6) suggest some we may question include:

- Assumptions about the roles of men and women
- Assumptions that take heterosexuality as the norm
- Assumptions of Western society being the norm
- The concept of "Eurocentric assumptions"
- Assumptions of research and studies done with more prosperous middle class are relevant to other economic and social groups
- Assumptions around religious or spiritual beliefs

Lifespan Development

A term we will use frequently in this chapter is that of "lifespan development".

Lifespan development is a branch of psychology which considers human growth and development across the whole lifespan of a human being. This can be described as studies which considers human growth and development across the whole lifespan of a human being. One thing you will notice is that these studies are not restricted to one field of academic study nor is there a unified theory.

One definition that may be helpful around lifespan development is

> The sequence of events and experiences in a life from birth until death, and the chain of personal states and encountered situations which influence, and are influenced by this sequence of events.
>
> (Runyan 1978, p. 570)

Hunter (2005) argues that life cycle can be reduced to a developmental model or models which outline the social and psychological change encountered as a person passes through the major stages of life. These stages being childhood, adolescence, mid-life, old age and eventually death. "Lifespan studies" is a broad perspective encompassing a number of academic disciplines including:

- Psychology
- Sociology
- History
- Anthropology
- Biology

According to Baltes (1987), there are seven main principles of the lifespan perspective which are as follows:

1   It is a lifelong process.
2   It is multidimensional and multidirectional.
3   The process shows plasticity – it can be affected and changed by life experience and circumstances.
4   It involves gains and losses.
5   It is an interactive process between the individual and their environment.
6   It is culturally and historically embedded.
7   It is a multidisciplinary field of study.

In today's often rapidly changing outlook and cultural changes, these points are very relevant and bring into question many of the previous theories and ideas which have been developed to understand what it means to be human and how we develop as human beings.

Key Theories and Concepts in Human Growth and Development

Aside of some key broad theories around human growth and development, there are also some concepts which affect and have challenged theorists and researchers in this field for decades. Some of the broad concepts we should consider include:

- **Active vs. passive:** This concept asks key questions such as do we take an active part in our development or are we completely at the mercy of our environment? Are we blank slates at birth and altered by events and environment? (Ryan and Edward 2000).

- **Critical vs. sensitive periods of development:** Are there critical periods or sensitive periods which impact on human growth and development? A critical period is a specific time during development when a particular event has its greatest impact (Fox 2014).

  Attachment theory highlights critical periods for a child's emotional development. Better understanding of human plasticity and resilience now tells us change is possible later in life despite significant deficits in early life.

- **Continuity vs. discontinuity in change:** Is development smooth and (continuous) throughout life or are there abrupt stages based (discontinuous)? Can our development be identified by discrete stages in which something has to occur before we can move to the next stage? Is childhood development abrupt and in stages? Is it different to adult development?

- **Stability vs. change:** Are we consistent and predictable over our lifespan or do we fluctuate in who we are and what we do over time? Are we a victim of our childhood and our genes? Current research has mainly drawn the conclusion that our development is characterised by both stability and change.

  There has always been strong debate over how much change is possible of over our lifespan. Baltes and Smith (2003) argues adults are able to change but the capacity is less than that of a child and diminishes over time. Kagan (2003) argues personality traits such as shyness have a genetic base but can be changed over time. There is a lot of evidence now pointing to personality and personality disorders having far more of a genetic base (Paris 2015, p. 45).

- **Nature vs. nurture:** A perennial issue which has been hotly debated over the years giving rise to such questions as, are we born this way or do we develop? Are we a victim of our genetic inheritance or environmental factors? Both are now recognised as shaping development. The question is how much do each play in development? The influence in modern research of concepts like "Epigenetics" plays an important role.

In the science of genetics, "epigenetics" is the study of cellular and physiological phenotypic trait variations that result from external or environmental factors that switch genes on and off and affect how cells are expressed (Moore 2015).

All the concepts we have highlighted here help to challenge and broaden our thinking around how we develop as human beings. As you can see, we cannot think too literally or state with absolute certainty that any one theory or idea is correct. Using the idea of flexibility helps us to continually learn and develop and understand what it is to be human and how we develop.

Human Physical Development

Dr. Arnold Lucius Gesell (1880–1961) was an American clinical psychologist, paediatrician and professor at Yale University. His research and contributions to the field of human development came through what he termed the Maturational Theory. Gesell was one of the first psychologists to systematically describe children's physical, social and emotional achievements and developmental stages. He believed that a child's growth and development are influenced by both their environment and genes. He called this process maturation, the process by which development is governed by intrinsic factors, principally the genes.

He based his theory on three major assumptions which were as follows:

- Development is orderly, sequential and predictable and builds on earlier learning, skills or behaviours
- Children develop individually and at their own pace, but every child follows the same sequence
- Certain aspects of development happen at specific times and can lead to states of equilibrium of disequilibrium

Gesell described a series of ten developmental milestones. These milestones are the following:

1 **Motor characteristics:** The development of physical movement and hand/eye coordination is clearly important in our development and encouraging plenty of physical activities is important for this milestone.
2 **Personal hygiene:** Attention to daily health routines such as eating, sleeping, bathing and instilling the importance of these activities at an early age is another important milestone.
3 **Emotional expression:** The encouragement of healthy expression of a range of affective attitudes in the right settings such as laughing, crying, assertion and anger.
4 **Fears and dreams:** The ability to deal with a range of emotions such as anxieties, hopes and fears. Being attentive, highlighting it is OK to have these states.
5 **Self and sex:** Development of confidence and positive relationships. We will be looking further into the self and intimate relationships as we go through the various stages of childhood and adult development.
6 **Interpersonal relations:** Again highlighting the importance of love and relationships at all levels, friends, family, peers and eventually intimate relationships. All very important factors in overall human growth and development across all age stages.
7 **Play and pastimes:** Recognition of the importance of play and encouragement of interests in reading, music, art, sport and more. The importance of play and recreation for children and adults is so important and often significantly underestimated in importance.
8 **School life:** Adjustment to school life and the educational environment is for many challenging and stressful, meeting new friends and developing a strong learning and eventually a strong work ethic.
9 **Ethical sense:** Development of a sense of what is good and bad. An appropriate response to instructions, punishment, praise and reason. Allowing space to consider consequences of behaviours and the development of a strong moral compass are all important factors for human beings interactions with others and overall existence in community and wider groups.
10 **Philosophical outlook:** Developing an ability to express thoughts on deeper emotive subjects such as war, death, religion and culture. Encourage discussion and awareness of major issues of the day.

We will now have a brief look at three major psychological theories which have influenced the developing ideas of human growth and development and discuss some of the major contributors to each of these major schools.

Psychodynamic Theory

In the early 20th century, **Sigmund Freud**proposed a set of ideas known as **psychodynamic theory.** The theory highlighted key ideas around human growth and development and aspects of personality theory. The psychodynamic theory is a view that explains personality in terms of conscious and unconscious forces. Psychodynamic theories commonly hold that childhood experiences shape personality.

Erik Homburger Erikson (1902–1994) was a German born American developmental psychologist and psychoanalyst known for his theory on psychosocial development in human beings. Erikson built upon Freud's work and identified eight separate stages of development across the lifespan. Erickson's model highlights the **social** context of development referred to as the **psychosocial** stages.

The model presents a useful template to chart the human lifespan and offers developmental stages faced throughout life. Each stage has a positive or negative outcome, though we tend not to be at either end of the spectrum. The outcome of the stage is determined by our environment, and the care giving strategies or experiences to which we are exposed.

Erickson's eight stages of psychosocial development are:

1   Trust vs. mistrust – age to 1
2   Autonomy vs. doubt – age 2–3
3   Initiative vs. guilt – age 4–5
4   Industry vs. inferiority – age 6–11
5   Identify vs. role confusion – ages 12–20
6   Intimacy vs. isolation – ages 20–40
7   Generativity vs. stagnation – ages 40–65
8   Ego integrity vs. despair – 65 years and over

Erickson believed that in each stage we face a crisis that needs to be resolved in order for us to develop socially and emotionally and move forward to the next stage. As you can see from the stages if a certain crisis is not resolved issues will continue to manifest themselves later in life from that stage such as feelings of mistrust of others or doubt in one's own abilities. A well-known term often cited from Erickson's stages is when someone is said to have an "inferiority complex".

Behaviourist Theory

Behaviourism is the view that the appropriate focus of psychology should be observable behaviour, without reference to inner states. In this view, behaviour provides the key to understanding human and non-human animals. Behaviourism emerged methodologically in the early 20th century as a reaction to what was termed "mentalistic" psychology, which often had difficulty making predictions that could be tested using rigorous experimental methods.

The primary tenet of methodological behaviourism, as expressed in the writings of Watson and others, is that psychology should only concern itself with observable events. There has been a drastic shift in behaviourist philosophies throughout the 1940s and 1950s and again since the 1980s.

A behaviourist explanation for learning is that humans and animals come to associate certain stimuli with their own behaviour. For instance, a child might associate praise with polite action; the praise reinforces the child's polite behaviour, and the child thereby learns (becomes conditioned) to act politely.

B.F. Skinner was a prolific author, publishing nearly 200 articles and more than 20 books. In a 2002 survey of psychologists, he was identified as the most influential 20th-century psychologist. **Radical behaviourism** is the concept purposed by B.F. Skinner that acknowledges the presence of private events – including cognition and emotions – but does not actually prompt that behaviour to take place.

While behaviourism is no longer a dominant school of thought, his work in operant conditioning remains still quite important and relevant today.

- Mental health professionals often utilise operant techniques when working with clients
- Teachers frequently use reinforcement and punishment to shape behaviour in the classroom
- Animal trainers rely heavily on these techniques to train dogs and other animals

Humanistic Theories

Key pioneers of this approach included **Carl Rogers** and **Abraham Maslow**.

Humanistic psychology, also often referred to as humanism, emerged during the 1950s as a reaction to the two approaches that dominated psychology at the time.

Sometimes called the third force in psychology, after the psychodynamic and behaviourist approaches.

Humanistic, humanism and humanist are terms in psychology relating to an approach which studies the whole person, and the uniqueness of each individual.

Human growth and development is studied from the point of view of the individuals subjective experience. The approach is important because it redirected psychology towards the study of the self. Essentially the humanistic approach considers human behaviour not only through the eyes of the observer, but through the eyes of the person doing the behaving. The fundamental belief of the humanistic approach is that people are innately good and that mental and social problems result from deviations from this natural tendency.

The humanistic approach states that the self is composed of concepts unique to ourselves. **The self-concept includes three components:**

> **Self-worth** or **self-esteem:** What we think about ourselves. Rogers believed feelings of self-worth developed in early childhood and were formed from the interaction of the child with the mother and father.

> **Self-image:** How we see ourselves, which is important to good psychological health. At a simple level, we might perceive ourselves as a good or bad person, beautiful or ugly. Essentially self-image has an effect on how a person thinks, feels and behaves in the world.

> **Ideal self:** This is the person who we would like to be. It consists of our goals and ambitions in life, and is dynamic – i.e. forever changing. The ideal self in childhood is not the ideal self in our teens or early or late adulthood.

Attachment Theory

Attachment theory is a psychological model that attempts to describe the dynamics of long-term interpersonal relationships between humans. Initially attachment is about a strong emotional tie that develops over time between an infant and its primary caregivers.

Attachments are welded in the heat of interaction (Maurer and Maurer 1988).

The following are some key characteristics around attachment theory:

- **Proximity maintenance:** There's a strong desire to be near the people we are attached to
- **Safe haven:** Caregiver/attachment figure is a safe haven for us to whom we have a tendency to return to for comfort and safety in the face of a fear or a threat
- **Secure base:** The attachment figure acts as a base of security from which the child can explore the surrounding environment
- **Separation distress:** Anxiety which often occurs during the absence of the attachment figure

There are a number of key phases in the development of attachment within infants described and developed by Schaffer and Emerson (1964) and Bowlby (1969):

- **Pre attachments** (indiscriminate social responsiveness) birth to two months old
- **Attachments in the making** (recognition of familiar people) two to seven months old
- **Specific or clear cut attachments** (separation protest and stranger anxiety) 7–24 months old
- **Multiple attachments** from eight months old

A number of types of attachment were developed and attributed to children, these would then relate to adults:

Type A – avoidant
Type B – securely attached
Type C – resistant or ambivalent
Type D – disorganised

You can find about more about these types of attachment by looking at Mary Ainsworth's work (Ainsworth et al. 1978).

Child Development

Piaget's Stages of Cognitive Development

Piaget believed a child's thinking passed through four separate stages. He emphasised the importance of maturation and the provision of a stimulating environment for children to explore.

Piaget has been, and continues to be, an important influence on how we think about children's thinking skills.

- **The sensory motor stage:** Birth to two years old – this stage consists of **six sub-stages** that also show significant gains in a child's thinking as they progress through infancy. Children are using their physical or motor skills and their senses to explore their world and develop their cognitive understandings. This stage fits well with many theories around child development.
- **The pre-operational stage:** Two to seven years old – in this stage children are less reliant upon senses and physical exploration. Their thinking is developing but still in a simplistic style and process. A classic example in this stage is where a child is shown two balls of dough exactly the same size. They will agree that the balls are the same size, but when one is flattened, they will usually tell you that one of them is now bigger.
- **The concrete operational stage:** 7–11 years old – this stage aligns with middle childhood, children are beginning to be able to demonstrate much more logical thinking, although they need concrete materials to help them reach the correct conclusions. In this stage, you will see children working on mathematical problems using blocks, counters or even their fingers to help them work out the answer.
- **The formal operational stage:** 11 years onwards – a final stage encompasses the rest of the individual's life. Piaget believed that once we reached the age of 12 we were capable of much more abstract thinking and able to solve problems in our heads.

Lev Vygotsky's Sociocultural Theory

This relates to both cognitive and social development. A Russian theorist who died in 1934, his work only found a broader audience in recent thinking around psychosocial development.

Vygotsky developed his theories around the same time as Piaget. He emphasised the importance of relationships and interactions between children and more knowledgeable peers and adults. Vygotsky believed that children's cognitive understanding could be enriched and deepened when they were **"scaffolded"** by a parent, teacher or peer (Berk 1996).

Vygotsky also saw children's thinking developing in stages, but he emphasised the social and cultural influences on a child's learning. Vygotsky also emphasised the role of language in the development of thinking processes. He saw the child's ability to think logically as developing in stages. He outlined four different stages of development.

- **Thinking in unordered heaps:** Preschool stage the start of conceptual thought with a lot of use of trail and error but with the start of some problem solving processes
- **Thinking in complex stages:** Starting to make connections between objects but not in a consistent manner
- **Thinking in concepts:** Starting to think in more abstract concepts
- **Thinking in true concepts:** Developing more mature thinking and starting to manipulate a number abstract concepts at one time

Vygotsky also identified four different stages of speech development these being:

1 **Primitive speech stage:** Birth to two years – the child is just learning to speak and imitating words and naming objects often responding emotionally with laughter and crying.

- **Naïve psychological stage:** Two to four years – here there is a realisation words are symbols for objects and there is a greater curiosity as to what objects are called.
- **Egocentric or private speech stage:** Four to seven years – children often talk aloud to themselves and often whilst performing tasks or problem solving. This "private speech" demonstrates the child's thinking.
- **Ingrowth or inner speech stage:** Eight years on – the outward private speech declines and the private speech becomes a lot more internalised. There is still some outward private speech when dealing with complex or unusual problems.

Adult Development

Becoming an adult. Adulthood usually covers the largest part of our lives, but the adult years of human development have attracted much less research over the years than childhood years. One reason for this apparent lack of interest in adulthood research can be down to a view that it is all over by adulthood. Some developmental psychologists tended to believe and take the view that the process of development is completed once we achieve our adult years (Durkin 1995).

It is true that stability and continuity of personality do occur in adulthood suggesting that development is a done deal. But there is more, in adult life there is a complex process of change and interplay between, the psychological, sociological and biological aspects of life which continue to shape who we are.

Transitions in Young Adult Life

- Periods of rapid growth/change/disruption disequilibrium are often known as transitions
- Transitions can be related to physiological changes, status or role changes, or changes in situations
- These are followed by periods of relative calm and consolidation

Looking at how young adults negotiate the difficult business of transition and finding a new adult identity, their identity James Marcia defined four different kinds of "identity status" found among adolescents/young adults.

1 **Identity diffusion:** Avoidance of commitment and indecision around major life decisions.
2 **Identity foreclosure:** An acceptance of others' values (parents, teachers) rather than self-determined goals.
3 **Moratorium:** Intense identity crisis as the individual struggles to make life decisions but is actively engaged in trying to make those decisions.

4   **Identity achievement:** The individual has resolved their crisis and made firm commitments on their terms based on their own thinking and decision making.

Young Adulthood – Problems Encountered

There are a range of issues any young adult can encounter, a few may include:

- Relationship difficulties
- Parenting difficulties
- Possible offending
- Drug and alcohol and other health and life issues
- Mental health issues
- Disabilities, learning, physical and psychological
- Chronic illness
- Coping as a carer for ageing parents

Daniel Levinson (1978) – **Seasons of a life** proposed there is an underlying order in the human life cycle, and although every individual life is unique, we all go through the same sequence, of four stages. From a study of 40 men, Levinson was able to construct a stage theory of development based on alternating periods of transition and stability. There are many questions and views on age range within our development especially around what is consider adolescence and also older age. Notice Levinson's age span and compare it with other theorists such as Erickson.

- Childhood and adolescence (0–22 years)
- Early adulthood (17–40 years)
- Middle adulthood (40–65 years)
- Older adulthood (60 and over years)

In this theory the **"structure changing"** periods of transition last four to five years and are times when the individual experiences inner crisis and conflict, questions the status quo and makes new choices to alter the pattern of his life. The **"structure-building"**periods of stability, lasting six or seven years, are geared towards con-solidation and the pursuit of new goals and values.

Critics suggest that stage models of the adult life such as Levinson's don't reflect either the diversity of individual experience or take account of the very changing world we are in today as it relates to areas such as:

- Gender
- Race
- Historical time and place
- Life events

Sugarman (2001) concludes that incorporating gender and race into the theory highlights that the content of the stages, Levinson suggests, is by no means universal, but that alternative phases of change and consolidation are a consistent feature of adult development.

Mid Adult Life Development

Adult human middle age can be considered a cultural construct. The concept of middle age is socially constructed. It came into use as an increasing lifespan led to new roles at midlife and hence this particular aspect of development has grown. As our health and well-being generally increase, hence there are a number of issues specific to this stage of human development.

Mid Adult Life – Presenting Issues

- Some physical decline
- A decline in fertility for women
- Fewer career options
- Adolescent children
- Empty nest syndrome
- The Bucket list syndrome
- Is this a halfway point?
- Assuming job and civic responsibilities
- Relinquishing job and civic responsibilities
- Becoming a parent or grandparent
- Becoming a carer
- Middle carer phenomenon

Middle adulthood can be seen as a time of both gains and losses. The span of middle adulthood can be defined chronologically, contextually or biologically. Most middle-aged people are in good physical, cognitive and emotional condition (depending on a number of factors). They have heavy responsibilities and multiple roles in middle age. It can be a time for taking stock and making decisions about the remaining years.

The "mid-life crisis" has entered popular mythology as a time when adults (particularly men) go through a sort of second adolescence. An increasing sense of one's own mortality and a fear of loss of opportunities which will not come again and perhaps being "left behind" by the contemporary (working) world has all helped develop the concept of mid-life crisis.

When it comes to mid-life is there a difference between the view we take of men getting old and women getting old? There are thoughts and views that there is a "double standard of ageing" causing women to seem less desirable as they lose their youthful appearance and often men being more desirable. For both men and women, anxiety about getting older can be heightened by a society view that places a premium on youth.

Values and Priorities

Fiske and Chiriboga (1990) asked the participants in their longitudinal study of adulthood a key question "What is your main purpose in life at the present time?" From the answers, they developed the following seven categories of values/priorities:

1   **Achievement and work:** Economic competence, rewards, success and social status
2   **Good personal relations:** Love and affection, happy marriage and friends

3   **Philosophical and religious:** Including concern with the meaning of existence and adherence to an ethical code
4   **Social service:** Helping others, community service, etc.
5   **Ease and contentment:** Simple comforts, security and relaxation
6   **Seeking enjoyment:** Recreation and exciting experiences
7   **Personal growth:** Self-improvement, being creative

Late Adult Life Development

In the late 20th and early 21st century, advances in nutrition and health care have extended the period of good health as well as extending the overall life expectancy which in turn has put a continued strain on many aspects of our health and social care services.

Some believe there is a prejudice against older people in Western cultures, referred to as ageism. The increase of senior citizens around the world especially in more economically developed countries could be considered a problem. The fact is, with the number of elderly people increasing, there will be a greater need for people to care for them.

It has also created a significant issue in other areas – pensions provision relied upon life expectancy at retirement being short but as life expectancy continues to become longer so therefore is the issue around pension provisions.

The term ageism was invoked to express concern about the condition and treatment of older people during the 1960s and 1970s. Butler defined ageism as

> a process of systematic stereotyping of and discrimination against people because they are old, just as racism and sexism accomplish this for skin colour and gender.
> (Butler and Lewis 1973, p. 20)

Seeing ageism as something that applies only to older people fosters a "them" and "us" view of "the elderly" as a minority group, different and separate from the rest of society. If old age is seen as inevitably accompanied by decrement and decline then it is not surprising if fear and ambivalence about ageing leads younger people to distance themselves from those who are older.

Coping with Late Adulthood

Toffler (1971) suggests that we can cope with large amounts of change, pressure, complexity and confusion provided at least one area of our life is relatively stable.

Toffler's Stability Zones

Toffler's concept is fairly simple. Stability zones are places or things that make you feel safe, relaxed and secure. Think of them as buffers – types of protection or defence – against the outside world. Our stability zones can make us feel safe. Something safe and familiar, something that doesn't change. These zones and the concept can greatly help in supporting people in old age.

Toffler details five stability zones, each can be stand-alone but often overlap.

1   People
2   Ideas
3   Places
4   Things
5   Organisations

People stability zones are sources of social support. They represent values and enduring relationships with others, for example, family, long-standing friends and colleagues.

Ideas that are stability zones could be a deeply felt religious belief or a strong personal and/or professional commitment to a philosophy, political ideology or cause.

Places of varying scale can comprise stability zones. They might be large scale (like a country) or small scale (e.g. a street or a particular room). "Home" is often a stability zone, a place with a comforting familiarity about it, perhaps where one grew up or has spent considerable time.

Things as stability zones take the form of favourite, familiar, comforting possessions.
    They might range from family heirlooms, through particular objects to favourite items of clothes.

Organisations as stability zones could be the work organisation, a professional body, a club, or any other organisation to which one belongs and with which one identifies.

Stability zones can overlap – "home" has elements of place, people and things, for example; "books" have elements of things and ideas; and "the work place" might have elements of all stability zones.

Conclusion

This chapter has examined the full lifespan development and considered some key and significant theories and approaches which over the decades has helped us understand what it means to be human and how we develop through our lives from birth to death. We have discussed some general theories which have helped us to critique and evaluate a range of concepts and ideas. We have discussed some broad psychological theories including psychodynamic, behaviourist and humanistic approaches to human growth and development.

We have gone on to consider some very influential theories such as attachment theory and childhood development theories before considering the various stages of adulthood. Hopefully you have seen from the areas we have covered that human growth and development is both complex and challenging in relation to out understanding and work around various ages.

Our lifespan development is both generally lengthy and complex with many theories and ideas having developed over the years. These theories and ideas continue to develop as the world changes. It is important to appreciate many of the theories that have already gone but also to always challenge and develop new ideas and concepts from ever changing and ever developing understanding of human growth and development.

Exercise – Life Course Reflections

Throughout this chapter, we will be considering our development as human beings across a life course from birth to death. Many things influence individual human growth and development. Take time to reflect on the following questions/statements.

Make some notes and keep this sheet to refer to and link it to different stages of development and you can reflect how these events and impacts have influenced your development and that of those around you (we do not develop and change in isolation – our development impacts those around us at many different levels).

- **Activity 1: Consider and note down two major events in your life.**

- One positive event –

- One negative event –

- How have these events impacted on your life and the course of your life and personal development?

- List down a couple of people who have influenced you in your life – consider how they have done this.

- What is the next major stage of your life and what barriers do you see in achieving that stage or goals in that stage?

```



```

- What are your strengths to achieving what you want to do in that next major stage?

```



```

References

Ainsworth, M.D.S., Blehar, M.C., Waters, E., & Wall, S., 1978. *Patterns of attachment: A psychological study of the strange situation*. Lawrence Erlbaum.

Allport, G.W., 1961. *Pattern and growth in personality*. Holt, Reinhart & Winston.

Baltes, P.B., 1987. Theoretical propositions of lifespan developmental psychology. *Developmental Psychology*, 23 (5), 611–626.

Baltes, P.B. and Smith, J., 2003. New frontiers in the future of aging: From successful aging of the young old to the dilemmas of the fourth age. Gerontology, 49 (2), pp. 123–135.

Beckett, C., and Taylor, H., 2019. *Human growth and development*. 4th ed. London: Sage.

Berk, L.E., 1996. *Child development*. London: Anchor Books.

Bowlby, J., 1969. Attachment and loss v. 3 (Vol. 1).

Butler, R.N., and Lewis, M.I., 1973. *Aging & mental health: positive psychosocial approaches*. Missouri: Mosby.

Durkin, K., 1995. *Developmental social psychology: From infancy to old age*. Blackwell Publishing.

Erickson, E., 1963. *Childhood and society*. 2nd ed. London: W.W. Norton.

Fiske, M., and Chiriboga, D.A., 1990. *Change and continuity in adult life*. San Francisco: Jossey-Bass.

Frankl, V.E., 1958. On logotherapy and existential analysis. *The American Journal of Psychoanalysis*, 18, 28–37.

Fox, N.A., 2014. What do we know about sensitive periods in human development and how do we know it? *Human Development*, 57 (4), 173–175.

Hunter, D.J., 2005. Gene–environment interactions in human diseases. Nature reviews genetics, 6 (4), pp. 287–298.

Jung, C.G., 1933. *Modern man in search of a soul*. Harcourt, Brace.

Kagan, J., 2003. Biology, context and developmental enquiry. *Annual Review of Psychology*, 54, 1–23.

Levinson, D., 1978. *The seasons of a man's life*. New York: Ballantine.

Maslow, A., 1968. *Toward a psychology of being*. 2nd ed. New York: Van Nostrand Reinhold.

Maurer, C., and Maurer, D., 1988. *The world of the newborn*. New York: Basic Books Inc.

Moore, D., 2015. *The developing genome*. Oxford: Oxford University Press.

Paris, J.A., 2015. A *concise guide to personality disorders*. Washington DC: American Psychological Society.

Pilgrim, D., 2017. *Key concepts in mental health*. 4th ed. London: Sage Publishing.

Rogers, C., 1962. *On becoming a person*. London: Constable Publishing.

Ryan, D., and Edward, L., 2000. Self-determination theory and the facilitation of intrinsic motivation, social development, and well-being. *American Psychologist*, 55 (1), 68–78.

Ryff, C., and Singer, B., 1998. The contours of positive human health. *Psychological Inquiry*, 9 (1), 1–28.

Schaffer, H.R., & Emerson, P.E., 1964. The development of social attachments in infancy. *Monographs of the society for research in child development*, 1–77.

Sugarman, L., 2001. *Life-span development: frameworks, accounts and strategies*. 2nd ed. Hove: Psychology Press.

Toffler, A., 1971. *Future shock*. New York: Bantam Books.

4 Current Issues in Health and Social Care

Jennifer Sanders, Lee Reynolds, and James Pike (with contributions from Ashleigh Moogan)

The chapter aims to:

- Developing an understanding of key issues in health and social care is essential to understanding current issues
- Developing research and academic skills are required to explore these issues
- A critical approach to the use of information discussing the key issues needs to be encouraged

Objectives

After reading this chapter, you should:

- Be aware of the key skills required for studying in higher education
- Understand how to search and evaluate literature
- Be able to discuss key issues in health and social care

After reading this chapter, you will know the meaning of the following terms: literature searching and evaluating, summarising, paraphrasing, citing, referencing, rights, justice, utilitarianism and deontology.

There is a Moment of Reflection at the end of the chapter to assist with developing your academic skills.

Introduction

Health and social care issues are often emotive and divisive, making newspaper headlines and trending on social media platforms. This media information is often what forms people's opinions on such issues, can be useful to gage the public views on a matter and in some instances be the stimuli for research or policy action. However, such sources are not scholarly and therefore have limited application to studying at higher education. The first part of this chapter will introduce how to search for and evaluate literature to include in academic assignments. The concept of reading for academic purposes will be explored, including how to appraise literature, and how to paraphrase and summarise these for write-up. Harvard citing and referencing format will also be outlined.

DOI: 10.4324/9781003079873-5

The second part of this chapter explores three contemporary issues in health and social care: assisted dying, mandatory childhood vaccinations and the use of technology in social care. Such complex and challenging issues require a philosophical and ethical exploration. Four key concepts and theories are briefly outlined to aid such examination (see Beauchamp and Childress, 2013, for further detail of these):

> Rights – Rights can be a source of protection: from oppression, unequal treatment, invasion of privacy, etc. Rights could also be an entitlement to something: confidentiality, autonomy, access. We have civil, legal and social rights. Rights can be problematic: individual v. communal interests, obligation v. right, which rights are priority?

> Justice – Related terms include fairness, equity, desert and entitlement. Within health and social care, distributive justice can be the focus with discussion focusing on individual needs, fair opportunity, and practicalities of allocation, priority setting and rationing.

> Utilitarianism – This theory, which falls under consequentialism, centres on the notion of the greatest good for the greatest number. Firstly, an act's rightness or wrongness is assessed by the consequences it produces. Secondly, the right act is one of utility – produces the maximum positive outcome.

> Deontology – This theory, also referred to as Kantian theory, focuses on duties. Firstly, the rightness or wrongness of an act is measured by its features rather than its consequences. Secondly, the motivation for the act is drawn from an individual's morality.

Discussion, of the three issues listed above, will outline the key issues, providing examples of how to incorporate the ideas of others and discuss these critically, through utilising the academic skills described.

Key Skills

In the first edition of this book, there are tips and guidance on getting started with assignments, writing skills, effective reading and note taking strategies. This chapter will focus on the skills of searching, evaluating paraphrasing, summarising, citing authors and referencing literature.

Literature Searching

Before searching for books, journal articles, reports or policy documents, it is key to identify what you know and what remains to be found out (Crème and Lea 2008; Ridley 2012). Rehearsing these ideas can offer key terms for effective literature searching. This might come in the form of a mind map or a free-writing exercise where useful ideas and search terms are extracted (Crème and Lea 2008; Smith 2013). This information can be used to adapt the parameters of the search for fewer, more specific results. Ridley (2012) offers further guidance for conducting and recording literature searches.

To decide whether a source is worth reading, the CRAAP test (Blakeslee 2004) could be applied:

- Current
- Reliable/accurate
- Authoritative
- Purposeful

If the source fails one aspect of the test, it does not mean that it cannot be used if it is meaningful or relevant to the point being made in the assessment. However, if the reason why it fails this test in some way undermines that point then it needs to be mentioned with that literature in the assessment. If the source fails on several counts, then consider other sources making the same point. While some sources are more academic and critical, some provide valuable contextual information such as policies, statistics that highlight the scale of issues, government reports or serious case reviews that examine the extent of problems or provision (Pears and Shields 2019).

Evaluating Literature

While sources appear valuable, it is important not to take their content at face value (Cottrell 2017). Not everything you read will be used in the assessment as more relevant and quality sources are uncovered as your understanding of the topic grows. Questions for evaluating literature include but are not limited to (Ridley 2012):

- What were the authors trying to achieve?
- What did the author conclude as being problematic, important or useful moving forward?
- Did the authors achieve what they set out to?
- Do their conclusions make sense based on what they did and what they have cited?

When writing assessments, answering these kinds of questions enable the reader to make decisions. Evaluating can involve identifying strengths or application to situations to demonstrate significance, so it is not necessarily about criticism. Additionally, evaluating does not mean locating a source arguing the opposite. Sometimes, literature misses relevant viewpoints, so evaluating may involve highlighting what the literature does not say rather than what it does (Ridley 2012).

Summarising Literature

Approaching literature with prepared questions creates ease in summarising key ideas in the form of answers. There are several linear and visual ways to record and re-hearse these (Crème and Lea 2008; Ridley 2012; Cottrell 2017).

The quantity and quality of notes taken from individual sources will depend on its perceived value. Information taken from literature should be meaningful and relevant to the point being made in the assessment, with anything else considered description.

For example, if the article discusses in depth the very problem or strategy being discussed in the assessment, this could be worth a couple of sentences, whereas other sources may not even be mentioned. Remember, it is not quantity of information that influences the considerations of the reader.

Paraphrasing

Paraphrasing is the rewording of ideas (Ridley 2012). Engaging in reading makes this easier as students identify what is important, problematic or useful moving forward to address issues related to the assignment brief. But how is this conveyed? Many paragraphs address one of those points. This position needs justifying by explaining why or how that is the case, demonstrated with an example that integrates another perspective, culminating in the impact of the problem, consideration, or strategy for those exemplified. This informs the reader's approach moving forward (Godfrey 2016).

In addition to using structure, language can be used to enable readers to access the point (Cottrell 2017). This involves using tentative language and third person pronouns to remove generalisations and subjectivity from the argument; subject specific words that enable the reader to identify what the paragraph is about; formal, but simple language, that signposts and shows the reader what direction the argument is taking.

Citing the Reading

Acknowledging the work of others demonstrates understanding and engagement with a wide range of reading (Pears and Shields 2019).

Citations are what references look like within the paragraph. Citations are used when positing a claim, reason, an example, or a way forward and its impact. Highlighted earlier, a variety of sources may be utilised. In the Harvard system, sources are cited using only the author's last name and year of publishing (Pears and Shields 2019). There are exceptions such as acts of parliament and YouTube videos, so be familiar with the institution's referencing guide. Citations can be used in two forms.

When the author's name is grammatically part of the sentence, this is **integral**.

> *Oldham (2020, p. 77) posits the importance of 'consulting institutional referencing guidance'.*

In **non-integral** citations, the author's name is not explicitly mentioned but the citation must be there. These tend to appear at the end of a clause or sentence.

> *Online reference generators are convenient but often inaccurate (Kessler and Van Ullen 2005).*

Imagine the contents of the brackets are not spoken when reading the sentence aloud, the sentence not making sense indicates that there is an issue with grammar or the citation placement, which needs revisiting.

Creating the Reference List

Citations require a matching entry in the reference list at the end of the assignment (Crème and Lea 2008; Pears and Shields 2019). Each item in this alphabetical list should contain information that enables the reader to locate the source (Pears and Shields 2019). It is important students locate their university's guide to referencing, because these often differ from online automatic reference generators, but Pears and Shields (2019) offer ideal introductory guidance. The exception is where the university subscribes to a generator using the university's template. Using Harvard, a reference begins with the author's last name, their first initials and the year in which it was published. The other information about the source depends on what type of source it is:

Book
Johnson, B. 2011. *Referencing Systems*. London: Seldom Press

Journal Article
Miller, F. 2019. Incorporating Sources. *Academic Haberdashery*. 8 (2) 45–56

Website
Pence, T. 2014. *Sorting Citations*. [Online] Available at: https://c1t4t1on.com [Accessed 12 November 2019]

Suggested further reading

Godfrey, J., 2016. *Writing for University*. 2nd ed. London: Palgrave.
Pears, R., and Shields, G., 2019. *Cite Them Right: The Essential Referencing Guide*. 11th ed. London: Red Glove Press.
Ridley, D., 2012. *The Literature Review: A Step-by-Step Guide for Students*. 2nd ed. London: SAGE.

Current Issues

Three key issues will now be briefly discussed, with suggestions of further reading provided. These discussions will demonstrate application of the CRAAP Test (Blakeslee 2004) and evaluation of literature. Summarising and paraphrasing of literature (Cottrell 2017) will provide insight into some of the key ethical issues that need consideration.

Assisted Dying

Assisted dying is an oft debated topic in healthcare and political spheres. The notion raises ethical dilemmas around autonomy, rights, and the role of medical professionals. There are a range of individuals – both professional and public – who may have differing perspectives on the issue. It can be the focus of news headlines, TV panel shows and documentaries. These can include comparisons to the legal practices in countries such as the Netherlands and United States, as well as stories of individuals travelling to access services like Dignitas in Switzerland.

Euthanasia and assisted suicide are illegal in England and Wales (NHS 2020), with prosecution policy being introduced to include the encouraging of or assisting in a suicide which happens abroad. Since 2002, there have been several attempts to introduce an assisted dying bill in England and Wales (House of Lords 2017). In session 2016–2017 the most recent attempt to introduce legislation failed to progress passed the first reading in the House of Lords. This proposed Assisted Dying Bill (2016) set the parameters of assisted dying to be enabling competent adults who are terminally ill to have assistance to end their own life by a qualified medical practitioner.

Before a discussion of arguments for and against an assisted dying legislation being introduced in England and Wales, some definitions and distinctions between alike concepts is needed to enable a full understanding of assisted dying:

> Euthanasia – the act of deliberately ending a person's life. This act can be classified as voluntary, provided at the request of a competent individual, or non-voluntary, provided for an incompetent individual.

> Assisted suicide – the act of deliberately assisting another to kill themselves, for example making arrangement for them to self-administer a lethal dose of drugs.

> Assisted dying – autonomous choice to die when terminally ill, aided by a doctor. This is often referred to as physician-assisted suicide.

An article by Haigh (2012) opens with distinguishing the different terms relating to assisted dying, whilst acknowledging that these terms are often used interchangeably. This needs to be taken into consideration when identifying terms to be used in literature searches and when appraising the relevance of literature found. Haigh goes on to outline some of the legislation relating to assisted dying/assisted suicide/euthanasia around the world. However, as the article was published in 2012 it lacks currency, as it does not cover developments such as the most recent bill proposals in England and Wales, and the very recent and controversial move to allow euthanasia for terminally ill children under 12 in the Netherlands (Care Not Killing 2020). Haigh continues to explore the legal position in England and Wales, referring to some high-profile cases, such as that of Debbie Purdy, which can be verified and explored along with other personal stories at the Campaign for Dignity in Dying website.

Haigh (2012) goes on to explore the evidence base of the assisted dying debate, acknowledging that whilst the issue is contentious with some strident opposition it is important to separate emotion and rhetoric from the evidence. It is for this reason that literature found through academic databases is more reliable than solely basing an argument on personal stories. An interesting aspect of Haigh's paper is that she identifies the arguments against assisted dying, then refutes these to frame her case for an assisted dying law in the United Kingdom. The key arguments she discusses are the 'slippery slope', money will be diverted from palliative care services, the laws of God will be compromised, trust will be eroded between patients and healthcare professionals, and access to high-quality palliative care will remove the need for assisted dying. Taking each in turn Haigh outlines the issues, identifies a lack of evidence to support the point or draws on empirical evidence which demonstrates the counter-argument. Within these discussions (see Haigh 2012), principles such as autonomy and justice provide an opportunity for ethical theories to be applied to aid understanding of the key issues relating to assisted dying.

Haigh (2012) ends her article by discussing the implications for nursing practice, an informed piece as professor of nursing at a UK university. Whilst the arguments in this article are supported by empirical evidence, it is acknowledged that generalisation of findings from one country to another should be cautious of possible cultural differences, particularly if that country has a form of assisted dying legislation in place.

Within the same year in the same professional magazine an article by Robinson and Scott (2012) was published, outlining arguments why assisted suicide must remain illegal in the United Kingdom. Like Haigh (2012), the article starts with definitions and current legal status in the United Kingdom. They go on to provide an overview of the debate, drawing on ethical concepts around rights, justice and consequentialism. The article then focuses on two issues supporting the notion assisted dying should not become legal: protection of vulnerable groups and assessment of mental capacity. These arguments are supported with empirical evidence, or critique is provided for research supporting the 'for' stance. Interestingly, several sources used are the same as those in Haigh's article. This demonstrates how the same piece of research can be used to support two opposing arguments by different authors, highlighting the importance of accessing and appraising the primary research yourself. Robinson and Scott conclude their article with an overview of guidance on how nurses should respond to questions or requests for an assisted suicide.

The publisher RCN has publicly taken a neutral stance on the debate around assisted dying legislation (2014), supported by the publication of these opposing articles. The purpose of both articles is to explore current issues affecting nursing practice, and therefore aimed at professionals and those studying such concepts. Whilst in practice the issue itself has not changed, it would be important to access empirical research conducted in recent years to ascertain if perceptions have altered over the past eight years, given the developments in legislation.

In sum, the articles by Haigh (2012) and Robinson and Scott (2012) provide a detailed overview of the assisted dying debate, supported by empirical evidence. Read in conjunction, they demonstrate the ethical dilemma of assisted dying and how research can be presented in a way to support or oppose key arguments. Therefore, to further one's understanding of the debate it is recommended to access the primary empirical research directly, including more up-to-date evidence from a wider range of publishing sources and authors.

Suggested further reading

Karsoho, H., Fishman, J.R., Wright, D.K., and Macdonald, M.E., 2016. Suffering and medicalization at the end of life: the case of physician-assisted dying. *Social Science and Medicine* [online], 170, 188–196. DOI: doi.org/10.1016/j.socscimed.2016.10.010

Wicks, E., 2020. Assisted dying reframed in the context of English law's approach to suicide. *Medical Law International* [online], 20 (4), 287–307. DOI: /doi-org.ntu.idm.oclc.org/10.1177/0968533220982637

Mandatory Childhood Vaccinations

In the United Kingdom, we have a free vaccination schedule for children which starts in infancy and continues throughout childhood. These vaccines are delivered by the NHS and whilst highly encouraged by all health professionals, they are not mandatory, and parents can refuse to have their children vaccinated if they wish to do so. The vaccines we use contain weakened or inactive parts of an antigen, to trigger our bodies into producing antibodies and creating an immune response. This means that if we come into contact with the antigen, our immune system already has the antibodies to fight it and we will not become sick (WHO 2020). As there are children with weaker immune systems that cannot receive the vaccinations, we rely on herd immunity, meaning if 95% of children are vaccinated, the whole population should remain safe and immune (NHS 2019).

However, there has been a recent decline in vaccination rates, which has allowed outbreaks of measles causing the United Kingdom to lose its 'measles-free' status just three years after eliminating the virus. 'Anti-vaxxers' and the concern sparked by the now discredited MMR and Autism paper are explanations for this. In response, the government pledged to develop a strategy to improve immunisation services, public health information and communication, as well as addressing parental safety fears (Ford 2019). In an interview at a Conservative Party Conference Health Secretary Matt Hancock disclosed advice had been sought and that making vaccinations mandatory was being considered. There is precedence for vaccinations to be compulsory, with the *Vaccination Act 1853* mandating the smallpox vaccination, with the disease being eradicated. Investigation by Gravagna et al. (2020) suggests there is currently over 100 countries across the world which have mandatory vaccinations, with the majority imposing penalties for non-compliance.

Isaacs, Kilham and Marshall (2004) provide an ethical exploration of whether childhood vaccinations should be mandatory. As vaccinations involve a mild form of the virus entering our body, there are concerns over the risk of harm. A risk v. benefits calculation is made, with consideration of the consequences of vaccination and non-vaccination. Herd immunity is an important outcome of vaccination, as a high level of vaccine uptake means those who cannot be vaccinated are protected. This is a utilitarian view of vaccination producing the greatest good for the greatest number. It is a strong argument for mandatory vaccinations, but there is also concern that compulsion to vaccinate could lead to protests and decline in uptake, as seen in the 19th century, over fears of infringing choice and autonomy.

Consideration of autonomy and choice leads to a debate around rights (Isaacs, Kilham and Marshall 2004). Children have a right to be protected. Communities have a right to be protected. Compulsory vaccinations would uphold these rights. But what about parental autonomy and rights? Here, exemptions based on medical, religious or philosophical grounds question the appropriateness of mandatory vaccinations. A consideration of the risk of harm again becomes prominent, drawing debate on the duties of parents and the state to protect children and communities. A rise in rates of preventable diseases could justify mandatory vaccinations, under the state's duty of care to the public. However, such compulsion can be seen as coercive and lead to a loss of trust in the state. Particularly when a decline in voluntary vaccinations may be linked to concerns around the safety of vaccinations encouraged by the state.

This concern of harm and impact of trust led Isaacs, Kilham and Marshall (2004) to conclude with alternatives to mandatory vaccinations. These centre around improving education and awareness to encourage vaccine uptake, possibility of inducements and exclusions to encourage vaccine uptake, and the notion of a 'no fault vaccine injury compensation scheme'. Whilst Isaacs, Kilham and Marshall provide good coverage of the arguments for and against mandatory vaccinations, one criticism is the lack of acknowledgement that children may not be vaccinated for reasons beyond safety concerns and exemptions.

Elliman and Bedford (2013, p. 1435) state that under immunised children comprise two main groups, one being 'those who are partially vaccinated because their parents have difficulties in accessing services or for other practical reasons'. Here, the argument that mandating vaccinations would lead to an increase in immunisation falls short, because it does not address the structural issues preventing uptake. In fact, mandating vaccinations could lead to widening inequalities in child health, where penalties would further negatively impact these already socially disadvantaged households.

Following an ethics discussion of the arguments for and against compulsory vaccinations, and the possible alternatives to mandates, it becomes clear that there are more fundamental issues to be addressed. There is hope that comprehensive strategy developed by the government, which includes the campaign Value of Vaccines, will address concerns and increase availability and accessibility leading to vaccine coverage which provides herd immunity (PHE n.d.).

Suggested further reading

Lasseter, G., Al-Janabi, H., Trotter, C.L., Carroll, F.E., and Christensen, H., 2018. The views of the general public on prioritising vaccinations programmes against childhood diseases: a qualitative study. *PLoS One* [online], 13 (6). DOI: https://doi.org/10.1371/journal.pone.0197374

Torracinta, L., Tanner, R., and Vanderslott, S., 2021. MMR vaccine attitude and uptake research in the United Kingdom: a critical review. *Vaccines* [online], 9 (4), 402–423. DOI: https://doi.org/10.3390/vaccines9040402

Technology in Social Care

The future of social care faces many challenges including an ageing population and a growing staffing shortfall. It may sound like science fiction, but could robots be the answer? Robots have been used in care settings in several countries, including Japan, Germany and the United Kingdom (Li 2015; Papadopoulos et al. 2021). Evidence suggests that robotic pets can reduce loneliness (Banks, Willoughby and Banks 2008). New research concluded in September 2020 purports to show that Pepper, a 'culturally competent' humanoid robot, has been shown to reduce loneliness and improve mental health among the elderly (Papadopoulos et al. 2021).

Many researchers have expressed concern about what replacing human carers with robots could mean, especially for quality of care (Folbre 2006; Sparrow and Sparrow 2006; Parks 2010; Sharkey 2011; Sharkey and Sharkey 2012a, 2012b). Prescott (2013) has responded and argued that the replacement of human carers by robots is not likely. Prescott argues that many opponents employ a 'slippery slope' form of argument, where a worst-case scenario is assumed. He argues that the worst-case scenario of older people being left with virtually no human contact and attended to almost solely by machines is highly unlikely. Robots would need to be advanced enough to be able to work unsupervised, and those responsible for care would have to consider it acceptable.

For Prescott, there are a number of 'defeaters' working against these conditions being met. Firstly, robots are not yet advanced enough, and so are more likely to be deployed in 'human-robot teams'. Secondly, because the number of human workers in care might be reduced, he argues that care roles should become more professional. Thirdly, Prescott argues that if human carers were relieved of more mundane duties, it would free up more time for meaningful social contact. Fourthly, as the computer-literate generations age, tomorrow's older people will be more culturally in tune with using technologies to stay connected to family. Lastly, he argues that older people themselves will have power to prevent the dystopian outcomes of fully robotised care due to growing electoral power.

The evidence, however, is not on Prescott's side that time freed up by introducing robots would likely be given over to increasing social interaction. As Duffy (2011) points out, care workplaces are victim to cost cutting and streamlining, which can mean the relational components of care (i.e., social interaction) are reduced. It seems a more likely outcome that the time freed up by introducing robots will simply be eliminated. This would follow the pattern of industry: where new technologies have increased the productivity of workers, they have often found themselves discharged rather than promoted to new less 'productive' roles (see Marx 1983).

Older people are already a significant electoral force. However, this has not led to meaningful change in a creaking social care system: the recommendations of the 2011 Dilnot Inquiry, advocating a maximum lifetime spend on care of £100,000 have been ignored for 10 years, and the latest *Green Paper*, commissioned in 2017, has been delayed six times.

Another perspective comes from Coeckelbergh (2010). He considers four arguments against the replacement of humans by robots in social care. Firstly, an AI system may be able to perform a series of tasks, but it cannot provide 'deep care' based on a genuine concern for the person. Secondly, it may be able to perform functions but cannot provide 'good' care since this necessarily requires contact with human beings. Thirdly, even if AI technologies could provide good care, they fundamentally violate the principle of privacy due to their monitoring functions, and so should be banned. Fourthly, AI assistive technologies provide 'fake' care: they are likely to 'fool' people by making people think they receive real care. Coeckelbergh argues that none of these are grounds to reject AI technologies, but instead pose serious questions about the care we already provide.

Firstly, if robotised care would lack an emotional connection, this is the case for much care that is provided by humans today. Arguably, day-to-day tasks completed by staff without any personal or emotional engagement is particularly undignifying and unethical. Coeckelbergh argues being treated like 'a thing' by a machine would be less morally degrading than to be treated like a thing by a human.

Secondly, Coeckelbergh argues that 'good' care should aim at promoting and preserving the dignity of the patients. It is quite plausible, he argues, that AI assistive technologies could play a role in achieving this care, and they cannot be dismissed out of hand. Regarding the argument about privacy, he argues that privacy cannot play top trumps and must always be balanced against other considerations. He argues that appropriate privacy measures could be designed into AI technologies. Lastly, he argues, concerns over 'fake' care are not significant because the vast majority will be well aware that they are not dealing with an AI.

Coeckelbergh concludes that the four arguments he examines are not strong ones against robots, but instead they

> force us to develop more systematic and comprehensive criteria for good care and rethink our existing practices of care. [...] We should not set the standards of care too high when evaluating the introduction of AI assistive technologies in health care, since otherwise we would have to reject many of our existing, low-tech health care practices (p. 189).

One possible criticism of Coeckelbergh's argument is that the line between technologies assisting human workers and the replacement of human workers is not so clear-cut. In the 19th century, the introduction of the machine loom revolutionised textile production, allowing one worker to produce what would have previously taken several. The machine loom still required a human worker, and so it did not 'replace' humans, but the increased productivity it brought led to workers being laid off. Was this replacing workers, or 'assistive technology'?

Suggested further reading

Coeckelbergh, M., 2010. Health Care, Capabilities, and AI Assistive Technologies. *Ethical Theory and Moral Practice* [online], 13 (2), 181–190. DOI: https://doi.org/10.1007/s10677-009-9186-2

Papadopoulos, C., Castro, N., Nigath, A., Davidson, R., Faulkes, N., Menicatti, R., Khaliq, A.A., Recchiuto, C., Battistuzzi, L., Randhawa, G., Merton, L., Kanoria, S., Chong, N-Y., Kamide, H., Hewson, D., and Sgorbissa, A., 2021. The CARESSES randomised controlled trial: exploring the health-related impact of culturally competent artificial intelligence embedded into socially assistive robots and tested in older adult care homes. *International Journal of Social Robotics* [online], 23 (1), 1–21. DOI: https://doi.org/10.1007/s12369-021-00781-x

Conclusion

The discussions above have started to outline the diverse perspectives of some current health and social care issues. These issues are very real, with perspectives influenced by experience, culture, legislation, etc. as well as the media. Discussions around ethics can often take place, and so some key theories and concepts have been identified to aid understanding and navigating such complex issues. When discussing health and social care issues in academic work, students are required to draw on the literature and research available to explore the issues, rather than relying on their personal opinions. A wide range of skills is needed for this: finding and understanding sources of information, incorporating these sources with critical thinking, utilising citation and referencing conventions.

When researching health and social care issues, students will come across a range of sources of information. Some of these will be considered more academic than others, for inclusion within formal academic work. But even those less academic sources can have their place in helping us understand the complexities and experiences of health and social care issues. Using the evaluation strategies outlined in this chapter will help you ascertain the utility of the sources. Take a moment to list as many sources as possible, and identify how they may or may not be used in academic work.

Moment of reflection

Table 4.1 provides some examples of when a range of different sources would and would not be used in academic work.

Summary of Main Points

You should be able to:

* Search and evaluate literature
* Produce evidence-based debates
* Understand key issues in health and social care

Table 4.1 Moment of reflection

Source of information	When it may be used	When it should not be used
Blog	• To provide a real-life perspective if about someone's experience • To show emotive nature of a topic • To demonstrate real issues	• As sole supporting evidence to a point in an assignment
News article	• To highlight the topical nature/public interest of an issue	• As sole supporting evidence to a point in an assignment
Information from.org website	• As examples of campaigns on an issue • To provide information from specialist charities/organisations	• As the only form of evidence for a particular issue • As the only source if assignment is supposed to be providing a balanced view • When there's a report available rather than just a webpage
Book or edited book	• To provide basic information about a concept • To provide definitions • Can be used as a gateway to access more reliable/academic sources	• As the source of research/evidence • Less so in Year 2 work, rarely in Year 3 work
Journal article	• As primary research/evidence • As a source providing a critique/evaluation/analysis of an issue	• May not be required in a reflective piece
Government report	• As primary research/evidence • As example of political nature/interest/importance	• May not be required in a reflective piece
Report by non-government organisation	• As primary research/evidence • As example of political nature/interest/importance	• If the report/account is biased and not appropriate for your purpose of including it

References

Assisted Dying Bill, 2016. HL Bill 42 [online]. Available at: https://publications.parliament.uk/pa/bills/lbill/2016-2017/0042/17042.pdf [Accessed 13 December 2020].

Banks, M.R., Willoughby L.M., and Banks W.A., 2008. Animal-assisted therapy and loneliness in nursing homes: use of robotic versus living dogs. *Journal of the American Medical Directors Association*, 9 (3), 173–177. 10.1016/j.jamda.2007.11.007

Beauchamp, T.L., and Childress, J.F., 2013. *Principles of biomedical ethics*. 7th ed. Oxford: Oxford University Press.

Blakeslee, S., 2004. The CRAAP test. *LOEX Quarterly* [online], 31 (3), 6–7. Available via: https://commons.emich.edu/loexquarterly/vol31/iss3/4 [Accessed 20 December 2020].

Care Not Killing, 2020. *Dutch to extend euthanasia to children of any age* [online]. London: Care Not Killing. Available at: https://www.carenotkilling.org.uk/articles/dutch-to-extend-euthanasia-to-children-of-any-age/. [Accessed 14 December 2020].

Coeckelbergh, M., 2010. Health care, capabilities, and AI assistive technologies. *Ethical Theory and Moral Practice* [online], 13 (2), 181–190. 10.1007/s10677-009-9186-2

Cottrell, S., 2017. *Critical thinking skills: developing effective argument and analysis*. 3rd ed. London: Palgrave.

Crème, P., and Lea, M.R., 2008. *Writing at university: a guide for students*. 3rd ed. Maidenhead: Open University Press.

Duffy, M., 2011. *Making care count: a century of gender, race and paid care work*. New Brunswick, NJ: Rutgers University Press.

Elliman, D., and Bedford, H., 2013. Should the UK introduce compulsory vaccination? *The Lancet* [online], 381 (9876), 1434–1435. 10.1016/ S0140-6736(13)60907-1

Folbre, N., 2006. Nursebots to the rescue? Immigration, automation, and care. *Globalizations* [online], 3 (3), 349–360. 10.1080/14747730600870217

Ford, S., 2019. *Loss of 'measles free' status by UK sparks widespread concerns* [online]. Nursing Times: Essex. Available at: https://www.nursingtimes.net/news/primary-care/loss-measles-free-status-uk-sparks-widespread-concerns-19-08-2019/ [Accessed 30 December 2020].

Godfrey, J., 2016. *Writing for university*. 2nd ed. London: Palgrave.

Gravagna, K., Becker, A., Valeris-Chacin, R., Mohammed, I., Tambe, S., Awan, F.A., Toomey, T.L., and Basta, N.E., 2020. Global assessment of national mandatory vaccination policies and consequences of non-compliance. *Vaccine* [online], 38 (49), 7865 – 7873. 10.1016/j.vaccine.2020.09.063

Haigh, C., 2012. Exploring the case for assisted dying in the UK. *Nursing Standard* [online], 26 (18), 33–39. 10.7748/ns2012.01.26.18.33.c8875

House of Lords, 2017. *Assisted dying legislation: North America and England and Wales* [online]. London: UK Parliament. Available at: https://lordslibrary.parliament.uk/research-briefings/lif-2017-0019/ [Accessed 13 December 2020].

Isaacs, D., Kilham, H.A., and Marshall, H., 2004. Should routine childhood immunization be compulsory? *Journal of Paediatrics and Child Health* [online], 40 (7), 392–396. 10.1111/j.1440-1754.2004.00399.x

Kessler, J., and Van Ullen, M.K., 2005. Citation generators: generating bibliographies for the next generation. The journal of academic librarianship, 31 (4), pp. 310–316.

Li, J., 2015. The benefit of being physically present: A survey of experimental works comparing copresent robots, telepresent robots and virtual agents. *International Journal of Human-Computer Studies* [online], 77, 23–37. 10.1016/j.ijhcs.2015.01.001

Marx, K., [1867] 1983. *Capital: volume 1*. London: Lawrence & Wishart.

National Health Service, 2019. *Why vaccination is safe and important* [online]. London: National Health Service. Available at: https://www.nhs.uk/conditions/vaccinations/why-vaccination-is-safe-and-important/ [Accessed 11 December 2020].

National Health Service. 2020. *Euthanasia and assisted suicide* [Online]. London: National Health Service. Available at: https://www.nhs.uk/conditions/euthanasia-and-assisted-suicide/ [Accessed 13 December 2020].

Papadopoulos, C., Castro, N., Nigath, A., Davidson, R., Faulkes, N., Menicatti, R., Khaliq, A.A., Recchiuto, C., Battistuzzi, L., Randhawa, G., Merton, L., Kanoria, S., Chong, N-Y., Kamide, H., Henson, D., and Sgorbissa, A., 2021. The CARESSES randomised controlled trial: exploring the health-related impact of culturally competent artificial intelligence embedded into socially assistive robots and tested in older adult care homes. *International Journal of Social Robotics* [online], 1–12. 10.1007/s12369-021-00781-x

Parks, J., 2010. Lifting the burden of women's care work: should robots replace the "human touch"? *Hypatia* [online], 25 (1), 100–120. 10.1111/j.1527-2001.2009.01086.x

Pears, R., and Shields, G., 2019. *Cite them right: the essential referencing guide*. 11th ed. London: Red Glove Press.

Prescott, T.J., 2013. *Sunny uplands or slippery slopes? The risks and benefits of using robots in care*. UKRE Workshop on *Robot Ethics* hosted by the University of Sheffield Adaptive Behaviour Research Group on March 2013 in Sheffield.

Ridley, D., 2012. The literature review: A step-by-step guide for students. London: Sage.

Robinson, V., and Scott, H., 2012. Why assisted suicide must remain illegal in the UK. *Nursing Standard* [online], 26 (18), 40–48. 10.7748/ns2012.01.26.18.40.c8874

Sharkey, N., and Sharkey, A., 2011. The eldercare factory. *Gerontology* [online], 58 (3), 282–288. 10.1159/000329483

Sharkey, A., and Sharkey, N., 2012a. Granny and the robots: Ethical issues in robot care for the elderly. *Ethics and Information Technology* [online], 14 (1), 27–40. 10.1007/s10676-010-9234-6

Sharkey, N., and Sharkey, A., 2012b. The crying shame of robot nannies: an ethical appraisal. *Interaction Studies* [online], 11 (2), 161–190. 10.1075/is.11.2.01sha

Smith, R.J., 2013. *Advantage study skills*. 2nd ed. S.L.: R1 Publications.

Sparrow, R., and Sparrow, L., 2006. In the hands of machines? The future of aged care. *Mind and Machines* [online], 16 (2), 141–161. 10.1007/s11023-006-9030-6

World Health Organisation, 2020. *How do vaccines work?* [online]. S.L.: World Health Organisation. Available at: https://www.who.int/news-room/feature-stories/detail/how-do-vaccines-work#:~:text=Vaccines%20contain%20weakened%20or%20inactive,rather%20than%20the%20antigen%20itself [Accessed 11 December 2020].

5 Working with People

Amy Allen

The chapter aims to:

- Explore how concepts of equality, human rights and diversity inform communications between professionals and service users
- Develop a range of communication skills and interventions used by practitioners in a range of settings
- Explain the importance of self-awareness when working with vulnerable people

Key terms:

Equality
Equity
Diversity
Therapeutic relationship

Introduction

The term 'health and social care' encompasses a wide range of different types of services which provide support for an infinite number of individual needs. Each setting has its own ways of working which suit the specific type of care being provided. However, there are some universal skills and values which are vital for ensuring high-quality care can be provided (Gee 2017). This chapter seeks to introduce these core skills and values to give a foundation upon which many other professional attributes can be developed. The chapter is entitled 'Working with People' because, at the most basic level, this what health and social care professionals seek to do – to be able to provide support to individuals, no matter their needs, characteristics, background or other factors.

This is such a key tenet of the caring professions that it forms the first standard of the Standards of Conduct, Performance and Ethics set out by the Health Care Professions Council (HCPC):

> **1. Promote and protect the interests of service users and carers**
> *Treat service users and carers with respect*
> 1.1 You must treat service users and carers as individuals, respecting their privacy and dignity.

DOI: 10.4324/9781003079873-6

1.2 You must work in partnership with service users and carers, involving them, where appropriate, in decisions about the care, treatment or other services to be provided.

1.3 You must encourage and help service users, where appropriate, to maintain their own health and well-being, and support them so they can make informed decisions.

Make sure you have consent

1.4 You must make sure that you have consent from service users or other appropriate authority before you provide care, treatment or other services.

Challenge discrimination

1.5 You must not discriminate against service users, carers or colleagues by allowing your personal views to affect your professional relationships or the care, treatment or other services that you provide.

1.6 You must challenge colleagues if you think that they have discriminated against, or are discriminating against, service users, carers and colleagues.

Maintain appropriate boundaries

1.7 You must keep your relationships with service users and carers professional.

(HCPC 2016, p. 5)

Caring professionals often meet service users at a time when they feel particularly vulnerable. They have come to a service for help and support with an issue (or often multiple issues) which are causing them distress. The initial interaction the service user has with a professional is often vital in ensuring that appropriate and effective care can be given (Gotlieb 2000; Komen 2015). Professionals need to rapidly build trust and rapport with the individual to enable them to 'open up' about what is causing them distress. If the individual feels uncomfortable or unwelcome, they are unlikely to feel safe to share personal information and may be deterred from using the service in the future (Neighbour 2018). Professionals must ensure that everyone who comes to the service feels equally welcome and supported, and this chapter aims to introduce the core values and skills needed to do this. The first section of this chapter explores some key concepts which professionals need to be aware of when ensuring they are providing high-quality care to all. The second section focuses on developing the practical skills needed to develop a therapeutic relationship. The third section explores some of the specific barriers experienced by those with a protected characteristic and how these can be overcome.

Discrimination, Marginalisation and Health Inequality

The Equality Act (2010) made it unlawful for any public body, organisation or workplace to discriminate against an individual because of any of any of nine protected characteristics. This law consolidated several existing pieces of legislation into one simpler act. It also made clear the responsibility of care providers to ensure they consider the impact of their policies and procedures on individuals with any of the nine protected characteristics.

The nine protected characteristics:

1   Age
2   Disability

3 Gender reassignment
4 Marriage and civil partnership
5 Pregnancy and maternity
6 Race
7 Religion or belief
8 Sex
9 Sexual orientation

(Equality Act, 2010)

The term discrimination describes the unfavourable treatment of an individual or group because of a protected characteristic (known as direct discrimination) or putting in place a rule or policy or way of doing things that has a worse impact on someone with a protected characteristic than someone without one, when this cannot be objectively justified (known as indirect discrimination).

Individuals or groups who experience discrimination can become marginalised in society. Marginalisation means being pushed out to the edges, in essence being made to feel like you do not belong in the society in which you live. Marginalised groups feel unwelcome or disadvantaged in their society to a point where they feel unable or unwilling to participate. Bradby et al. (2020) found that service users from minority groups felt services were dismissive of their concerns. In response, these service users often withdrew from the services or sought alternative provision which prioritised their needs more effectively. This experience of marginalisation and a lack of understanding of individual needs creates a barrier to seeking further help. If those in marginalised groups do not feel cared for or welcomed by health care services, they will not seek medical care when they need it which can lead to further deterioration in health status, worsening existing health inequalities. For this reason, it is vital that services actively seek to engage with marginalised groups and ensure they remove the barriers which have deter them from seeking help in the past.

Equality, Equity or Removing Barriers?

The term 'equality' is used freely in the media, in educational settings and in general conversation. However, its meaning is often unclear (Thompson 2018). Does it mean treating everyone the same? Let's explore the meaning of 'equality' by also discussing two other interrelated terms – 'equity' and 'removing barriers'. Figure 5.1 illustrates the difference between the words equality and equity. If all three baseball fans were treated equally (each being given the same box), then one fan still cannot see the game. However, if we use those same resources, we can create equity so that all three fans can watch. We can see that making our society fair and accessible for all does not mean treating everyone the same, it is about providing support or tools to those who need them to ensure everyone has an equal opportunity to participate.

There is also a third way to ensure all three fans in this image can participate though – by removing the barrier which is creating the inequality. In this example, the solid wooden fence could be replaced by a wire fence so all three fans can see through it, removing the need for the boxes. This removal of barriers is the ultimate goal in achieving equality of opportunity. Rather than those who are at a specific disadvantage having to seek support to achieve equity, we redesign to remove the barriers which cause the disadvantage. Thompson (2018) therefore defines equality as meaning 'equal fairness'.

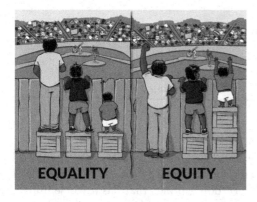

Figure 5.1 Equality vs. equity.

Source: https://interactioninstitute.org/illustrating-equality-vs-equity/

Another way to explore this concept is to look at the word 'disabled'. This term implies that an individual is unable to do something. However, it is often the environment, not the individual where the disabling barriers exist. For example, an individual may have an impairment which means they need to use a wheelchair, but it is the lack of ramps which disables them from entering a building. This is what is referred to as the social model of disability – the barriers and attitudes of society prevent someone with an impairment from participating, not the individual themselves (Goering 2015).

Professional Self-Awareness

Often, we can be unaware of how our behaviour impacts on others. It is easy to unknowingly make someone feel you are not listening with a simple gesture such as a yawn. Whilst in everyday life this can be socially uncomfortable, in a care setting it can be much more problematic. A vulnerable individual may have taken a lot of time to build up the confidence to seek help, if their first interaction with a professional makes them feel devalued, judged or unwelcome, they are unlikely to continue to seek support. This can lead to them becoming more vulnerable. By contrast, if a service user feels listened to, valued and respected, they are much more likely to engage with the support available leading to a more positive outcome.

Professionals working in the caring industries must regularly reflect on their own practice to develop self-awareness (Jasper and Rosser 2013). Being aware of how our gestures, words and actions impact on a service user helps us to develop our skills. Although we are unaware of them, our unconscious biases can influence the quality of care we provide (Matarozzi et al. 2017). Self-awareness also involves becoming aware of our private beliefs or prejudices and how these may be affecting our professional behaviour. This is often an uncomfortable process but it can be an important step towards ensuring we are not acting in a way which disadvantages anyone (Neighbour 2018).

Developing professional self-awareness can be a formal or informal process and can be done individually or as part of a professional group of peers (Trafford 2017). Exercises for developing professional self-awareness include:

- Writing reflective accounts of interactions with service users to evaluate their efficacy and impact

- Participating in role-plays or simulated interactions to practice or develop therapeutic communication skills
- Discussing or reflecting on ethical issues related to the professional setting to explore the impact of personally held beliefs on professional decision-making
- Seeking feedback from service users or peers to identify areas for development

Developing the Interpersonal Skills Employed by Practitioners to Engage with Service Users in a Range of Settings

In our daily lives, we communicate in a variety of different ways. We naturally adapt the style and content of our speech to match the audience and purpose. Certain words, phrases and behaviours are expected in a social situation, but would not be acceptable in a more formal setting. In developing advanced interpersonal communication skills, such as counselling skills, a professional seeks to become aware of how they are communicating and how this may influence an interaction (Beesley 2017).

What Is a Therapeutic Relationship?

All care should be person-centred and tailored to meet the needs of the individual. This is difficult to do without first understanding that individual's needs. A therapeutic relationship is one in which a professional actively seeks to engage with an individual to explore their needs and provide support using a person-centred approach (Egan and Reese 2020). It is a broad term which can be used to describe the relationship between the service user and the professional in a variety of contexts. The term 'therapeutic relationship' can describe many types of caring, professional relationships. Such relationships are distinct from personal relationships as they are formal in nature, with boundaries and a clear purpose.

The therapeutic relationship is one of mutual respect, with the client seen as the expert on their own needs and circumstances. Using this approach, Egan and Reese identified three outcome-focused goals of the therapeutic relationship:

1 Life enhancing outcomes for the service user
2 Learning how to help oneself
3 Developing a prevention mentality

Each of these requires the empowerment of the service user to take an active role in the process of change. The building and maintaining of a professional relationship can therefore be vital in enabling meaningful change for the individual.

Beginnings

At the beginning of any therapeutic relationship, it is important to establish purpose, boundaries and expectations (Nelson-Jones 2013). You may be meeting with a service user who is reluctant to accept help or does not understand why they need to engage with you. Starting with a clear introduction can help to build their confidence in your and avoid misunderstandings about how you can help. Whilst the introduction you give will be different in every role or service, there are a few fundamental points which should be included.

At the beginning of the first meeting, it is important to introduce yourself and your role. Often service users are referred to a new setting without understanding why. People with complex needs may see lots of health and social care professionals in many different settings so identifying who does what can be confusing. Ensure that you state your name clearly and explain your role, including the reasons you feel the meeting is needed (Boyd and Dare 2014). Making the purpose of the meeting clear upfront can also help the session to be more meaningful as it enables the service user to focus on the aspect you are there to help with.

Explaining the boundaries of the therapeutic relationship is also an important initial step. It is often important for the service user to understand whether the session is confidential and what exceptions there may be to this confidentiality. Other boundaries may include whether or not the service user can contact you outside of your arranged meeting times, whether others can join the session (for example a partner or family member) and where meetings can take place (Moss 2020).

Perhaps the most important part of the introduction is to set mutual expectations for the session or series of sessions. Be sure the ask the service user what they would like to achieve during your time together. You may have conflicting aims, the service user may feel that they wish to focus on a different aspect of their care to the one you feel should be the key focus. By discussing what each party wishes to achieve in the session, you can ensure that the time spent together is meaningful and productive. Setting expectations is an important part of this negotiation. It is not uncommon for a service user to have unrealistic expectations of what a service can offer. By talking about what they expect and what you are able to deliver, you can avoid conflict later on and set an agenda which is mutually beneficial (Morrison 2014). You may find that the service user is not happy with the purpose of the meeting and does not wish to continue, such decisions must be respected.

Activity 1   Skills

Whilst you are practicing these skills, it can be a good idea to develop a set of notes to help you to remember all the information needed in a first meeting.

Imagine you are a social worker meeting a service user for the first time to discuss how you can support them. Create a set of notes of what you might say to introduce yourself and explain the purpose of your meetings.

Make sure you include the following key points:

- Introduce yourself and your role
- Explain the purpose of the meeting
- Explain confidentiality (and it's limits)
- Encourage the service user to introduce themselves and their expectations of the meeting

Building the Relationship

There are many skills which an effective communicator uses to develop a therapeutic relationship. When used appropriately, these help to build trust with the service user and help to ensure that meetings are productive and client-focused. Together, this group of skills is often referred to as active listening (Moss 2020). Using active listening skills signals emotional awareness which can help to reduce distress and develop the therapeutic relationship (Bodie et al. 2015). Some of these valuable skills are introduced in Table 5.1.

Table 5.1 Skills

Positioning	The layout of a room and the positioning of the seating can be important in ensuring that a service user feels comfortable and able to talk. The space between the professional and the client should be sufficient that personal space is not invaded and that the interaction does not feel intimidating. On the other hand, too much distance can become a barrier to communication.
	Different cultures have different distances at which they feel comfortable (Sorokowska et al. 2017). Where possible, a professional should allow a service user to moderate the interpersonal space so they feel comfortable.
	Often reducing physical barriers can also help to build trust, for example avoiding having a large desk between the two parties.
Body language	Professionals must be aware at all times of the non-verbal signals we are sending to service users through our body language and facial expressions. Adopting an open body posture, avoiding crossed arms and facing the service user send signals that they have our full attention and we are listening.
Tone, pace and volume	An individual's tone of voice can influence the meaning of what is being communicated. The same words can be perceived as aggressive if shouted or soothing if whispered. To create a calm and supportive environment in which a service user feels comfortable to talk, it is important that the professional uses a calm and clear voice. It can take practice to develop a voice which conveys care and support, especially if a professional naturally speaks quickly or loudly.
Open questions	When building a therapeutic relationship with a service user, a professional seeks to encourage them to say as much as possible about their situation, their feelings or their needs so they can provide appropriate support. One way to do this is through the use of open questions. Open questions are those which require a fuller answer and cannot be answered with one word such as 'yes' or 'no'. Asking open questions invites the service user to follow their own path in explaining things, rather than restricting them to answering in a specific way. This helps a session to be more client-centred (Royal College of Nursing 2021).
	Examples of open questions include:
	'Tell me how you have been feeling this week' 'What do you think we should discuss today?' 'What are your main concerns?' 'Describe the situation in your own words'

(Continued)

Table 5.1 (Continued)

Closed questions	Whilst closed questions restrict the service users' answers, they can be useful for clarifying certain points (Semyonov-Tal and Lewin-Epstein 2021). Closed questions can be used carefully to check understanding or present a choice. Examples may include: 'Did that happen today?' 'How old were you when that happened?' 'Are you happy to continue with this session?'
Mirroring	An advanced skill, which should be used subtly and sparingly is mirroring. This technique can be a way of overcoming barriers and building a connection with a service user. Here, the professional mirrors the posture or gestures of the service user. For example, if the service user is leaning back with crossed arms, the professional could adopt this posture briefly, then slowly move to a more open posture. Doing this can encourage the service user to do the same thing which can help them to feel more open and engaged.
Reflection of content or feelings	The professional can make the service user aware of a key point or feeling by using reflection. For example, if the service user begins to cry, the counsellor may say 'You're feeling sad'. This shows understanding and acceptance of the feelings being expressed. This skill must be used sensitively though to avoid making assumptions (Geldard, Geldard and Foo 2019).
Paraphrasing	Paraphrasing can be vital for checking understanding and showing that a professional has listened. The professional gives a brief summary of what the service user has said and asks the service users if they have understood correctly. This helps to avoid misunderstandings before proceeding further.
Challenging	Challenging is another advanced skill that should be used with care. Here, the professional questions the words used or the beliefs held by the service user about a particular subject. The aim is to encourage the service user to think from another perspective, not to devalue what has been said. For example, if a service user says 'I'm not good at anything', a professional could challenge this by highlighting something they are good at to show this broad and harmful sentiment to be untrue. Another example of challenging involves exploring contradictions for example if the individual's non-verbal behaviour does not match with what they are saying (Geldard, Geldard and Foo 2019). For example, 'You say this was a fun experience but talking about it seems to make you anxious, why is that?'
Probing	Probing questions encourage the service user to give more detail about what has been said or think more deeply about it. Example of probing questions include: 'Tell me what happened before/after that' 'How did that make you feel?' 'What are your thoughts on what happened?' 'Tell me more about that'
Revisiting	Often a service user may mention something which seems important but, in trying to explain lots of things at once, brushes over it quickly. As professionals should try to avoid interrupting as much as possible, it can be useful to make a note of these things and revisit them later in the session. This is referred to as revisiting as the professional is going back to something mentioned earlier to gain more detail or understand how it relates to the conversation.

Endings

The way an interaction is concluded can be as important as the way it is begun (Neslon-Jones 2013). In most health and care settings, interactions are limited to appointment slots with strict timings. To ensure an interaction does not end abruptly, it is useful to signpost to the service user that the session is coming to an end. This can help the service user to ensure that they have covered all the points they wished to discuss. The next step is to summarise what has been discussed to ensure there is agreement about the key points and the meaning both parties will be taking away from the interaction. This helps to ensure that nothing has been missed and that there is no misunderstanding. This summary should lead to a clear set of actions. These could be things that the professional is going to do (for example a referral form), or things the service user will do (for example regular breathing exercises). There may also be discussion about meeting again and what purpose the next meeting will have. Finally, it is important to value what has taken place. Often interactions between service users and professionals involve the sharing of deeply personal information which can leave an individual feeling vulnerable or exposed. It is vital to take time to acknowledge this, to thank the service user for their time and to reassure them that what has said will remain confidential (Moss 2020).

Considerations when Working with People with Specific Characteristics

Whilst each service user's needs are unique, there are some of the factors a professional may need to consider when working with individuals with certain characteristics. The following section will explore some of the barriers experienced by people with specific protected characteristics and introduce ways in which these barriers can be overcome. First, gender and sexuality are discussed, followed by race and ethnicity. Whilst these are just some of the protected characteristics covered by the Equality Act (2010), it is hoped that they demonstrate some of the complexities of overcoming health inequalities for all.

Gender and Sexuality

The LGBT Foundation (2022) conducted a survey exploring the experiences of accessing primary health care services for people in the LGBTQ+ community. They found that 41% of respondents felt their GP surgery did not meet their needs as an LGBTQ+ individual and 12% had experienced discrimination based on their gender identity or sexuality in the past year. This may be due to a lack of services aimed specifically at the LGBTQ+ community and the feeling that existing services are designed from a heteronormative perspective, which do not welcome or consider the needs of people who are not heterosexual or cisgendered, leading to further marginalisation (McDermott 2021; Scott 2021).

A lack of awareness amongst primary care staff can add extra burden to non-binary and transgender individuals who feel obligated to educate the professionals they meet about their gender and needs. Professionals may place unnecessary emphasis on gender-related issues once they know an individual is non-binary or transgender which, although well-meaning, can lead to further reluctance to access primary care in the future (Vincent 2020). Specific awareness training aimed at supporting mental health practitioners to talk comfortably about issues related to sexuality and gender can be beneficial and have a positive impact on outcomes for LGBTQ+ service users experiencing self-harm or suicidal tendencies (Hughes, Rawlings and McDermott 2018).

Professionals should check how a service user would like to be addressed. An individual's preferred name and pronoun may differ from their legal name used official paperwork such as a referral form. Professionals must be sure to use the gender pronoun that each individual prefers (for example 'he', 'she' or 'they'). It is vital that professionals do not make assumptions about the sexuality of service users. For example, assuming a female service user is in a heterosexual relationship by referring to their partner as 'he'. Such examples of unconscious bias can make the service user feel the professional is making a judgement and create a barrier to forming a trusting relationship.

Race and Ethnicity

Both interpersonal and structural racism still have a negative impact on the opportunities of people from ethnic minorities within the United Kingdom. Experiencing racism significantly increases the chances of developing mental illnesses (Kwate and Goodman 2015; Williams and Etkins 2021). Experiencing racism has also been linked to hypertension and chronic stress (Brondolo et al. 2011). The recent COVID-19 pandemic highlighted the impact of health inequalities. The pandemic disproportionately affected ethnic minority communities, who experienced significantly higher infection and mortality rates than their white counterparts.

MacPherson (1999, p. 49) used the following statement to define institutional racism in the Stephen Lawrence Enquiry:

> The collective failure of an organisation to provide an appropriate and professional service to people because of their colour, culture, or ethnic origin. It can be seen or detected in processes, attitudes and behaviour which amount to discrimination through unwitting prejudice, ignorance, thoughtlessness and racist stereotyping which disadvantage minority ethnic people. It persists because of the failure of the organisation openly and adequately to recognise and address its existence and causes by policy, example and leadership. Without recognition and action to eliminate such racism it can prevail as part of the ethos or culture of the organisation. It is a corrosive disease.

This stirring definition also provides a template for how institutional racism can be overcome to reduce inequalities and ensure equity of opportunity. Eliminating institutional racism requires a systematic review of procedures and practice at every level of an organisation. There must be an ongoing, active dialogue between practitioners, public bodies and the communities served by an organisation to identify barriers to access and overcome these effectively (Bhui et al. 2018).

Memon et al. (2016) found that a lack of flexibility within current mental health care provision was often a barrier to seeking mental health support amongst ethnic minorities. Participants felt that the service provider did not recognise or could not respond to their individual needs in a rigid system designed for the majority, not for individual needs. It is therefore vital that practitioners take time to understand the individual needs and concerns of minority ethnic service users and develop strategies for providing culturally sensitive and individually tailored care.

People from an ethnic minority are less likely to trust a medical practitioner than their white counterparts which can lead to reluctance to seek help or follow medical advice, further compounding health inequalities (Campos-Castillo 2015). Lack of trust contributes to other health behaviours such as vaccine hesitancy. COVID-19 vaccine rates were lower amongst minority ethnic groups in the United Kingdom. Razai et al. (2021) argue that trust in medical professionals amongst ethic minorities has been eroded by discrimination, institutional racism, past unethical medical research in black populations and cultural insensitivity. Rebuilding this trust will be complex but necessary if we are to reduce health inequalities.

Complex Needs and Intersectionality

Whilst understanding the barriers and issues faced by people within individual groups or characteristic is helpful in improving practice, it does not show the full picture. People are complex, belonging to multiple 'groups', having multiple 'characteristics' and multiple social roles or identities. For example, and individual can belong to an ethnic minority, the LGBTQ+ community and have a disability or impairment. The term intersectionality describes the complexity of being an individual with multiple facets to their identity and encourages us to explore the way that these different facets interact to shape the individual (Romero 2018).

Unfortunately, having multiple protected characteristics can create further barriers to well-being within our current care systems. People of colour within the LGBTQ+ community are six times more likely to experience discrimination in a primary care setting than their white counterparts (LGBT Foundation 2022). Whilst the expectation of stigma amongst black transgender youths led to reluctance to access health care services (Goldenberg et al. 2019)

Practitioners must take a holistic approach to understanding the multifaceted lives of those under their care and explore the factors which are influencing the individual's well-being.

Conclusion

The ability to work with people from all walks of life is a vital skill for health and social care professionals. Creating an inclusive and welcoming environment for all which takes into account the barriers cause by the intersection of identities, such as gender, race and disability ensures that good quality care can be provided. Whilst this seems like a simple premise, there are still those in our society who feel marginalised or excluded from seeking the support they are entitled to. By developing their communication skills and building therapeutic relationships with service users, professionals can play a vital role in overcoming these inequalities.

This chapter has provided an introduction to the core principles and skills needed to engage with service users in any health or care setting. The role of the Equality Act (2010) has been used to provide a framework for exploring the challenges of working with a diverse and varied population. The practical skills required for developing a therapeutic relationship have been introduced and their importance in relation to providing person-centred care has been discussed. Finally, specific challenges and barriers faced by people with protected characteristics and concept of inter-sectionality have been explored.

References

Beesley, P., 2017. *Developing your communication skills in social work.* London: SAGE Publications.

Bhui, K., Nazroo, J., Francis, J., Halvorsrud, K., and Rhodes, J., 2018. *The impact of racism on mental health* [online]. Oxford: The Synergi Collaborative Centre. Available at: https://synergicollaborativecentre.co.uk/wp-content/uploads/2017/11/The-impact-of-racism-on-mental-health-briefing-paper-1.pdf [Accessed 30 May 2022].

Bodie, G.D., Vickery, A.J., Cannava, K., and Jones, S.M., 2015. The role of "active listening" in informal helping conversations: impact on perceptions of listener helpfulness, sensitivity, and supportiveness and discloser emotional improvement. *Western Journal of Communication*, 79 (2), 151–173.

Boyd, C., and Dare, J., 2014. *Communication skills for nurses.* Chichester: Wiley Blackwell.

Bradby, H., Lindenmeyer, A., Phillimore, J., Padilla, B., and Brand, T., 2020. 'If there were doctors who could understand our problems, I would already be better': dissatisfactory health care and marginalisation in superdiverse neighbourhoods. *Sociology of Health and Illness*, 42(4), 739–757.

Brondolo, E., Love, E.E., Pencille, M., Schoenthaler, A., and Ogedegbe, G., 2011. Racism and hypertension: a review of the empirical evidence and implications for clinical practice. *American Journal of Hypertension*, 24 (5), 518–529.

Campos-Castillo, C., 2015. Racial and ethnic differences in trust in sources of health information: a generalized distrust in physicians. In: Kronenfeld, J.J., ed. *Education, social factors, and health beliefs in health and health care services.* Bingley, UK: Emerald, 2015, 163–186.

Egan, G., and Reese, R., 2020. *The skilled helper.* 3rd ed. Andover: Cengage Learning.

Equality Act, 2010. *The Stationery Office Limited.* London.

Gee, R., 2017. Contemplating 'career' across disciplines. In: Barnard, A., ed. *Developing professional practice in health and social care.* London: Routledge, 2017, 180–198.

Geldard, K., Geldard, D., & Foo, R.Y., 2019. *Counselling adolescents: The proactive approach for young people.* Sage.

Goering, S., 2015. Rethinking disability: the social model of disability and chronic disease. *Current reviews in musculoskeletal medicine*, 8 (2), 134–138.

Goldenberg, T., Jadwin-Cakmak, L., Popoff, E., Reisner, S.L., Campbell, B.A., and Harper, G.W., 2019. Stigma, gender affirmation, and primary healthcare use among black transgender youth. *Journal of Adolescent Health*, 65 (4), 483–490.

Gotlieb, J.B., 2000. Understanding the effects of nurses, patients' hospital rooms, and patients' perception of control on the perceived quality of a hospital. *Health Marketing Quarterly*, 18 (1–2), 1–14.

Health Care Professions Council, 2016. *Standards of conduct, performance and ethics* [online]. London: Health Care Professions Council. Available at: https://www.hcpc-uk.org/globalassets/resources/standards/standards-of-conduct-performance-and-ethics.pdf [Accessed 30 May 2022].

Hughes, E., Rawlings, V., and McDermott, E., 2018. Mental health staff perceptions and practice regarding self-harm, suicidality and help-seeking in LGBTQ youth: findings from a cross-sectional survey in the UK. *Issues in Mental Health Nursing*, 39 (1), 30–36.

Jasper, M., and Rosser, M., 2013. Reflection and reflective practice. In: Rosser, M., Jasper, M., and Mooney, J., eds. *Professional development, reflection and decision-making in nursing and health care*. 2nd ed. Chichester, West Sussex, UK: Wiley-Blackwell, 2013, 41–82.

Komen, I., Šepac, M., and Vujičić, M., 2015. Music, emotions and first impression perceptions of a healthcare institutions' quality: an experimental investigation. *Ekonomski Vjesnik/ Econviews*, 28 (S), 71–90.

Kwate, N.O.A., and Goodman, M.S., 2015. Cross-sectional and longitudinal effects of racism on mental health among residents of Black neighborhoods in New York City. *American Journal of Public Health (1971)*, 105 (4), 711–718.

LGBT foundation, 2022. *Pride in practice: LGBT patient experience survey 2021* [online]. Manchester: LGBT Foundation. Available at: https://drive.google.com/file/d/ 1-gFPdpjB8mfFtgdAti-4PH0pPB7fcow1/view [Accessed 10 May 2022].

MacPherson, W., 1999. *The Stephen Lawrence enquiry* [online]. London: UK Parliament. Available at: https://assets.publishing.service.gov.uk/government/uploads/system/uploads/ attachment_data/file/277111/4262.pdf [Accessed 30 May 2022].

Mattarozzi, K., Colonnello, V., De Gioia, F., and Todorov, A., 2017. I care, even after the first impression: facial appearance-based evaluations in healthcare context. *Social Science & Medicine*, 182, 68–72.

McDermott, E., Eastham, R., Hughes, E., Pattinson, E., Johnson, K., Davis, S., Pryjmachuk, S., Mateus, C., and Jenzen, O., 2021. Explaining effective mental health support for LGBTQ+ youth: a meta-narrative review. *SSM - Mental Health*, 1, 100004.

Mermon, A., Taylor, K., Mohebati, L.M., Sundin, J., Cooper, M., Scanlon, T., and de Visser, R., 2016. Perceived barriers to accessing mental health services among black and minority ethnic (BME) communities: a qualitative study in Southeast England. *BMJ Open* [online], 16 (6), e012337. 10.1136/bmjopen-2016-012337

Morrison, J., 2014. *The first interview*. 4th ed. New York: Guildford press.

Moss, B., 2020. *Communication skills in nursing, health & social care*. 5th ed. London: SAGE Publications.

Neighbour, R., 2018. *The inner consultation: how to develop an effective and intuitive consulting style*. 2nd ed. Boca Raton, FL: CRC Press.

Nelson-Jones, R., 2013. *Introduction to counselling skills*. 4th ed. London: SAGE Publications.

Razai, M.S., Osama, T., McKechnie, D.G.J., and Majeed, A., 2021. Covid-19 vaccine hesitancy among ethnic minority groups. *BMJ (Clinical Research Ed)* [online], 372, n513. 10.1136/bmj.n513

Romero, M., 2018. *Introducing intersectionality*. Cambridge: Polity.

Royal College of Nursing, 2021. *Asking effective questions* [online]. London: Royal College of Nursing. Available at: https://www.rcn.org.uk/clinical-topics/supporting-behaviour-change/ asking-effective-questions [Accessed 29 April 2022].

Scott, A., 2021. LGBTQ critical condition?: the Journal of the Health Visitors' Association. *Community Practitioner*, 94 (6), 40–43.

Semyonov-Tal, K., and Lewin-Epstein, N., 2021. The importance of combining open-ended and closed-ended questions when conducting patient satisfaction surveys in hospitals. *Health Policy OPEN* [online], 2, n100033. 10.1016/j.hpopen.2021.100033

Sorokowska, A., Sorokowski, P., Hilpert, P., Cantarero, K., Frackowiak, T., Ahmadi, K., Alghraibeh, A.M., Aryeetey, R., Bertoni, A., Bettache, K., and Blumen, S., 2017. Preferred interpersonal distances: a global comparison. *Journal of Cross-Cultural Psychology*, 48 (4), 577–592.

Thompson, N., 2018. *Promoting equality: working with diversity and difference.* 4th ed. London: Red Globe Press.

Trafford, S., 2017. Reflective writing for professional practice. In: Barnard, A., ed. *Developing professional practice in health and social care.* London: Routledge, 2017, 169–179.

Vincent, B., 2020. Views of the clinic: non-binary perceptions and experiences of general health services. In: Vincent, B., ed. *Non-binary genders: navigating communities, identities, and healthcare.* Bristol: Bristol University Press, 2020, 133–168.

Williams, D.R., and Etkins, O.S., 2021. Racism and mental health. *World Psychiatry*, 20 (2), 194–195.

6 Social Policy in Health and Social Care

Chris Towers and Richard Machin

After reading this chapter, you should be able to:

- Understand what social policy is
- Consider diverse ways of knowing social policy and reflect on how you and different people may come to understand it
- Describe and discuss different perspectives

Introduction

This chapter starts by outlining what social policy is before considering not just different perspectives but broader concerns about how we come to know the subject, including through the most contemporary of themes, the COVID-19 pandemic. In this part of the chapter Richard Machin guides you through how social policy played a critical part in the management of the pandemic. The chapter continues with an exploration of what social policy is before focusing on different ways of knowing the subject, including through the use of film. Chris Towers focuses on the work of film-maker Ken Loach, used by the writers in the classroom. This medium of film brings not just broad issues of policy to the fore, but specific issues such as conditionality.

What Is Social Policy?

Social policy is all around us even if you may not be always aware of it. Social policies may seem remote, not relevant to everyday life but questions of policy focus on matters such as health care, income, education, child, and elderly care and have relevance to you at all stages of the life course. Social policies are dynamic, they shape lives and effect both the providers and users of health and social care services. Social policies are acts of parliament, but also the broad actions of non-government agencies, such as charities and policies enacted through the courts.

If you are interested in the welfare and well-being of different groups in society, social policy will be of interest to you. The impact of social policies can be felt everywhere: in our homes, communities, and workplaces. Social policy is concerned with the way society is structured and the extent to which human needs are met and social justice is promoted. Our discussion of social policy inevitably leads us

DOI: 10.4324/9781003079873-7

to think about the decisions made by national government in areas such as health, education, housing, and social security. However, the focus of social policy should not be limited to what governments do, although we should certainly hold them to account and critically analyse how their decisions respond to social need and problems. Social policy also considers the ways in which local authorities, voluntary agencies, and private organisations organise and arrange their services. These decisions can be pragmatic, based on the capacity of organisations and what funding is available.

In this way, social policy is a very broad topic and is interested in economics (particularly how resources are allocated and distributed), how the media reports on social issues and groups in society. The subject also lends itself to questions of ideology. Ideologies are belief systems, they are groups of ideas and proport their own ideas on how we should live, and the choices governments and others can make (McLellan 1986; Roberts 2004; Hoffman and Graham 2004). Those on the so-called 'left wing' tend to favour governments doing more to support people with the provision of social security, or welfare benefits, so that they can buy food and other goods. Then there are 'right wingers', aligned broadly to the Conservative Party, who may be in favour of less government or state support. However, as Spicker (2021) argues this is never straight forward, as in some circumstances Conservatives can be supportive of state support and the Labour Party not always supportive of it.

Social policy requires us not only to reflect on theoretical concepts around human need and resource allocation, but to also think about times in our lives where we have been particularly affected by policy. This may be when we have needed to claim welfare benefits, relied on the National Health Service, or had a housing-related issue. Of course, people who are eligible for health and social care services are equally impacted by social policy. This includes children and young people, people with mental health problems, people experiencing poverty-related issues and people who have come to the United Kingdom from abroad. The lives of all these groups of people are enormously affected by policy decisions made on a national and local level, and we should develop a clear understanding of this if we are to work effectively with service users. Such groups can be marginalised and struggle to gain support through social policies (Bochel et al. 2008). Groups can be marginalised along lines of race or ethnicity (Phillips and Williams 2021), disability and age, with reference to disabled children (Goodley and Runswick-Cole 2011) or social class and gender (Brown, Ellis and Smith 2020) with overlapping discriminations that compound each sense of marginalisation. Following the economic crisis of 2008–2010, the UK government resolutely imposed austerity measures which included significant reductions in funding to public services (such as local government, the police and youth services) and cuts to welfare benefits. The regressive impact of these polices has been highlighted and Pierson (2016, p. 1) has made the links between post-2010 policy and 'marginalisation, poverty, powerlessness and isolation'.

Whilst policy making may or may not be relevant to the needs of such groups or fail to counter processes of marginalisation these realities can exist alongside wider debates. Over the last few years, social policy has dominated the news, whether this is discussions about Brexit, university tuition fees, the impact of social media or

Table 6.1 Beveridge's Giants (Hudson et al. 2015)

Beveridge's Giant	Key issues	Welfare pillar
Want	Insufficient income	Social security
Idleness	Lack of employment opportunities	Employment
Squalor	Poor-quality housing	Housing
Ignorance	Inadequate educational opportunities	Education
Disease	Limited access to health care	Health

the Black Lives Matter movement. All these issues demand careful consideration of what we want society to look like, how and where money should be spent, how we can protect the most vulnerable in society, and how discriminatory systems should be challenged and reshaped. Of course, these are not new issues and Hudson et al. (2015) state that the five traditional 'pillars' of social policy: social security, employment, housing, education, and health, can be traced back to the inception of the British welfare state. The 1942 Beveridge report identified five significant problems that the UK population was facing to be addressed through the foundation of the welfare state: want, ignorance, squalor, idleness, and disease. These terms are now outdated of course, but Table 6.1 illustrates how Beveridge's 'Five Giants' translate to the five welfare pillars of social policy:

Below is a summary of the main issues that the five welfare pillars of social policy are concerned with:

Social security policy: In a UK setting social security policy refers to providing financial support to people at key times in life, primarily through the payment of cash benefits. This may be because of unemployment, disability, incapacity for work, old age, or to help with childcare and housing costs. Social security policy has a variety of aims including protecting income, reducing poverty, redistributing income, and encouraging the return to employment.

Employment policy: Employment policy aims to support people in work and to encourage the unemployed to find work. There can be tensions between protecting the rights of employees (e.g., through the minimum wage and access to employment tribunals) and giving freedoms to employers (e.g., through flexible working conditions such as zero hours contracts). Employment policy is concerned with health and safety in the workplace, working conditions and challenging discrimination. 'Welfare to Work' policies have become increasingly prominent, supporting the long-term unemployed to develop skills and secure employment, although critics argue that these have had limited success in moving people into work (Jordan 2018).

Housing policy: Housing policy is concerned with the provision of accommodation which is, of course, a basic need. In the United Kingdom, there are three main types of housing tenure: owner occupation and the private and social rented sectors (primarily local authority and housing association properties). Housing policy focuses on the supply/demand, cost, security, and allocation of accommodation. There has been a significant increase in homelessness since 2010 and many commentators argue that decisions made by policy makers have contributed to increased levels of homelessness and that more needs to be done to provide affordable housing and ensure people have an adequate income to pay for accommodation.

Education policy: Education policy focuses on the organisation and delivery of learning and teaching. Alcock and May (2014) state that there is often a tension in education policy: some policy makers subscribe to the view that education is primarily about the acquisition of knowledge, and others argue the focus should be on the development of skills. Education policy focuses on early years provision, compulsory education, further and higher education and lifelong learning.

Health policy: Health policy focuses on the health and medical care of the population. Much of the focus is on the National Health Service (NHS) and the provision of primary care (GPs and community services) and secondary care (hospitals and specialists). Health policy also looks at public health (promoting healthy lifestyle choices and protecting against threats to health), medical research, private health care, and health inequalities. Much debate in this policy area centres on the cost of health care and access to services.

It is important to emphasise that contemporary social policy is not only concerned with the five traditional welfare pillars, although they have rightly demanded attention for many decades. Social policy explores how society responds to social problems and need, and of course, this changes over time. In addition to the five welfare pillars identified above, social policy focuses on issues such as crime, transport, immigration, and environmental policy. These policy areas should not be seen as separate from one another and the people that we work with in the health and social care sector will be affected by many overlapping areas of social policy which simultaneously affect and shape their lives.

Social Policy and COVID-19

It is important to make links between some of the more theoretical social policy concepts and how social policy works in action. We will now explore the impact of the COVID-19 pandemic to demonstrate the huge impact of social policy. We will look at how the UK government made policy decisions in each of the five main areas of social policy during the pandemic:

Social security: When the COVID-19 pandemic took hold in the United Kingdom in the early months of 2020, the government announced £7 billion of additional funding for the social security system. The government recognised that the pandemic had huge economic and health costs and made several important changes to key welfare benefits. Universal Credit is the main means-tested benefit in the United Kingdom and the government uprated the payment by £20 per week from April 2020 to October 2021. Universal Credit has been a controversial benefit with many people arguing that too many people have their benefit stopped (or sanctioned) if they are judged not to comply with the conditions set out in a claimant commitment.

The government temporarily stopped all sanctions during the first lockdown in March 2020 and allocated an extra £1 billion to help people living in the private rented sector were struggling to pay the rent. In the first two months of the lockdown, an unprecedented 2.5 million people made claims for Universal Credit. Many people claim social security benefits because they are unfit for work (Employment Support Allowance) or have long-term health problems or disabilities (Personal Independence Payment). Entitlement to these benefits usually requires a claimant to attend a medical and to have regular reviews but the government suspended these during the pandemic.

The government moved quickly to respond to the COVID-19 crisis and 59% of the additional funding went to people in the lowest quartile of incomes. However, critics argue that in the ten years leading up to the pandemic the UK government's programme of welfare reform downsized the social security system to unacceptable levels (Machin 2021). The emergency COVID-19 social security measures removed some of the sharp edges from the system but exposed its weaknesses, especially for some key claimant groups such as women, disabled people, and people from some minority ethnic groups. The marginalisation and social exclusion which social policy can create were clearly exposed.

Employment: The COVID-19 pandemic sent a shockwave through the United Kingdom's employment market. The government realised that they needed to act quickly to try to protect jobs and compensate earnings. In March 2020, the Coronavirus Job Retention Scheme (CJRS) was established to provide financial support to employees who could not work because of the pandemic. Where employees were unable to work and were 'furloughed' the government initially paid 80% of wages, up to a maximum of £2,500 per month. The government planned that the CJRS would last for three months, but the ongoing impact of the pandemic meant that the scheme was extended until the end of September 2021.

In the decade leading up to the pandemic successive governments had argued that there needed to be a reduction in government spending. However, in response to the pandemic the UK government recognised the urgent need to introduce policies which would protect jobs and incomes and spent unprecedented amounts to support these aims. The scope of the CJRS was extraordinary; it subsidised the wages of 9.6 million employees, approximately one-third of the entire workforce. It has been praised for providing support for the low-paid young employees, and those working for small businesses. However, criticism have been aimed at the policy for sustaining unviable jobs and not targeting sectors most in need of support (Pope, Dalton and Tetlow 2020).

Housing: The main concerns of housing policy are to ensure that people can access appropriate and affordable housing and to implement strategies to reduce homelessness. However, many people in the housing sector have highlighted a 'housing crisis' in the United Kingdom. Since 2010, there has been a 141% increase in the number of people who are rough sleeping, although there has been a slight decrease in numbers since 2017 (Gov.uk 2020). There has also been a marked increase in the numbers of people presenting as homeless to their local authority. There are several key drivers for these worrying trends. They include insecurity in the private rented sector, a lack of appropriate housing in the social rented sector, and changes to welfare benefits (particularly the rollout of universal credit and reductions in the level of housing support).

The COVID-19 pandemic demonstrated the power of social policy to decisively respond to a deep-rooted social problem such as rough sleeping, providing there is the political will and financial resources. On 26 March 2020, the UK government instructed local authorities to 'bring in' rough sleepers by the weekend to make sure they were safe and stop the transmission of COVID-19. Through the 'Everyone In' policy, the government provided local authorities with £3.2 million to accommodate rough sleepers in accommodation such as hotel rooms, student accommodation and Bed and Breakfasts, and to provide medical care and food. In the first month of this policy local authorities in England had offered accommodation to 90% of rough sleepers, and 'Everyone In' was recognised as an important measure to protect rough sleepers during the pandemic.

An important element of social policy is to carefully scrutinise government policy and hold policy makers to account. The 'Everyone In' Initiative has been acknowledged as a successful policy; swift and clear government action responded to the public health needs of an incredibly vulnerable population in society. 'Everyone In' worked alongside other policies such as the temporary increase in levels of welfare benefits and a moratorium on evictions. However, the government has been criticised for subsequent mixed messages about rough sleeping. Concern has been raised about a lack of support for non-UK nationals, and a lack of clarity about measures which should be taken to prevent rough sleeping in the first place (Fitzpatrick et al. 2020). Rough sleeping remains a significant policy concern; new people have started to sleep rough during the pandemic, new vulnerabilities are exposed as result of financial insecurity, and affordable accommodation remains elusive for many groups in society.

Education: The COVID-19 pandemic has demonstrated the critical role that education places in the well-being and development of children and young peoples' lives and stimulated important debate about the direction of education policy and educational inequality. Research by the International Literacy Centre at University College London shows that at the start of the pandemic staff at primary schools were not only focusing on teaching pupils, but were also engaged in doorstep welfare checks, distributing emergency food provisions, delivering resources to students, and liaising with social services. This research argues that lessons need to be learnt from the pandemic and that education policy should direct additional funding to schools in deprived areas to recognise their role in meeting not only the educational needs of pupils, but also broader health and welfare needs (International Literacy Centre 2020).

The UK government has argued that schools should be the 'engines of social mobility', circumstances of birth should not dictate the quality of education received and subsequent life chances (Gov.uk 2016). However, even before the COVID-19 outbreak research indicated that by the time pupils take their Gerenal Certificate of Secondary Education disadvantaged children are on average one and a half years of learning behind other pupils. There is compelling evidence that educational inequalities have widened during the pandemic. The Institute for Fiscal Studies (2020) report that following the initial March 2020 lockdown, 64% of secondary school pupils in state schools from the richest households were offered active help (such as online teaching) compared to 47% from the poorest fifth of households. Children from the poorest fifth of households spent an average of 4.5 hours a day on educational activities compared with 5.8 hours day for children from the highest-income quintile of families.

The Education Policy Institute (2020) argue that post-pandemic education policy needs a significant shift in direction. This includes a temporary suspension of Ofsted inspections, a 'Teacher Volunteer Scheme' to encourage retired/inactive teachers to return to schools to help disadvantaged children, and a doubling of the pupil premium.

Health: 'Health is related to how we organise our affairs in society' (Marmot 2016, p. 30); we can judge how well a society is doing by looking at the health of the population. More than any other event in recent times, the COVID-19 pandemic has stretched our health systems and challenged policy makers. The pandemic has emphasised how central health policy decisions are to all our lives; key areas of concern include access to services, health care costs and preventing the spread of communicable disease.

Immediate policy responses were required to respond to the pandemic, and immense longer-term challenges have been created. In line with countries around the world, the UK government imposed a series of local and national lockdowns to slow the spread of coronavirus. These lockdowns were broadly supported by the public (Skinner 2021) but had a serious impact on the economy, education, and social and mental well-being of the population. The UK government introduced the test, track, and trace system to ensure that anyone with COVID-19 symptoms could be tested and to allow the recent contacts of anyone with a positive test to be traced and, if necessary, to self-isolate. The appropriateness of a centralised and privatised test, track and trace scheme was questioned with critics arguing that a policy of this nature would be more effective if administered on a local level under the jurisdiction of directors of public health. The decision to prioritise intensive care capacity through the building of five emergency 'Nightingale' hospitals was challenged as these new facilities were largely unused (Day 2020).

COVID-19 has created a series of longer-term health policy issues. The NHS has overseen the rollout of the most significant vaccination programme in UK history. The pandemic has created a huge backlog of non-COVID-19 related care and treatment; this will take years rather than months to address (Ham, 2020). It has been estimated that up to 10 million people will require new or additional mental health support as a direct result of the pandemic; 1.5 million of these cases are for children and young people under the age of 18 (Centre for Mental Health, 2020). Policy makers must address long-standing recruitment and retention issues in the health service and tackle health inequalities based on income, ethnicity, and gender. The pandemic has further exposed the urgent need for the effective integration of health and social care services. An effective joined-up approach has proved elusive for successive governments and had led to the introduction of a £12 billion a-year tax rise to respond to NHS backlogs and fund the reform of social care.

Different Ways of Knowing Social Policy

Whilst you may know social policy in your own ways, through lived experience of the pandemic or being out of work or homeless or indeed needing childcare you may also know it through film, television, or the internet. Knowing social policies through the visual image is helpful as it can cross linguistic or cultural barriers, including through the work of film directors such as Ken Loach. Chris Towers reflects here on the use of film in the classroom.

Introducing the Films of Ken Loach

Film can create and stimulate learning, drawing out the experience of learners and help them to relate the subject to what they see and hear in the classroom (van de Watering et al. 2008; Coutts, Gilliard and Biglin 2011; Perkin and Linamarin-Garcia 2012; Befit 2015, p. 103). Various films of Ken Loach have been employed but, in this chapter, I focus films in particular on, the perhaps seminal, 'Cathy Come Home' I (1965), 'It's a Free World' (2007), and 'I Daniel Blake' (2012).

Film is a useful teaching resource and can be influential on many levels, mediating experiences, providing metaphors and meanings, signs and symbols that can convey understanding in many ways (Champoux 1999). Film has been shown to enhance experiential learning and as a way of getting students to consider issues of diversity, religion, race, and social class (Villalba and Redmond 2008). We can see how some of these issues of social policy have been played out through some of Loach's films

Cathy Come Home, was significant in that it brought issues of homelessness to the public imagination. Shown on the BBC in 1965, it attracted a very wide audience and its seminal nature made it an important work to bring to students. The film was influential and depicted the plight of a young family experiencing unemployment and subsequent homelessness. It showed the father unable to accompany his wife into a shelter and its impact was so strong it led, in 1967, to the foundation of the charity 'Crisis' (Fitzpatrick and Pawson 2016). Our teaching of social policy, seeking to draw out the 'lived experience' of social issues such a homelessness, was complimented by this film screening.

Loach's 2007 film *It's a Free World* was written by Paul Laverty and directed by Loach. The film has resonance in that it depicts issues of importance within contemporary Britain, the emotive issues of race and identity entangled with issues of gender, social class, power and social exclusion. Students needed to understand these issues in the classroom, particularly ideas associated with intersectionality (Crenshaw 1991; Collins 1998; Cole 2009; Schulz and Mullings cited in Viruell-Feuentes et al. 2012). Students can struggle with such a concept and the depiction of this in film allows the student to literally 'see' and 'hear' intersectionality in action. Inviting responses to the film's students reflected a depth of impact upon them, such as when one student said:

> I attended for the love of learning and to express joy at emergent understanding of social policies. I was particularly animated about the dilemmas facing both migrants and the young graduate females.

In keeping with showing films of a contemporary nature, '**I Daniel Blake**' was chosen for just as 'It's a free world' highlighted the complexities of ethnicity, race, social class, and gender, this film showed issues in the modern 'gig' economy. The film was thus able to draw light towards the complex, dialectic relationship between structure and agency. It was important to let the students struggle with those relationships, to see how one impacts on the other and this film captured the essence of that struggle. *I, Daniel Blake* is Ken Loach's welfare state polemic that is blunt, dignified and brutally moving (Bradshaw 2016). The film is a fictional story of a middle-aged widower in the north-east who cannot work or get benefits after his near fatal heart attack in this 'modern social relist fiction' (Bradshaw 2016).

Blake is caught in the perfect storm of bureaucratic misery told to rest by the NHS consultant, presenting as quite well at the Department of Work and Pensions he is assessed as not being entitled to sickness benefit. The modest income from Job Seeker's allowance is conditional on his exhaustive searching for work and attending CV workshops. In his naivety, Blake is open about his inattention to work, so is humiliatingly labelled a scrounger. His online application without access to a computer, smartphone or internet is relegated to public library access and the repetition from the computer freezing. The new friend of Daniel is Katie the quick-tempered single mother of two who has been relocated to Newcastle from London. Daniel fixes up Katie's dilapidated flat and shows he likes work. The scene in the foodbank and Jobcentre offices are the *mise-end-scene* of the story telling of a filmic conditional welfare. Student responses told me something of how they responded, showing reflective attitudes towards the issues and the depictions:

> People's perceptions of people on benefits are wrong – not everyone has made the choice.
>
> A lot of the people are desperate for work as well as support. (Student A)
>
> Choices are both constrained and structured but mainly constrained by the people at the top. (Student B)
>
> It took me back to when I worked as an agency worker. This film showed how hard it is, working long hours with no insurance, low pay and benefits.

Another student expressed a range of responses to the film

> the film, it's a free world gave us the chance to explore issues about emigration, sexual abuse, illegal employment and exploitation. The other good thing about the film today was that it highlighted matters concerning the assignment in another module and I hope (lecturer 1) and (lecturer 2) will buy you a coffee for making their jobs ten times earlier. But more than that, I would love if possible if we can have special days for films like this one.

There have been various studies suggesting emotional engagement through exposure to film. Film has evoked particular emotions such as fear and anger (Fernandez et al. 2012) but a range of other more complex emotions have been observed in our students, from resentment or confusion, to loss or despair. We found that emotion plays a part in students learning, indeed it has been recognised that teachers need to manage emotions in the classroom in order to be effective, what can be called 'emotion work' (Tsang 2011, p. 1313, cited in Gallant 2013) or 'emotional labour' (Gallant 2013). Students, teachers and other practitioners can both use emotion to mediate or develop understanding and transfer knowledge. Lewis and Tierney (2013) identified how the emotional interactions in a diverse, inner city classroom stimulated learning, transforming understandings.

Reflective Learning in the Classroom

Students have frequently been confused as they watch and take aboard Loach's work but, in a sense, this has been positive, learning to get to know the world as not as a set of dualities but as complex interplays and tensions embodied through lead characters who have struggled with those very same complexities. The lead character, Angie, in a '*It's a free world*' showed compassion and brutality as she tried to marry the needs of her son, the need to earn a living and to have some sort of moral compass. She wanted to find work for the migrants to enable herself to thrive or simply survive but in doing so was both abused and abuser as she was victim to sexist bosses, oppressive to migrants but also responsive to them, all at the same time. Students became emotionally involved in these dilemmas but were both confused and delighted by these complexities. This accords with Shaimaa (2009) who suggests that these questions arise from a process whereby the student as audience is pulled into the issues in passionate engagement with the issues.

Conclusion

This chapter has considered different ways of knowing social policy, from the personal lived experience, be that through the pandemic or through particularly experiences of housing or health, education, or employment. It has also asked you to consider other ways of knowing policies, including film. There are diverse ways of knowing what social policy is and different experiences or perspectives. Policies shape lives or have the potential to and the exploration of issues around the COVID-19 pandemic have exemplified this. So also has the visual image and films, also explored through this chapter. and film, and in this case the work of Loach, has focused students' hearts and minds on the issues. Loach's work has consistently drawn out the lived experience and highlighted the issues of power and control but so too have those lived experience that many of you will know either directly or indirectly through friends and family. The case study examples, and reflections have hopefully served this understanding and encouraged you to take this understanding further.

Summary of Main Points

You should be able to:

- Understand what social policy is and how it can shape lives
- Be aware of different perspectives in social policy
- Be aware of how policies can affect lives but also of the difficulties services may have in delivering care given people's different wants, needs, opportunities and inequalities

References

Alcock, P., and May, M., 2014. *Social policy in Britain*. 4th ed. New York: Palgrave Macmillan.
Befit, S., 2015. Assessment innovation and student experience: a new assessment challenge and call for a multi-perspective approach to assessment research. *Assessment and Evaluation in Higher Education*, 40 (1), 103–119.

Bochel, C., Bochel, H., Somerville, P., and Worley, C., 2008. Marginalised or enabled voices? 'User participation' in policy and practice. *Social Policy and Society*, 7 (2), 201–210.

Bradshaw, P., 2016. *The Jungle Book* review – spectacular revival of Disney's family favorite. *Guardian* [online], 12 May. Available via: https://www.theguardian.com/film/2016/apr/12/the-jungle-book-review

Brown, K., Ellis, K., and Smith, K., 2020. *Vulnerability as lived experience in women, vulnerability and welfare service systems*. London: Routledge.

Champoux, J.E., 1999. Film as a teaching resource. *Journal of Management Inquiry*, 2 (8), 206–217.

Cole, E., 2009. Intersectionality and research in intersectionality. *The American Psychologist*, 64 (3), 170–180.

Collins, P.H., 1998. It's all in the family: intersections of gender, race and nation. *Hypatia*, 13 (3), 62–82.

Coutts, R., Gilliard, W., and Biglin, R., 2011. Evidence for the impact of assessment on mood and motivation in first – year students. *Studies in Higher Education*, 36 (3), 291–300.

Crenshaw, K., 1991. Mapping the margins: intersectionality, identity politics and violence and women of colour. *Stanford Law Review*, 43 (6), 1241–1299.

Day, M., 2020. Covid-19: Nightingale hospitals set to shut down after seeing few patients. *BMJ*, 2020 (369), 1860.

Education Policy Institute, 2020. *Preventing the disadvantage gap from increasing during and after the Covid-19 pandemic* [online]. London: Education Policy Institute. Available at: https://epi.org.uk/publications-and-research/disadvantage-gap-covid-19/

Fernandez, C., Pascual, J.C., Soler, J., Elices, M., Maria, J., Portella, M.J., and Fernández-Abascal, E., 2012. Physiological responses induced by emotion-eliciting films. *Applied Psychophysiology and Biofeedback*, 37, 73–79.

Fitzpatrick, S., and Pawson, H., 2016. Fifty years since 'Cathy Come Home': critical reflections on the UK homelessness 'safety net'. *International Journal of Housing Policy*, 16 (4), 543–555.

Fitzpatrick, S., Watts, B., and Simms, R., 2020. *Homelessness monitor England 2020: COVID-19 crisis response briefing*. London: Crisis.

Gallant, A., 2013. Advances in research on teaching. In: Newberry, M., Gallant, A., and Riley, P., eds. *Emotion and school: understanding how the hidden curriculum influences relationships, leaderships, teaching and learning*. 18th ed. Bingley: Emerald Group Publishing Limited, 163–181.

Goodley, D., and Runswick-Cole, K., 2011. Problematising policy: conceptions of 'child', 'disabled' and 'parents' in social policy in England. *International Journal of Inclusive Education*, 15 (1), 71–85.

Hoffman, J., and Graham, P., 2004. *Introduction to political ideologies*. Great Britain: Pearson.

Hudson, J., Kuhner, S., and Lowe, S., 2015. *The short guide to social policy*. 2nd ed. Bristol: Policy Press.

Institute for Fiscal Studies, 2020. *Learning during the lockdown: real-time data on children's experiences during home learning*. London: Institute for Fiscal Studies. Available at: https://ifs.org.uk/uploads/Edited_Final-BN288%20Learning%20during%20the%20lockdown.pdf

International Literacy Centre, 2020. *Responding to COVID-19, briefing note 3: resetting educational priorities in challenging times* [online]. London: UCL. Available at: https://discovery.ucl.ac.uk/id/eprint/10111679/1/Moss_Briefing%20Note%203%20Responding%20to%20COVID-19%20system%20change_final.pdf

Jordon, J., 2018. Welfare grunters and workfare monsters? An empirical review of the operation of two UK 'work programme' centres. *Journal of Social Policy* [online], 47 (3), 583–601. 10.1017/S0047279417000629

Lewis, C., and Tierney, J.D., 2013. Mobilizing emotion in an urban classroom: producing identities and transforming signs in a race-related discussion. *Curriculum and Instruction*, 24 (3), 289–304.

Machin, R., 2021. COVID-19 and the temporary transformation of the UK social security system. *Critical Social Policy* [online], 26101832098679. 10.1177/026101832 0986793

Marmot, M., 2016. *The health gap: the challenge of an unequal world*. London: Bloomsbury.

McLellan, D., 1986. *Ideology*. Minnesota: University of Minnesota Press.

Ministry of Housing, Communities & Local Government, 2020. *Official statistics: rough sleeping snapshot in England: autumn 2019* [online]. London: GOV.UK. Available at: https://www.gov.uk/government/statistics/rough-sleeping-snapshot-in-england-autumn-2019

Perkin, R., and Linamarin-Garcia, L., 2012. Academic emotions and student engagement. In: Christenson, S.L., Rashly, A.L., and Wiley, C. eds. *Handbook of research on student engagement*. London: Springer, 259–282.

Phillips, C., and Williams, F., 2021. Sleepwalking into the 'post-racial': social policy and research-led teaching. *Social Policy and Society*, 21 (1), 1–16.

Pierson, J., 2016. *Tackling poverty and social exclusion: promoting social justice in social work*. 3rd ed. London; New York: Routledge.

Pope, T., Dalton, G., and Tetlow, G., 2020. *The coronavirus job retention scheme: how has it been used and what will happen when it ends?* [online]. London: Institute for Government. Available at: https://www.instituteforgovernment.org.uk/sites/default/files/publications/coronavirus-job-retention-scheme_0.pdf

Roberts, A., 2004. The state of socialism: a note on terminology. *Cambridge University Press* [online], 63 (2), 349–366. 10.2307/3185732

Shaimaa, C., 2009. The power of perspective: teaching social policy with documentary film. *Journal of Teaching in Social Work*, 29, 85–100.

Skinner, G., 2021. *Most Britons continue to say they are following coronavirus rules; almost half believe lockdown measures are not strict enough* [online]. London: Ipsos MORI. Available at: https://www.ipsos.com/en-uk/most-britons-continue-say-they-are-following-coronavirus-rules-almost-half-believe-lockdown

Spicker, P., 2021. *An introduction to social policy* [online]. UK: Spicker.uk. Available at: http://www.spicker.uk [Accessed 4 October 2021].

UK, G., 2016. National minimum wage and national living wage rates. URL: www.gov.uk/national-minimum-wage-rates

Van de Watering, G., Gijbels, D., Dochy, F., and Van der Rijt, J., 2008. Students' assessment preferences, perceptions and their relationship to study. *Higher Education*, 56 (6), 645–658.

Villalba, J.A., and Redmond, R.E., 2008. Crash: using a popular film as an experiential learning activity in a multi-cultural counselling course. *Counselor Education and Supervision*, 47 (4), 264–276.

Viruell-Fuentes, E.A., Miranda, P.Y., and Abdulrahim, S., 2012. More than culture: structural racism, intersectionality theory, and immigrant health. *Social Science Medicine*, 75 (12), 2099–2106.

7 Professional Practice and Work-Based Learning

Dolores Ellidge, Jessica Arnold, Monique Duncan, and Dani Shepherd

This chapter aims to support readers to:

- Develop knowledge and understanding of professionalism in practice and key knowledge and experience essential for graduate roles
- Understand benefits and opportunities for work-based learning
- Reflect on personal strengths and limitations and create a personal development plan
- Gain insight into career options with a degree in health and social care

Introduction

Health and social care services are reliant on a broad range of job roles and specialities. At the heart of these is the desire to provide a high-quality service through provision of professional practice underpinned by evidence and expertise. There are a myriad of concepts related to effective professional practice, far too many to cover in a single chapter therefore the aim is to consider the concepts of vulnerability, risk and safeguarding in relation to both service users and professional accountability. Further information regarding professional practice can be found in professional websites such as the Nursing and Midwifery Council, SCIE or The Health and Care Professionals Council and in the book edited by Barnard 'Developing Professional Practice in Health and Social Care'.

Students gaining theoretical knowledge in their journey through their degree is only part of the knowledge required for professional practice. Gaining knowledge through experience provides students with greater understanding of working in health and social care and enables them to develop key skills required for graduate practice and consequently has the potential to increase their employability. The second part of this chapter focuses on work-based learning, that is learning through hands-on experience in the workplace. The chapter considers skills such as time management, organisation, stress management and how to use opportunities in university to develop these skills which are transferable to work-based learning opportunities and future practice.

Exploration of Risk, Vulnerability and Resilience in Relation to Service Users and Practitioners

Risk, vulnerability and resilience are key concepts in promoting health and well-being and safeguarding service users and practitioners. The concepts will be considered

DOI: 10.4324/9781003079873-8

separately however in reality they entwine in service delivery which is underpinned by legislation such as the Equality Act 2010 and professional practice regulation and guidance such as the Code for Nurses and Midwives (NMC 2018).

As a concept, risk is part of our everyday life – in childhood we are taught to assess risk and make decisions which reduce risk. Risk is the likelihood that a person will be harmed, and our comprehension of risk and the potential consequences is impacted by our experiences, our social networks, our ability and our perception of the risk versus the reward – that is, is the potential outcome more beneficial than the potential loss or harm? Giddens (1999) suggests that society has developed the concept of risk in response to consideration of safety. Within health and social care practice the assessment of risk is key to the safety and well-being of service users and staff which supports Gidden's theory. This focus on safety can be in the context of risks in the care environment, treatment or procedures and within the remit of safeguarding those who are identified as vulnerable to risk.

Vulnerability is a concept which you will all be familiar with and which is well-recognised in health and social care. It can be defined as susceptibility to physical, emotional or social harm (Heaslip 2013) which can be short term, due to a change in circumstances such as acute illness, or long term. Vulnerability incorporates both the potential for harm and actuality of being exposed to harm. At times we can all feel vulnerable; having a long-term health condition such as asthma and experiencing a pandemic, having someone your own age die or feeling out of your depth at work. These examples of vulnerability tend to affect that one aspect of our lives and with time feelings of vulnerability reduce. For other people vulnerability will be linked to a risk of harm or not having their needs met and in addition, may not have the capacity to meet their own needs. Examples of this would be babies and young children and people with dementia. A further example is young migrants seeking asylum who Bradby et al. (2019) identify are vulnerable due to traumatic experiences and limited social support. This personalisation of vulnerability includes individual perception and there can be a difference in how people perceive someone to be vulnerable, for example, the individual themselves, their family or support network and health and social care practitioners who may identify different vulnerabilities to risk than the individual themselves. There can be situations where an individual does not feel vulnerable and makes a decision to remain in what others perceive to be a risky situation such as an elderly person continuing to live at home following several falls or where mental health conditions such as Generalised Anxiety Disorder or Obsessive Compulsive Disorder can result in people perceiving themselves to be at risk to a degree which others do not recognise or understand. As practitioners we need to be aware of the range of factors which may contribute to people feeling vulnerable or being identified as vulnerable and strategies which can support them.

Resilience is a factor which can impact on an individual's vulnerability. It is described as 'the ability to persevere and thrive in the face of exposure to adverse situations' (Rogerson and Ermes, 2008, p. 1). An individual's innate resilience can be a product of upbringing and experience. Cohn et al. (2009, p. 362) support this suggesting that ego resilience is a 'personality trait that reflects an individual's ability to adapt to changing environments'. They identify the ability to adapt is linked to life outcomes such as childhood behaviour, interpersonal skills and mood responses to tragic life events. A key factor in building and maintaining resilience is attention to self and self-care (McCray, Palmer and Chmiel 2016) however an individual's capacity for self-care is impacted by availability of resources and sense of well-being (Cohn et al. 2014). The next section of the chapter will build on this discussion to consider risk, vulnerability and resilience in the context of professional practice.

All health and social care professionals have a duty of care to safeguard and protect every service user in their care. Through robust training to become autonomous professionals, each carer is bound by a code of conduct relevant to their particular discipline. In addition, care professionals acquire a fundamental set of skills which allows them to recognise signs and indicators of abuse or vulnerability in service users. These are, broadly speaking, observational and communication skills. Effective communication is considered essential to elicit the information required to undertake any assessment of concerns which a patient may have or make an assessment of possible abuse. If, for example, a service user makes a disclosure to a health or social care professional, there is a professional duty to question the disclosure and the situation as a whole in order to judge whether or not the service user is at immediate risk. As Sheldon and Hilaire (2015) point out, effective communication between health and social care workers and service users is paramount to the service user's safety. It must be understood that the role of the health and social care professional is vital in deciding how to proceed and report concerns to the local social care safeguarding organisation. However, it is also important to state that the health and social care professional's responsibility is not to investigate possible abuse, but to gather sufficient information to refer to the appropriate agency in order to protect the service user from harm. Fennell (2016) points to factors which may impinge upon a professional's confidence to initiate a referral; a lack of familiarity with the referral procedure can be especially disabling. In addition to this, professionals do need assurance that a receiving social care agency will investigate the concerns raised. When concerns relate to organisational safeguarding, there continues to be apprehension surrounding whistleblowing and fear of repercussions for the reporting individual. Moreover, there can be anxiety that if no action is taken by managers, no change will actually occur despite 'speaking out'. Kelly and Jones describe this as 'organisational silence' (2013, p. 186).

As a qualified practitioner, responsive leadership is essential. For example, a nurse must be able to 'Act without delay if you believe that there is a risk to patient safety' as clearly stated in the Nursing and Midwifery Code (NMC) (2018, p. 14). The professional standards of practice and behaviour for nurses, midwives and nursing associates are all embedded within the NMC Code. Operating as leaders within health and social care, it is crucial that all qualified professionals ensure they take all reasonable steps to protect people who are 'vulnerable or at risk of harm, neglect or abuse' (NMC 2018). The proficiency and confidence of newly qualified practitioners need to improve continually so that skills can be mastered for even greater ability and proficiency. Such skills can be discussed through clinical and managerial supervision in the workplace and through reflective practice. With support and experience, practitioners are able to refer service users to the appropriate safeguarding agency and ensure organisational protocol is followed if a concern has been identified by a service user. As summarised by the Department of Health (DoH) in 2006, leadership is primarily focused on providing a role model which promotes good quality and safe care. Professionalism must therefore be inclusive of safeguarding practices within all work contexts. Further information on escalating concerns and supervision can be found in the chapter on *Managing Health and Social Care.*

Care assistants are now expected to achieve a standardised level of knowledge of and training for safeguarding; this is mandatory in qualifying for the Care Certificate, formulated by Health Education England, Skills for Care and Skills for Health in 2015. With this qualification, a professional is deemed accountable and sufficiently competent to raise the alarm if needed in relation to safeguarding of a service user (Cavendish 2013).

Sheldon and Hilaire (2015) recognise that nurses develop communication skills throughout their training and that this is a continual process when working as a professional beyond graduation. They also acknowledge that communication skills can be practised through simulation by students in seminars, and that this builds the necessary skills and confidence to work in health and social care settings (Sheldon and Hilaire, 2015). Simulated practice amongst peers combined with inquiry-based learning and examination of case scenarios also draws upon and tests students' knowledge base regarding safeguarding. Prior to work placements, all students should receive safeguarding training which provides them with at least a basic knowledge of types of abuse and their role as a health or social care student in responding to concerns which may be raised by patients. Clarke (2015) asserts that the student's role on placement is to be an 'alerter' and communicate concerns to a qualified professional within the work setting. By building on prior experience, most health and social care students accrue the knowledge and confidence necessary for professional conduct. Undergraduate courses provide opportunities for students to gain valuable skills during a mandatory work placement. On this occasion, students will learn through experience how to process information, communicate effectively with a service user who has raised a concern or disclosed information, respond effectively and proceed to communicate concerns to the qualified professional to whom they are accountable. With time, a student's confidence should continue to grow beyond graduation as they enter the health or social care workforce and consolidate their knowledge, skills and experience.

Service User Engagement

According to the Social Care Institute for Excellence (SCIE) (2007) the participation of service users has increasingly become an important part of social care. The involvement of service users ensures a holistic approach is given which enhances the service users' experience and quality of care, as staff will be required to have training around participating cultures. It is reassuring that service users are being focused on and involved in their care, as they know what they need and how their needs may be met. Yet, it also shifts the dynamic between staff and service users – allowing them to take responsibility for their own care and being treated as an individual.

Within health and social care settings, the concept of choice and risk must be considered, when service users are involved in their own care. The approach to 'choice and risk' is to ensure individuals can live their lives as independent and full as possible, which others may take for granted, and part of this approach is to support service users to consider the consequence of an action and the likelihood of any harm from it. Thus, enhances the benefits of independence, well-being and choice (Department of Health 2007).

To enhance engagement, communication is vital, however non-verbal communication is just as important. Egan (1975 cited in Stickley 2011) created the acronym SOLER, which stands for 'sit squarely', 'open posture', 'lean towards the other', 'eye contact',

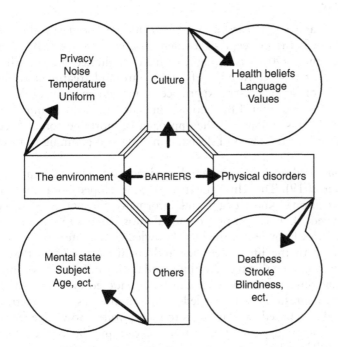

Figure 7.1 The environment, culture, physical disorders, other (Crouch 2016).

'relax'. SOLER is widely recognised in practice – especially nursing, however this is developed in the model SURETY; 'sit at an angle', 'uncrossed legs and arms', 'relax', 'eye contact', 'touch', 'your intuition' (Stickley 2011). The SURETY model allows professionals to think about non-verbal communication skills in a therapeutic setting, which avoids inhibition and allows service users to express themselves (Figure 7.1).

The effectiveness and employment of non-verbal communication implies that you are interested and paying attention. However, Crouch (2016) highlights there can be barriers which can affect this such as environmental and cultural barriers, age-related barriers and the mental capacity of an individual. The included image identifies key barriers to communication, for example, culture or physical disorders. Crouch (2016) suggests language is important as it ensures that the professional and service user can understand each other. An interpreter may assist with this communication process however it is suggested that language difficulties lead to poor quality assessment and management. Ensuring the correct environment is used is another important aspect of communication; a room being too cold or too hot, or within a noisy environment could hinder the communication between a professional and service user.

The focus of this collaborative approach in health and social care can be expanded from individual care to the development and delivery of services. The Offender Health Collaborative (see NHS England 2015) suggests that collaboration is 'the process by which people who are using or have used a service become involved in the planning, development and delivery of that service'. Arnstein's (2019) ladder of participation highlights that individuals and communities can be service users, service developers and, where power is devolved, they can contribute to or lead initiatives.

Evidence-Based Practice

It is essential that health and social care practice is evidence based (Brotherton and Parker 2013). Although the concept of Evidence-Based Practice (EBP) has been more popular since the 1990s it is thought to have originated much earlier and is founded in the belief that knowledge of health care and treatment is enhanced by consideration of service user experience alongside more traditional evidence. Muhrer (2012) states that EBP should 'include the values and preferences of the individual'. This element of the approach supports person-centred care where the service user is at the heart of decision-making and planning to meet their needs.

EBP incorporates robust and up-to-date research evidence with clinical expertise (Wakefield and Olleveant 2019). This clinical expertise is developed both through formal education (propositional knowledge) and informally through experience (non-propositional knowledge). This non-propositional knowledge is thought to be the basis of professional craft knowledge; the tacit knowledge of professionals and personal knowledge linked to the life experience and cognitive resources that a person brings to the situation to enable them to think and perform. Rycroft-Malone et al. (2003) propose that this craft knowledge can be considered evidence if it is articulated, scrutinised, contested and verified by communities of practice. Therefore to be truly evidence-based care, it needs to incorporate knowledge from; research evidence, clinical practice, patients, clients and carers and the local context (Rycroft-Malone et al. 2003). Clinical expertise develops through experience and enables experienced practitioners to utilise critical thinking in an intuitive way to support effective and responsive decision-making and early identification of concerns or deterioration of service users' condition as well as decreasing the chance of error (Payne 2015).

Although there are some limitations regarding EBP such as evidence may not be available to support all individual circumstances, the benefits of the approach may be seen to outweigh them. Benefits of EBP for service users include prevention of harm and decrease in unnecessary interventions (Dahm et al. 2010) as well as improvements in decision-making in complex situations (Muhrer 2012). For services EBP can result in more effective use of resources and practitioner accountability. However, Wakefield and Olleveant's study (2019) identified that practitioners may be unable to fully engage with EBP due to a range of factors such as lack of time, access to best evidence and for some practitioners, a lack of skills to seek out this evidence to support them to remain up to date in their practice.

Work-Based Learning

Work-based learning (WBL) has been widely acknowledged and recognised for the vital part it plays within continuous and future development of existing skills. The term WBL is used to describe an assortment of approaches by which students can learn through work (Lemanski, Mewis and Overton, 2011), developing practical skills that cannot be taught in a classroom, including extra curriculum activities in an academic setting. WBL is widely used throughout Higher Education, which enables students to gain an insight and experience within their chosen career or a field they are interested in after graduating (Figure 7.2).

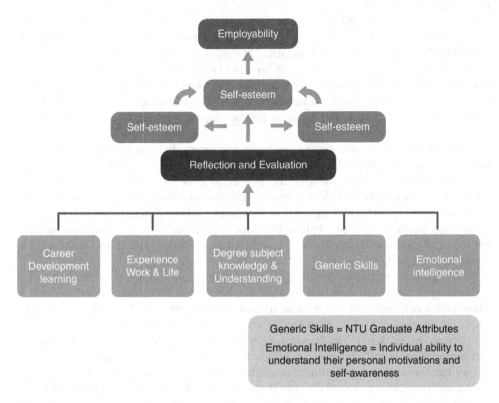

Figure 7.2 Skills.
Source: Pool and Sewell (2007).

As WBL merges practice with theory it is an experience which employers value and look for when recruiting graduates (Cottrell 2015). WBL boosts knowledge with experiences which allows students to keep updated with the changes that happen within organisations, such as changes in policies and legislation, as well as practical changes, for example manual handling training – as the techniques change over the years. Raelin (2008) highlights, it has been recognised that there are as many opportunities for learning in the workplace as there are in the classrooms therefore it is important that students embrace opportunities for WBL through completion of work-based placements or volunteering. Although ideally this experience would be within the sector of health and social care, all placements and volunteering have the potential to support students to develop transferable skills. In recent years universities have strived to improve student's opportunities to engage in WBL by embedding career guidance into their degree programmes, establishing links with employing organisations and increasing opportunities for WBL placements.

WBL and Time Management; Skills for Study and Practice

A skill which is important to supporting WBL is time management. Research suggests effective time management skills, including planning, organisation and prioritisation, stress management, are fundamental skills which helps to; meet work or studying demands, reduce stress and improve performance (Grissom, Loeb and Mitani 2015). Time management helps people to organise their professional lives as well as personal lives. The National Centre for Education Statistics (MacDonald 2018), report that mature students are the new majority in the classrooms which reinforces the importance of a professional work and personal life balance for students and their need to use interventions to build stronger and positive relationships between time management and desired outcomes such as degree classification and readiness for their preferred graduate role.

Organisational skills are key to studying and preparing yourself for assessment submission or attending placement, voluntary or paid work. Studying provides a great opportunity to learn these skills, and experience of meeting submission and other course deadlines can demonstrate your organisation and time management skills to potential employers as well as supporting future practice. Studying can be demanding particularly when balancing work experience or employment alongside, but the practical experience allows an insight into a working lifestyle and what will be expected from you.

With regard to academic deadlines or upcoming presentations, approaching tasks with plenty of time may seem like a simple tip, but alongside having self-awareness of when you work best will enable you to manage the time you have better. For example, if you know you work better in the evening then planning out time in the morning to do work may not be your most productive decision, and if your student accommodation is full and noisy towards the evenings then you may find that the library may be a better environment to enable you to avoid distractions. Doubling up with another student as a study buddy is also a good idea, as breaking a commitment to study with someone is harder than breaking the commitment to yourself. As well as helping you to be motivated, using a study buddy has been shown to diminish social barriers between students in the cohort, have a positive impact on academic achievement and it instils confidence in students to share concerns or questions they may have (Thalluri, O'Flaherty and Shepherd 2014).

McMillan and Weyers (2007), put forward that by looking at the assignment in advance, realistically evaluating when you are able to spend time on the assignment and taking into consideration other commitments, will put you in good stead and aid the structuring process. Breaking tasks down into achievable chunks such as daily or weekly objectives may also help balance time, alongside making tasks seem more manageable or achievable. Increased engagement and focus were also found to be a positive implication of breaking down tasks, with students finding that tasks seemed more 'do-able' when approached this way, alongside feeling they had clear instructions on what needed to be completed before ticking off and moving on to the next task (Table 7.1).

Activity 1   Think about your deadlines; are you prepared for them? Complete the table below, to support you in planning your assignments.

Table 7.1 Planning

Modules:							
Assignment Due Date:							
Grade wanting to Achieve?							
Date to read assignment brief by:							
Date to get resources by:							
Date to get complete plan by:							
Date to complete draft by:							
Comments							

Activity 2   Reflect on your planning; how has it made you feel? What else can you do to manage your time effectively?

Please also remember to reflect on the process when your feedback is received as this can impact on your perceptions of the effectiveness of your planning and the impact on your feedback and grade. This is a brief example from a final year student:

'I am pleased I have managed to complete my portfolio a week before it's due date. This has allowed me time to focus on my weaker areas: to proofread my work, to check my grammar and ensure all my references are cited and referenced correctly. To manage my time better, I could have prioritised part A, and started earlier so it does not feel I had to rush other parts of my portfolio'.

Post feedback: 'leaving extra time to proofread really improved feedback on my citations and references and my grammar is improving too. I was right; feedback for the rushed parts showed there were some areas which were less well developed'.

This section has focused on using time management skills to support you in work and study. Other information to support you to develop academic skills such as finding and evaluating sources, paraphrasing or citing and referencing can be found in the *Current Issues in Health and Social Care* chapter in this book.

WBL and Skills for Professional Practice

WBL supports undergraduate students to develop knowledge and understanding of key professional skills such as accountability and autonomy. Being in placement provides opportunities for students to observe these qualities and skills in practice and reflect on how this experience can support their own development.

Accountability is an essential part of health and social care practice and is therefore important in the workplace and personal life. Caulfield (2005) highlights being accountable means being responsible, and consequently taking the blame and being accountable for your actions when something goes wrong however it can also be seen as individual's responsibility regarding their behaviours and decisions, including whether or not to take action.

Darling-Hammond (1988, see Levine 1988) elaborates that governments create professional bodies and structures to warrant competence and auspicious practice in occupations that serve the public. Professionals and students must comply with their governing body's code of conduct; that is regulations outlining the rules, responsibilities and practices for an individual or organisation. In the field of health and social care the wide range of professions and roles has resulted in multiple governing bodies such as the NMC, General Dental Council (GDC) and Health and Care Professions Council (HCPC), who regulates 15 healthcare professions including dieticians, occupational therapists and social workers (HCPC 2021). The governing body's main duties are to ensure high standards are maintained by health and social care professionals: to uphold an up-to-date register of professionals; set and maintain standards for education, training and conduct, and investigate and act when their standards are not met or a professional's fitness to practise is questioned.

Accountability is important for everyone, including students when on placement and when studying at university. Students should adhere to their university's student code of conduct and code of behaviour whether on campus, in placement or in the community, and when in placement students should also follow the organisations' policies and protocols. In placement, students are accountable for practising within their sphere of competence. For example, if a practitioner delegates a task which is not within your knowledge, skills or experience, it is the student's responsibility to refuse and explain it is beyond their competence or role. It is the professional's responsibility to know the student's level of knowledge and skills and what tasks they are able to complete safely and effectively.

Accountability and Autonomy are interlinked. The term 'Autonomy' can be used interchangeably with the word 'independent' and has been identified as a fundamental factor in the values of healthcare ethics and professional practice (Baykara and Sahinoglu, 2014; Maier, 2014, cited in Zolkefli, Mumin and Idris 2020). Accountability translates to being responsible for your own actions which are essential for autonomy and decision-making within a professional role. Autonomy is a legal requirement in professional codes of conduct and is also often included in person specifications for job roles as health and social care professionals are required to have 'the ability to make decisions rather than being influenced by someone else or told what to do' (The Nursing Board for Brunei 2013 cited in Zolkefli, Mumin and Idris 2020).

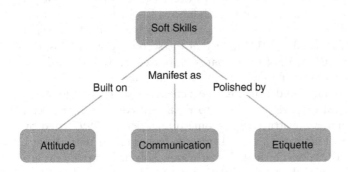

Figure 7.3 Progress.
Source: Ramesh 2010.

When in practice, most roles are autonomous, meaning it is your judgement and competence that determines decisions that need to be made, putting your own personal values and interests aside, and instead use your professional knowledge, without being influenced or instructed to do so. In addition, autonomy requires skills and attitudes which enable independent working without supervision. 'Soft skills' as illustrated in the diagram by Ramesh (2010) are those skills that are transferable, and which characterise how you interact with others. Doyle (2020) suggests these skills can be used regardless of your job role and similarly to autonomy, when applying for jobs they are requirements seen in person specifications, and which can also be recognised as problem-solving, teamwork, communication, motivation. These non-subject-specific skills impact people's performance within the workplace and are seen to be essential skills for graduate roles (Figure 7.3).

As students progress through their degree programme, they are supported and encouraged to engage in independent learning. The skills developed through independent learning are transferable to the workplace, enabling you to act and make decisions within your sphere of knowledge, to self-manage your workload and to communicate and question to ensure understanding of task and timescales.

Managing Stress

Faulkner (2017) identified that mental health within the United Kingdom (UK) was deteriorating and in 2018 they reported that 75% of adults in the UK had experienced high levels of stress and feelings of being unable to cope at some point in their lives (MHF 2018). The age group most vulnerable to stress was identified as 18–24 years – the age of a large proportion of undergraduate students (Caleb and Barden 2019). In addition, it is established that health care practitioners experience psychological ill-health in relation to workload and have higher levels of stress than other occupations (Michie and Williams 2003) therefore students who learn about stress and its management during their university experience will be able to transfer their knowledge, experience and coping mechanisms to the workplace. Further information on reducing stress and preventing burnout can be found in the *Managing Health and Social Care* chapter.

There are two types of stress often discussed in research, also known as the stress paradox. Eustress is described by Kupriyanov and Zhdanov (2014), as a type of stress that heightens an individual's ability to adapt to stressful situations, usually after the instance has occurred. Li, Cao and Li (2016) infer that the second type, distress, is a term used to refer to the negative form of stress that is more frequently discussed and may have negative impacts on an individual's health or well-being.

Eustress is primarily short term and can often be beneficial, by encouraging the individual to strive to not just achieve goals, but to push and consider if they can accomplish more, encouraging a constructive outcome (Quick, et al., 1997 cited by Nelson and Simmons, 2003). Eustress is seen to bring challenges rather than threats, whereby once the issue or occasion i.e. first day at a new job has started, the individual may no longer feel stressed and the situation may be remembered as a positive experience. Eustress can be described as pleasurably undertaking experiences with excitement or brief anxiety without the impact of fear (Harris, 1970 cited by Le Fevre, Matheny and Kolt, 2003).

Distress can be seen as a threat, rather than just a challenge and when an individual is under prolonged or severe stress, a heightened level of anxiety may present in the individual. Distress can be described as feeling unpleasant and can lead to mental health problems, with Rudland, Golding and Wilkinson (2019), adding that chronic stress is often related to sickness such as depression and the term 'stress' is commonly associated with unfortunate or disadvantageous outcomes such as job loss leading to financial difficulty.

Rudland, Golding and Wilkinson (2019) also infer that a level of stress may promote resilience and growth to overcome problems and that associating stress with negative outcomes may only add to the impact felt. This is concurred by Li, Cao and Li (2016), who add that the theory of eustress is often unrecognised and denote that the lack of understanding of eustress and its possible positive impacts on learning may limit an individual's ability to work through distress (Table 7.2).

Activity 3   Eustress and distress

From the table below, look at the issue or incident and decide which would be classed as positive/motivating (Eustress) and which would be classed as long-term or severe (Distress).

Table 7.2 Eustress and distress

Eustress	Issue/incident	Distress
	Starting a New Job	
	Family Bereavement	
	First Date	
	Injury or Illness	

(*Continued*)

Table 7.2 (Continued)

Eustress	Issue/incident	Distress
	Academic Presentation	
	Wedding Day	
	Financial Difficulty	
	Retirement	
	Buying a House	
	Relationship Breakdown	
	Academic Deadline	

The incidents that would be classed as Eustress are starting a new job; a first date; an academic presentation; wedding day nerves; buying a house or another academic deadline. They would be seen to reside in this category due to being short term. The incidents such as family bereavement; injury or illness; financial difficulty; retirement or relationship breakdown would reside in the distress category due to often bringing prolonged feelings of anxiety or negativity. There are various support services students can access via the university itself such as student well-being, library services and personal tutors, however there are also specific services such as a place of worship, the National Bereavement Service, Citizen's Advice Bureau or Stepchange Debt Charity.

Effective time management can decrease student stress. Misra and McKean (2000, cited by Adams and Blair 2019) undertook research that found that stress may be reduced by better time management skills. Haycock (1993, cited by Kachgal, Hansen and Nutter 2001) infers that between 25 and 50% of students experience academic procrastination during university, so for students who feel task or time management is not their strongest skill, you are not alone! Adams and Blair (2019) highlight that the improvement of time management skills can have positive effects on academic performance, so it is worth taking a look to see if productivity may be improved.

Personal Development

As identified earlier in the chapter alongside academic achievements such as degree classification, employers are looking for more from potential employees, but what does that mean for you as a student? Imagine yourself and another student both working at the same academic level and aiming to apply for similar jobs, what attributes or experience could you provide evidence of to make you stand out to a potential employer? For instance, think of a work-experience placement as a paid job, being professional and showing willingness to learn may make the placement an opportunity to network and make contacts. Additionally, the impression you make on your placement mentor could be the difference between them offering you voluntary work to gain experience after the placement ends or even keeping you in mind for a paid position after you have achieved your degree.

Volunteering in the area you intend to build a career in shows willingness to help others and personal motivation without the financial incentive. Furthermore, volunteering is highlighted by Wilson and Musick (1999), as having a possible positive impact on an individual's mental health (providing they do not feel overburdened), due to the self-validation that arises from helping another individual. Finally, volunteering can also be seen as a low commitment method of ensuring you understand the responsibilities of your future career path to ensure it is what you expected and that it is still the career you would like to continue to pursue.

Similarly, there are various opportunities on campus for students to get involved with that would make a Curriculum Vitae (CV) stand out and some are paid roles. Mentoring, for example, is a paid opportunity in which second and third year students utilise their skills to help new students settle into university life, alongside being able to signpost students towards support services if required. Undertaking the role as a mentor can boost students' confidence and communication skills as you will support students studying a module you have completed and use your experience to contribute to discussions, support learning and retention of knowledge.

Taking on the role of a course representative may seem daunting, however providing a channel to bridge the gap between students and lecturers is extremely important, and the contribution may result in positive changes to the course. Whilst this opportunity is unpaid, the workload is low and entails gathering information from students termly and feeding back in termly meetings. You can contribute at a level which works for you and the commitment to broadening communication between students and tutors and potentially improving the course you are studying looks great on any CV. Coincidentally, getting to know the staff team and being engaged, forthcoming and recognisable could also be advantageous in ways such as being thought of when opportunities arise that staff are aware of your interest or are suitable for you. Preparation for graduate-level roles is explored further in the *Leadership in Health and Social Care* chapter.

Conclusion

Being a health and social care practitioner requires a broad range of knowledge and skills and whilst completing a degree provides a solid foundation for graduate practice it is essential that alongside this, students need to have opportunities to develop attributes and to apply theory to practice which will support them to prepare for graduate roles. Having knowledge and understanding of core concepts which underpin practice in health and social care such as vulnerability, risk, accountability and evidence-based practice will provide a firm foundation for students practice in the field.

To be able to stand out from other applicants whilst seeking graduate job roles, students need to be able to demonstrate they have sector specific experience and a range of transferable skills. Students need to be proactive in seeking opportunities whilst studying, within the university life such as mentor or student rep roles and in the workplace through work experience placements or volunteering. These experiences will boost students' employability and support students to gain valuable insights into health and social care practice. Proactively engaging with the university's employability team will also support students to access opportunities and develop their self-presentation to support successful graduate employment.

References

Adams, R., and Blair, E., 2019. Impact of time management behaviors on undergraduate engineering students' performance. *SAGE Open* [online], 9 (1). 10.1177/2158244018824506 [Accessed 11 March 2021].

Aeon, B., and Aguinis, H., 2017. It's about time: New perspectives and insights on time management. *Academy of Management Perspectives* [online], 31(4), 309–330. 10.5465/amp.2016.0166 [Accessed 4 March 2021].

Arnstein, S.R., 2019. A ladder of citizen participation. *Journal of the American Planning Association* [online], 85 (1), 24–34. 10.1080/01944363.2018.1559388

Barnard, A., 2017. The current context and climate of professionals: Definitions and history. In: Barnard, A., ed. *Developing professional practice in health and social care*. London: Routledge, 2017, 7–30.

Baykara, Z.G., and Şahinoğlu, S., 2014. An evaluation of nurses' professional autonomy in Turkey. Nursing ethics, 21(4), pp. 447–460.

Bradby, H., Liabo, K., Ingold, A., and Roberts, H., 2019. Visibility, resilience, vulnerability in young migrants. *Health* [online], 23 (5), 553–550. 10.1177/1363459317739441

Brotherton, G., and Parker, S., eds. 2013. *Your foundation in health and social care*. London: Sage.

Caleb, R., and Barden, N., 2019. Higher education in the twenty-first century: changes and challenges for mental well-being. In Barden, N., and Caleb, R., eds. *Student mental health and wellbeing in higher education a practical guide*. London: Sage, 2019, 3–17.

Caulfield, H., 2005. Accountability. Oxford: Blackwell Pub.

Caulfield, H., 2011. *Vital notes for nurses: Accountability*. 1st ed. [e-book] Oxford: Blackwell Publishing. Available at: https://books.google.co.uk/books?id=jpo2IxcGZMkC&printsec=frontcover&source=gbs_ge_summary_r&cad=0#v=onepage&q&f=false [Accessed 7 March 2021].

Cavendish, C., 2013. *The Cavendish Review. An independent review into healthcare assistants and support workers in the NHS and social care setting* [online]. London: UK Government. Available at: https://assets.publishing.service.gov.uk/government/uploads/system/uploads/attachment_data/file/236212/Cavendish_Review.pdf [Accessed 24 April 2021].

Clarke, P., 2015. Student nurses on placement – collaborations or challenges. *The Journal of Adult Protection*, 17 (5), 287–295.

Cohn, M., Fredrickson, B.L., Brown, S.L., Mikels, J.A., and Conway, A.M., 2009. Happiness unpacked: Positive emotions increase life satisfaction by building resilience. *Emotion* [online], 9 (3), 361–368. 10.1037/a0015952

Cottrell, S., 2015. *Skills for success: Personal development and employability*. 3rd ed. London: Palgrave.

Crouch, A., 2016. Communication skills for holistic health assessment. Vital Notes for Nurses: Health Assessment, pp. 128–147.

Crouch, A., 2021. Communication skills for holistic health assessment. In: Crouch, A., and Meurier, C., ed. *Vital notes for nurses: Health assessment* [online]. Oxford: Blackwell Publishing, 2021, 128–132. Available at: https://onlinelibrary.wiley.com/doi/book/10.1002/9781119302728 [Accessed 15 April 2021].

Cohn, A., Fehr, E., and Maréchal, M.A., 2014. Business culture and dishonesty in the banking industry. Nature, 516(7529).

Dahm, K.T., Brurberg, K.G., Jamtvedt, G., and Hagen, K.B., 2010. Advice to rest in bed versus advice to stay active for acute low-back pain and sciatica. *Cochrane Database of Systematic Reviews* [online], 6. Available via: http://onlinelibrary.wiley.com/doi/10.1002/14651858.CD007612.pub2/full (Accessed 14 April 2021).

Darling-Hammond, L., 1988. Accountability for professional practice. In: Levine, M., ed. *Professional practice schools: Building a model* [online]. Washington D.C: Educational

Issues Department, 1988, 71–74. Available at: https://files.eric.ed.gov/fulltext/ED313344. pdf#page=77 [Accessed 27 February 2021].

Department of Health, 2006. *Modernising nursing careers, setting the direction* [online]. London: HMSO. Available at: http://www.nursingleadership.org.uk/publications/ settingthedirection.pdf [Accessed on 25 March 2021].

Department of Health, 2007. *Independence, choice and risk: A guide to supported decision making* [online]. London: Scie.org.uk. Available at: https://www.scie.org.uk/publications/adul tsafeguardinglondon/files/independence-choiceandrisk.pdf?res=true [Accessed 15 April 2021].

Doyle, A., 2020. *What are soft skills?* [online]. New York: The Balance Careers. Available at: https://www.thebalancecareers.com/what-are-soft-skills-2060852#what-are-soft-skills [Accessed 15 April 2021].

Duignan, J., 2006. Placement and adding value to the academic performance of undergraduates: reconfiguring the architecture – an empirical investigation. *Journal of Vocational Education & Training* [online], 55 (3), 335–350. Available via: https://www.tandfonline.com/doi/abs/ 10.1080/13636820300200233 [Accessed 22 February 2021].

Eade, D., n.d. *Success for all: Closing the graduate employment gap* [online]. Nottingham: Slideplayer. Available at: https://slideplayer.com/slide/15739631/ [Accessed 13 February 2021].

Egan, G., (1975). The Skilled Helper: A Systematic Approach to Effective Helping. Pacific Grove CA, Brooks/Cole.

Emanuel, E.J., and Emanuel, L.L., 1996. What is accountability in health care?. *Annals of Internal Medicine*, 124 (2), 229–239. 10.7326/0003-4819-124-2-199601150-00007

England, N.H.S., 2015. Liaison and diversion manager and practitioner resources service user involvement. Offender Health Collaborative, available at: www.england.nhs.uk/ commissioning/wp-content/uploads/sites/12/2015/10/ohc-paper-06.pdf (accessed 8 June 2019).

Faulkner, A., 2017. Survivor research and Mad Studies: the role and value of experiential knowledge in mental health research. Disability & Society, 32(4), pp. 500–520.

Fennell, K., 2016. Call of Duty: an exploration of the factors influencing NHS professionals to report adult protection concerns. *The Journal of Adult Protection* [online], 18 (3), 161–171. 10.1108/JAP-11-2015-0034

Giddens, A., 1999. Risk and responsibility. The Modern Law Revie [online], 62 (1), 1–10. Available via: https://onlinelibrary.wiley.com/doi/epdf/10.1111/1468-2230.00188?saml_ referrer [Accessed 1 February 2021].

Grissom, J.A., Loeb, S., and Mitani, H., 2015. Principal time management skills: Exploring patterns in principals' time use, job stress and perceived effectiveness. *Journal of Educational Administration* [online], 53 (6), 773–793. 10.1108/JEA-09-2014-0117 [Accessed 11 May 2021].

Haycock, L.A., 1993. The cognitive mediation of procrastination: An investigation of the relationship between procrastination and self-efficacy beliefs: University of Minnesota.

HCPC, 2021. *Who we regulate* [online]. London: HCPC. Available at: https://www.hcpc-uk. org/about-us/who-we-regulate/ [Accessed 21 May 2021].

Heaslip, V., 2013. Understanding vulnerability. In: Heaslip, V., and Ryden, J., eds. *Understanding vulnerability: A nursing and healthcare approach*. 1st ed. Chichester: John Wiley & Sons, Incorporated, 2013, 6–27.

Health and Safety Executive, n.d. *Who regulates health care* [online]. London: Hse.gov.uk. Available at: https://www.hse.gov.uk/healthservices/arrangements.htm [Accessed 13 February 2021].

Kachgal, M., Hansen, S., and Nutter, K., 2001. Academic procrastination prevention/intervention: Strategies and recommendations. *Journal of Developmental Education* [online], 25 (1), 14. Available via: https://search.proquest.com/openview/2162f67a685051ae284bb700ae6fb37f/ 1?pq-origsite=gscholar&cbl=47765 [Accessed 17 March 2021].

Kelly, D., and Jones, A., 2013. When care is needed: the role of whistle-blowing in promoting best standards from an individual and organisational perspective. *Quality in Ageing and Older Adults* [online], 14 (3), 180–191. 10.1108/QAOA-05-2013-0010 [Accessed 24 April 2021].

Kupriyanov, R., and Zhdanov, R., 2014. The eustress concept: problems and outlooks. *World Journal of Medical Sciences* [online], 11 (2), 179–185. Available via: http://www.idosi.org/wjms/11(2)14/6.pdf [Accessed 5 March 2021].

Lemanski, T., Mewis, R., and Overton, T., 2011. *An introduction to work-based learning.* [ebook]. Hull: Higher Education Academy. Available at: https://s3.eu-west-2.amazonaws.com/assets.creode.advancehe-document-manager/documents/hea/private/work_based_learning_1568036792.pdf [Accessed 15 February 2021].

Le Fevre, M., Matheny, J., and Kolt, G.S., 2003. Eustress, distress, and interpretation in occupational stress. Journal of managerial psychology.

Li, C., Cao, J., and Li, T., 2016. Eustress or distress: an empirical study of perceived stress in everyday college life. In: 2016 ACM International Joint Conference on Pervasive and Ubiquitous Computing: Adjunct (UbiComp '16) [online]. Available at: https://dl.acm.org/doi/10.1145/2968219.2968309 [Accessed 5 March 2021].

MacDonald, K., 2018. A review of the literature: the needs of non-traditional students in postsecondary education. *Strategic Enrolment Management Quarterly* [online], 5 (4), 159–164. Available at: https://onlinelibrary.wiley.com/doi/abs/10.1002/sem3.20115 [Accessed 4 March 2021].

McCray, J., Palmer, A., and Chmiel, N., 2014. Building resilience in health and social care teams. *Personnel Review* [online], 45 (6), 1132–1155. Available via: https://www.emerald.com/insight/publication/issn/0048-3486/vol/45/iss/6 [Accessed 24 April 2021].

McGowan, B., 2006. Who do they think they are? Undergraduate perceptions of the definition of supernumerary status and how it works in practice. *Journal of Clinical Nursing* [online], 15 (9), 1099–1105. Available via: https://onlinelibrary.wiley.com/doi/abs/10.1111/j.1365-2702.2005.01478.x [Accessed 5 March 2021].

Michie, S., and Williams, S., 2003. Reducing work related psychological ill health and sickness absence: A systematic literature review. *Occupational and Environmental Medicine* [online], 60, 3–9. Available via: https://www.ncbi.nlm.nih.gov/pmc/articles/PMC1740370/ [Accessed 23 April 2021].

McMillan, K., and Weyers, J., 2007. *How to write essays and assignments* [online]. Essex: Pearson Education Limited. Available at: https://books.google.co.uk/books?hl=en&lr=&id=1dUxbE49RbEC&oi=fnd&pg=PA11&dq=breaking+down+assignments&ots=_TJJs6VO1Z0&sig=nIHeLWT6fGoTr1MBSmEz4drkhBg&redir_esc=y#v=onepage&q&f=false [Accessed 17 March 2021].

Muhrer, J., 2012. Making evidence-based health care relevant for patients. *The Journal of Nurse Practitioners* [online], 8 (1), 51–52. Available via: https://search.proquest.com/docview/1507211601?accountid=14693&rfr_id=info%3Axri%2Fsid%3Aprimo [Accessed 24 September 2019].

NHS England, n.d. *Involving people in their own health and care.* London: NHS England. Available at: https://www.england.nhs.uk/wp-content/uploads/2017/04/ppp-involving-people-health-care-guidance.pdf [Accessed 27 April 2021].

NMC, 2018. *The Code: Professional standards of practice and behaviour for nurses, midwives and nursing associates* [online]. London: NMC. Available at: https://www.nmc.org.uk/globalassets/sitedocuments/nmc-publications/nmc-code.pdf [Accessed 01 February 2021].

Payne, L.K., 2015. Toward a theory of intuitive decision-making in Nursing. *Nursing Science Quarterly* [online], 28 (3), 223–228. 10.1177/0894318415585618

Phillips, S., 2012. Work based learning in health and social care. *British Journal of Nursing* [online], 21 (15), 918. Available via: https://www.magonlinelibrary.com/doi/pdf/10.12968/bjon.2012.21.15.918 [Accessed 01 November 2020].

Pool, L.D., and Sewell, P., 2007. The key to employability: developing a practical model of graduate employability. Education + Training.

Raelin, J., 2008. *Work-based learning: Bridging knowledge and action in the workplace.* [eBook]. San Francisco: Jossey-Bass, 1–7. Available via: https://books.google.co.uk/books?id=WXpn_GRvBV4C&printsec=frontcover&source=gbs_ge_summary_r&cad=0#v=onepage&q&f=false [Accessed 12 February 2021].

Ramesh, G., and Ramesh, M., 2010. *The ace of soft skills: Attitude, communication and etiquette for success* [eBook]. India: Pearson Education. Available via: https://books.google.co.uk/books?id=EdBuMdH4us8C&printsec=frontcover&source=gbs_ge_summary_r&cad=0#v=onepage&q&f=false [Accessed 15 April 2021].

Rogerson, M., and Emes, C., 2008. Fostering resilience within an adult day Support Program. *Activities, Adaptation & Aging* [online], 32 (1), 1–18. 10.1080/01924780802039220

Royal College of Nursing, 2021. *Clinical safeguarding* [online]. London: Royal College of Nursing. Available at: https://www.rcn.org.uk/clinical-topics/safeguarding 2021 [Accessed 01 April 2021].

Rudland, J., Golding, C., and Wilkinson, T., 2019. The stress paradox: how stress can be good for learning. *Medical Education* [online], 54 (1), 40–45. 10.1111/medu.13830 [Accessed 5 March 2021].

Rycroft-Malone, J., Seers, K., Titchen, A., Harvey, G., Kitson, A., and McCormack, B., 2003. What counts as evidence in evidence-based practice. *Nurse and Healthcare Management and Policy* [online], 47 (1), 89–91. Available via: https://onlinelibrary-wiley-com.libezproxy.open.ac.uk/doi/pdfdirect/10.1111/j.1365-2648.2004.03068.x [Accessed 27 April 2021].

Sheldon, L., and Hilaire, D., 2015. Development of communication skills in healthcare: Perspectives of new graduate nursing education. *Journal of Nursing Education and Practice* [online], 5 (7), 30–37. 10.5430/jnep.v5n7p30

Stickley, T., 2011. From SOLER to SURETY for effective non-verbal communication. *Nurse Education in Practice* [online], 11 (6), 395–398. Available via: https://www.sciencedirect.com/science/article/pii/S1471595311000618#bib7 [Accessed 15 April 2021].

Thalluri, J., O'Flaherty, J., and Shepherd, P., 2014. Classmate peer-coaching: "A Study Buddy Support scheme". *Journal of Peer Learning* [online], 8 (7), 92–104. Available via: https://ro.uow.edu.au/cgi/viewcontent.cgi?referer=https://scholar.google.co.uk/&httpsredir=1&article=1097&context=ajpl [Accessed 17 March 2021].

Wakefield, A., and Olleveant, N., 2019. Evidence-based practice and the importance of research. In: Burns, D., ed. *Foundations of adult nursing.* London: Sage, 2019.

Wareing, M., Chadwick, K., and Baggs, H., 2014. Student satisfaction with work-based learning: evaluation of a foundation degree health & social care programme. *Semantic Scholar* [online], 2 (2), 65–79. 10.11120/PBLH.2014.00034 [Accessed 01 November 2020].

WHO, 2017. *Facilitating evidence-based practice in nursing and midwifery in the WHO European Region* [online]. Europe: World Health Organization. Available at: https://www.euro.who.int/__data/assets/pdf_file/0017/348020/WH06_EBP_report_complete.pdf?ua=1 [Accessed 3 September 2020].

Wilson, J., and Musick, M., 1999. The effects of volunteering on the volunteer. *Law and Contemporary Problems* [online], 62 (4), 141. Available via: https://scholarship.law.duke.edu/cgi/viewcontent.cgi?article=1150&context=lcp [Accessed 18 March 2021].

Zolkefli, Z.H.H., Mumin, K.H., and Idris, D.R., 2020. Autonomy and its impact on midwifery practice. *British Journal of Midwifery* [online], 28 (2), 120–129. Available via: https://www.magonlinelibrary.com/doi/pdfplus/10.12968/bjom.2020.28.2.120?casa_token=O3VEXzVmOMIAAAAA:-m1gt9t5_Xj7k3M7P7oTIQ4zUls_a4Ntuc5WCSF78LImd3dOEc21GuU2YSrpEaT-dIV3R6UIDbVV_Q [Accessed 24 April 2021].

Part II

8 Health, Social Care and Crime

Jennifer Sanders

The chapter aims to:

- provide an understanding of issues facing criminal justice agencies
- examine the explanation for, and impact of, criminal behaviour
- challenge contemporary approaches of responding to criminal behaviour

Objectives

After reading this chapter you should be able to:

1 Understand the purpose of, and issues relating to, key agencies in our criminal justice system
2 Outline explanations of criminal behaviour and the impact it can have
3 Discuss the ways in which criminal behaviour is responded to

After reading this chapter you will know the meaning of the following terms: police, prison, restorative justice, multifactorial theory, bounded rationality, situational crime prevention
There is a Moment of Reflection at the end of the chapter.

Introduction

Like many health and social care issues, criminal and anti-social behaviour often make news headlines. It is this media portrayal of crime which influences our perceptions of criminal justice agencies such as the police and prisons. A quick search of news articles produces negative headlines such as 'We exposed undercover policing scandal', 'A case of police doing nothing for too long', 'Killer on loose after escaping prison'. News articles can also draw attention to some of the systemic issues which need addressing, as well as highlight the dangers of individuals taking the law into their own hands. Some examples will be provided in this chapter.

This chapter will briefly explore the function of the police and prison service, exploring some of the key issues continuing to affect the delivery of public trust in such bodies. The process of restorative justice will be discussed, as an effective way to respond to and address criminal behaviour and make amends. A broader overview of the criminal justice system can be found in the first edition of this book. The focus of this chapter will then turn to exploring some of the crimes

DOI: 10.4324/9781003079873-10

which often make news headlines, exploring explanations for, impact of and responses to these crimes.

The process of reporting crimes through news media, and the retweeting or sharing across social media platforms, moulds our perceptions of perpetrators and what is the 'right' response to crime. Sensationalised headlines, focusing on serious but rare crimes and creating a character to fear, such as the 'Yorkshire Ripper' or 'Moors Murderers', can skew our perceptions of likelihood of victimisation. Often there are calls for harsher punishments, longer sentences and criticism of alternatives to prison such as the use of community sanctions. The reporting of individuals being released early from prison also fuels the misconception that they are now 'free' and that justice hasn't been served.

Lack of trust in the police and increased use of social media has given rise to a different form of policing, in the shape of 'paedophile hunters'. However popular such vigilante groups are, there are concerns of hindering investigations and they do make devastating mistakes (see case of Darren Kelly: Tonkin 2016). Arguably, the most effective way to respond to crime is to address the causes of crime. This involves understanding the biological, psychological, sociological and other factors that may influence and impact on an individual. As this chapter will demonstrate, responses need to be preventative not just reactive, and draw on the wider health and social care sector, not just traditional criminal justice agencies and practices.

The Criminal Justice System

There are a number of good textbooks which provide a descriptive overview of the criminal justice system in England and Wales, as well as outlining key policy and legislation developments (e.g., Davies 2015). In this section, the focus is on two key agencies and aspects of the criminal justice system, highlighting two key issues: race and sex. The alternative practice of restorative justice will also be introduced.

Police

There are 43 police forces in England and Wales, which operate independently from political interference, and apply the rule of law with minimal force to result in public cooperation. Police duty is to protect the public, and their powers are to investigate crime, to prevent crime and to 'dispose' of criminal cases. In the last decade there have been major reforms to policing in England and Wales, which were provided by the *Police and Social Responsibility Act (2011)*. The purpose of these reforms was to make police more accountable to their local communities. An overview of policing governance, operation and powers in England and Wales can be found in House of commons briefing papers (see Brown 2020a and 2020b).

Whilst there is law and policy to follow, limited resources mean police judgement and discretion of enforcement is required. Such in-the-moment decision-making is common in most health and social care roles. However, there have been instances that indicate such discretion is abused within police work, with prejudice and stereotyping impacting on decision-making (Rowe 2017). Instances such as the Brixton Riots and the murder of Stephen Lawrence have led to accusations of institutional racism, fuelled by the media response (Neal 2003). Statistics show Black people are stopped and searched considerably more than White people – 38 for every 1,000 compared to

4 for every 1,000 (Home Office 2020a). Measures of ethnic breakdown show 7.3% identified as BME (Home Office 2020b). A lack of cultural diversity could explain racism in police culture, and should be the focus of change (Rowe 2017).

Another commonly noted aspect of police culture is sexism. Females account for just 31% of police officers across England and Wales (Home Office 2020b). Traditionally, policing is seen as a male occupation, with connotations of action, danger and strength associated with being masculine. Such hegemonic masculinity is reinforced through media and political rhetoric (Rowe 2017). There have been initiatives to boost equality in the force, and this is reflected in the number of female police officers increasing every year since 2010 (Home Office 2020b). However, experiences of bias and prejudice across probation, training, deployment and progression due to identifying characteristics such as sex are still experienced (Zempi 2020).

In addition to internal police relations, misogyny has impacted on police decision-making in response to sexual offences and domestic violence. Over recent years, there has been legislation and work around victim rights in relation to these crimes, which may have improved the training and attitudes of police officers (Myhill 2019). One area where police response is still problematic is sexual violence against men. Enduring hegemonic masculinity perceives male rape victims as subordinate. Javaid (2018) explored police attitudes and conceptualisation of male rape, finding police are unlikely to take male rape seriously. Some reasons for this include police insensitivity, enduring rape myths (e.g., 'men cannot be raped'), lack of training and lack of choice in responding police/forensic staff. Recently McKee, Mueller-Johnson and Strang (2020) evaluated the impact of a training programme on police attitudes towards victims of rape. Overall, they found a positive change in terms of the reduction in rape myth acceptance. Although there are limitations to the study with work still to be done, it does suggest training may be the appropriate and effective way to address enduring rape myths and attitudes towards rape victims within the police.

Suggested Further Reading

Bryant, R., and Bryant, S., 2020. *Blackstone's handbook for policing students.* Oxford: Oxford University Press.
Rowe, M., 2017. *Introduction to policing.* 3rd ed. London: Sage.

Prison

There are 117 prisons in England and Wales, with adult male prisons categorised as trainer, local, high security or open. Of the 12 adult female prisons, two are classified as open (Beard 2019). The current prison population in England and Wales is approximately 79,453, and in May 2020 49% (57) of prisons were overcrowded. Since 1900 the prison population has quadrupled, and we now have the highest rate amongst Western European countries (Sturge 2020).

There are four perceived purposes of prison (Gauke 2018):

Protecting the public by taking away the free liberties of criminals.

Deter the individual from committing crime again, in order to avoid the restrictions and removal of liberties.

Encourage the individual to reflect on their behaviour and change their ways through **rehabilitation**.

A feeling of **justice and retribution** for the victim and society.

The high prison population, overcrowding, poor living conditions, high levels of violence and understaffing constitute what is referred to as the 'penal crisis' (Cavadino et al. 2019). There is also concern regarding the demographics of the prison population.

The BAME community is over-represented in the prison population, with 27% compared to just 13% of the general population (Sturge 2020). Of particular concern is the over-representation of black people. It has been outlined above how black people are disproportionately of interest to the police. Racial bias occurs at other stages of the criminal justice system – charging, bail, and plea decisions, sentencing – contributes to the over-representation in prison (Cavadino et al. 2019). The Lammy Review (2017) identified several ways BAME individuals had a differential experience in prison. They were less likely to have mental health concerns identified, less likely to have a prison job or engage in offender behaviour programmes and report higher rates of victimisation from staff. Stereotyping and prejudicial views by the prison staff contribute to this discrimination. As with the police, a key issue to address is the lack of diversity in prison staff and leadership. HMPPS has stated its commitment to tackling this racial disparity through recruitment targets and revisions in prison office application tests, development of probation workforce reform strategy, launching initiatives with requirements for BAME representation on panels and new coaching programmes (Ministry of Justice 2020a).

Women are under-represented in the criminal justice system, accounting for less than 5% of the prison population. However, this is one of the highest rates of women's imprisonment in Western Europe. Although few in number, the experience and impact of prison for women is concerning. Among female prisoners, 84% are in for non-violent offences, they are largely (63%) on sentences of six months or less, and 48% are reconvicted within one year of release. There has been a consistent call for a reduction in the use of custodial sentences for women. Prison is deemed an inappropriate response due to the vulnerability of women – often victims of abuse and trauma, care-leavers, with addiction and/or mental health issues – and the inability to address complex causes of offending behaviour. Imprisoning women can also have a negative effect on the children they are primary caregivers for (Prison Reform Trust 2017). In 2007 Baroness Corston conducted a review of women in the criminal justice system, highlighting these vulnerabilities and proposing 43 recommendations to bring about radical change. Sadly, despite government support few recommendations have been implemented (see Corston 2007).

Influenced by the Corston Report, the Ministry of Justice (2018) developed the Female Offender Strategy with the aim to intervene earlier, increase the use of community solutions and improve the conditions for those in custody. The prison estate was designed for men, and women therefore have a more painful experience (Crewe, Hulley and Wright 2017). Research has demonstrated that where custodial sentences are used, it is key that the gender-specific needs of women are incorporated (see Jewkes et al. 2019). This includes considering the location and physical environment of prisons, alongside trauma- and gender-informed policies, practices and opportunities. The proposal of Residential Women's Centres in the Female Offender Strategy was a step towards this women-centred approach. In January 2021, in a commitment to improve conditions, it was announced that 500 new prison places for women were being built (Ministry of Justice 2021). This has been met with the criticism that funding could be better spent on women's centres and community support to address complex issues thus preventing entry into the criminal justice system, rather than increasing the female prison population (Sarraf 2021). To date, less than half of the strategy's recommendations have been achieved (Prison Reform Trust 2021). Like female prisoners, transgender prisoners are experiencing a more painful experience. This is an issue gaining increased media, research and political attention, regarding placement and treatment (e.g., Shaw 2020; Gorden et al. 2017; Beard 2018). It is anticipated policy and strategy will need to develop for a transgender-centred approach too.

Suggested Further Reading

Cavadino, M., Dignan, J., and Mair, G., 2013. *The penal system: an introduction.* 5th ed. London: Sage.
Scott, D., and Flynn, N., 2014. *Prisons and punishment: the essentials.* 2nd ed. London: Sage.

Restorative Justice

Restorative practice is a process which can be used in a range of settings, with a focus on building relationships, preventing conflict and repairing harm. There are six principles of restorative practice (Restorative Justice Council 2016):

Restoration – address needs and build resilience

Voluntarism – participation is voluntary by all involved

Impartiality – practitioners must remain impartial and ensure non-discriminatory practice

Safety – creating a safe space to express emotions

Accessibility – inclusive of any diversity needs

Empowerment – supporting individuals to make their own informed choices and ways to move forward

When used in criminal justice, restorative practice is referred to a restorative justice. Both victims and offenders need to agree to participate, and the offender must have admitted his guilt. The process involves the victim and offender communicating within a controlled environment, discussing the impact of the crime, holding the offender accountable and supporting them to make amends. A longitudinal study evaluating three restorative justice schemes found high levels of victim satisfaction rate, a reduction in offending and economic advantages (Shapland, Robinson and Sorsby 2011).

There are various types of restorative justice in operation in the UK (CPS 2019):

Direct or indirect restorative justice processes – communication guided by a facilitated to agree how best to repair the harm caused

Community conferencing – involves the whole community to resolve harm caused, useful in anti-social behaviour cases

Referral Order panels – part of a young person's order, where they attend a panel to discuss the factors contributing to their offence

Mediation – mediator runs a meeting to enable parties in dispute to come to an agreement

The CPS outlines that restorative justice can occur at any stage of the criminal justice process. The practice is seen most with children and young people, as a means of diverting them from crime or as part of their order on conviction. With adult offenders, restorative justice is usually part of a conditional caution. In these circumstances restorative justice is available to all victims and they should be contacted to seek their views on willingness to participate. The CSEW (ONS 2019a) indicates that between 2011 and 2019, on average only 6.4% of victims were offered the opportunity to meet the offender. Of these victims, on average 33.35% accepted this offer. Although low uptake, research indicates positive outcomes across several measures for victims who engaged with restorative justice: 57% reported improved health and well-being, 55% reported feeling safer, 62% reported being able to cope better and 68% felt better informed and empowered (Watson 2020). Such high victim satisfaction raises the question of why restorative justice is not used more. It may be that police and prosecutors involved do not understand the utility of restorative justice, reducing the likelihood of it being offered, or the victim being sufficiently informed of the process to accept the offer. It may also be an issue of when restorative justice is offered: too soon following the crime and a victim may not have recovered from the trauma to participate, but if too much time has passed since the offence they may not wish to revisit the traumatic experience (CPS 2019). The application of restorative justice will be discussed further in the next section.

Suggested Further Reading

Van Ness, D. W., Heetderks Strong, K., 2015. *Restoring justice: an introduction to restorative justice.* London: Routledge.
Wallis, P., 2014. *Understanding restorative justice: how empathy closes the gap created by crime.* Bristol: Policy Press.

Exploring Criminal Behaviour

This section will explore possible explanations, impacts and responses to sexual offences, theft, robbery and burglary.

Sexual Offences

The *Sex Offences Act 2003* is the law which legislates against a vast range of contact (e.g., rape) and non-contact offences (e.g., possession of indecent images of children), as well as prostitution and recent inclusion of 'upskirting' i.e., taking pictures under a person's clothing. In addition, the *Criminal Justice and Courts Act 2015* legislates against revenge porn, another act which is sexual in nature. The CSEW (ONS 2018) estimated that approximately 700,000 adults had experienced sexual assault in the last year. Police statistics indicate 150,847 sexual offences occurred in the year ending March 2018, but it is estimated fewer than 17% of victims report incidents of rape. Of these recorded offences, only 6% resulted in a charge or summons, with around 77% resulting in conviction. Those with sexual convictions account for 18% of the prison population (Ministry of Justice 2020b).

Sexual violence can have a range of psychological and physical effects on a survivor (The Survivors Trust 2019). These may include feelings of guilt, shame, confusion, fear and many more. Individuals may experience PTSD and other disorders or have a range of other reactions including substance misuse, self-injury and relationship problems. The CPS (2020) identify issues, needs and barriers particular groups of people who have been victim of sexual violence may experience. In addition to the assault itself, reporting the crime and pursuing criminal proceedings can cause further distress. Thomas (2013) provides an overview of how police handling of sexual offences has been criticised, and how secondary victimisation and victim blaming has been seen in court. The *Youth Justice and Criminal Evidence Act 1999* was introduced to address these issues, as well as introduce several special measures which can be implemented to make the experience less traumatic, these include:

Screens to shield the witness from the defendant

A live video link to enable the witness to give evidence from a separate room
Giving evidence by a video-recorded interview

There are many theories which attempt to explain how and why individuals sexually offend (see Ward, Polaschek, and Busch 2006). Multifactorial theories focus on how a range of factors interact to explain the behaviour. One comprehensive theory is Ward and Beech's (2016) Integrated Theory of Sexual Offending (ITSO), which can explain the cause of a range of sexual offending behaviours. This theory identifies how biological (e.g., genetics, neurobiology) and ecological (e.g., psychological vulnerabilities, environment) factors influence our neuropsychological functioning. The biological factors could be a genetic predisposition to sexual offending behaviour, link to the evolutionary need to reproduce, manifesting as coercion and force, or relates to deficits in brain development. The ecological factors capture the personal, social and cultural circumstances which an individual experience. These influence our motivational/emotional, action selection and control, and perception and memory systems. The interlocking of these neuropsychological functions creates clinical symptoms (e.g., emotional problems, cognitive distortions) which lead to sexual offending action. In turn, this action impacts on the biological and environmental factors leading to maintenance and escalation of sexual offending behaviour. Although comprehensive, this is a general theory of sexual offending. As such, it may not explain the behaviour of individuals with conditions such as ASD, where diagnostic symptomology may provide insight (see Allely and Creaby-Attwood 2016).

The Sentencing Council (2013) sets out the range of sentences applied to each type of sexual offence. These sentences include imprisonment, community orders and fines. In addition, the *Sex Offences Act 2003* details notification requirements and civil orders which can be applied to monitor and manage those with sexual convictions and protect the public. The Notification Requirements, known as the 'sex offenders register', are imposed automatically for a fixed or indefinite period for certain sexual convictions in England and Wales (Beard 2017). Notification Requirements can also be applied if the disposal was a conditional discharge, caution or hospital admission. Offenders are required to provide the police with up-to-date personal information (i.e., name, date of birth, national insurance number, address, passport and bank details). They also need to notify police of any travel. This 'register' is not publicly available, but under the child sex offender disclosure scheme parents, carers and guardians can ask police if someone they know has a record for child sexual offences.

Sexual Harm Prevention Orders (SHPOs) and Sexual Risk Orders (SROs) are the civil orders available to manage those with sexual convictions or who pose a risk of harm (Beard 2017). SHPOs restrict individuals from certain activities for a fixed period or until further notice. Such prohibited activities could include some employment opportunities (e.g., working with children) or particular activities on the internet. SROs do not require an individual to have a sexual conviction, instead they are imposed if there is a belief they pose a risk of harm to the public. Prohibitions may include contact with a particular child, or visiting a particular location previously associated with sexual conduct towards a child.

Whilst these sentences and civil orders may protect the public, and provide punishment for sexual offending behaviour, they do not fully address the complex and interacting factors known to cause and reinforce the behaviours. Rehabilitation, where treatment programmes address the complex interplay of factors contributing to sexual offending, would seem more appropriate (see Craissati 2018). A recent review of the Ministry of Justice's prison-based SOTP identified problems in regards to reducing reoffending and safeguarding the public (see Mews, Di Bella and Purver 2017). As a result, it was abolished and replaced with two programmes which address the different needs of each offender, although the effectiveness of these programmes is yet to be evaluated (McCartan, Hoggett and Kemshall, 2018). Charities like Safer Living Foundation are increasingly providing initiatives and opportunities to engage those with sexual offence convictions in the community to reduce reoffending (Blagden and Winder 2019).

In addition to punitive and rehabilitative measures, restorative justice has been considered as a useful tool to reduce reoffending. Whilst there may be concern of re-traumatisation, there has been high levels of victim satisfaction reported and rates of reoffending declining (JUSTICE 2019). As outlined earlier, restorative justice enables a dialogue between offender and victim, enabling accountability and reparation of harm caused. Restorative justice gives victims of sexual violence a voice, which is not heard in the criminal justice process if their allegations do not result in trial and conviction. In the wake of Jimmy Saville, Rolf Harris and Harvey Weinstein allegations and convictions, there has been a movement for victims of sexual assault to be empowered to speak out. Social media enabled this with #MeToo. Peleg-Koriat and Klar-Chalamish (2020) explored the public's views of #MeToo and restorative justice in sexual offence cases. Both had high levels of support, focusing on the nature of #MeToo increasing the discussion of sexual offences and restorative justice enabling coping and healing on the victim's terms.

The emotive nature of sexual offences, low levels of prosecution and lack of confidence in the police have led to a rise in 'paedophile hunters'. Paedophile hunters are groups of individuals who pose as children online, engage in sexually explicit conversations with an adult with the purpose of arranging a meeting. Upon arrival, the adult is confronted by the paedophile hunters who are recording, and often live streaming on social media, the encounter and probing the adult to admit to their online behaviours and intentions to have sexual contact with the child they thought they were meeting. Whilst paedophile hunters may purport they are aiding police and protecting children, there is concern their unregulated actions could hamper criminal proceedings (Purshouse 2020). There are several areas of concern: the way 'evidence' is collected and the public sharing of a target's personal information; misuse of citizen's arrest and entrapment; and a breach of human rights. There is also the concern of mistakes and use of violence, as was the case in the murder of Darren Kelly. Darren thought he was meeting a woman he had been exchanging messages with on a dating app. Instead, he was confronted by 'hunters' who proceeded to chase and stab him to death (Tonkin 2016). There are sadly several cases of mistaken identity or violence from paedophile hunters, questioning whether there should be regulation of such vigilantism.

Suggested Further Reading

Lievesley, R., Hocken, K., Elliott, H., Winder, B., Blagden, N., and Banyard, P., 2018. *Sexual crime and prevention.* Basingstoke: Palgrave Macmillan.
Ward, T., Polaschek, DLL., and Busch, AR., 2006. *Theories of sexual offending.* Oxford: Wiley-Blackwell.

Theft, Robbery Burglary

The *Theft Act* 1968 provides the following definitions:

> Theft – 'dishonestly appropriating property belonging to another with the intention of permanently depriving the other of it'
>
> Robbery – 'A person is guilty of robbery if he steals, and immediately before or at the time of doing so, and in order to do so, he uses force on any person or puts or seeks to put any person in fear of being then and there subjected to force'
>
> Burglary – 'person is guilty of burglary if he enters any building or part of a building as a trespasser and with intent ... or having entered any building or part of a building as a trespasser he steals or attempts to steal anything in the building or that part of it or inflicts or attempts to inflict on any person therein any grievous bodily harm'

Long-term trends indicate that overall theft has been declining since 1995, although there has been an 11% increase in the last two years. There has also been a rise of 11% in robberies in the last two years. Burglary offences had been rising, however the last year saw a decrease of 4% (ONS 2019b). There are several explanations for why individuals may engage in stealing behaviour.

Exploring the psychopathology of shoplifting sees a myriad of explanations. Research has identified links with kleptomania, depression, eating disorders, personality disorders and substance abuse. Such criminal behaviour is also justified through neutralisation: the idea there is no victim. Other justifications relate to negative views of 'the system', perception of few consequences and survival needs. As such, there have been attempts to categorise shoplifters (Gavin 2019).

Similarly, there have been attempts to identify types of street robbery. Goodwill et al. (2012) confirmed four types of robbery styles:

Blitz – high levels of violence and surprise, but little interaction with victim, substance abuse

Confrontation – use of weapon, verbal threats to persuade victim to comply, physical violence if necessary

Con – involves planning, interacts with victim to seem amicable and distracts victim

Snatch – opportunistic and impulsive, with low level interaction with victim

Research exploring the decision-making of burglars consistently finds that, whilst they exploit opportunities, target appraisal is rational and skilful (Taylor 2013). Rational choice theory asserts that individuals engage in criminal behaviour which maximises gains whilst minimising risks. Often heuristics and cues are utilised to aid quick decision-making, referred to as 'bounded rationality' (see Newburn 2017). Applied to burglary, these may be visual cues to indicate affluence, occupancy, ease of access and security. In addition to this risk-reward analysis, there is suggestion that morality is entwined in decision-making. Neutralisation techniques are drawn upon, allowing burglars to balance their self-concept as a moral person and the immoral criminal behaviour they commit. These techniques (denial of responsibility, denial of injury, denial of the victim, condemnation of the condemners, defence of necessity and justification by compromise) form a moral code which influences a burglar's target appraisal, modus operandi and items stolen (Taylor 2013).

In addition to exploring decisions, research has sought to understand the self-reported motivations and offence gains for burglars (Taylor 2016). The perceived gains of burglary are often financial and material. Strain theory supports that criminal behaviour, such as burglary, occurs when legitimate ways of attaining goals and meeting needs are not available (see Newburn 2017). Burglary can also lead to achievement of primary human goods (PHGs), which are life, knowledge, excellence in play, excellence in work, excellence in agency, inner peace, relatedness, community, spirituality, pleasure and creativity. Taylor (2016) analysed the accounts of burglars, applying a framework which sought to explain how such criminal activity can meet the offenders' PHGs. Taylor was able to conclude that burglary was an instrumental means to achieving these PHGs, which were not attainable by pro-social means.

Burglary can impact the victim financially in several ways: loss of cash and stolen goods, repairs to damage caused, increased insurance premiums, investment in security measures and loss of earnings if time off work has been required as a result of the crime. In addition, investigation and prosecution costs are incurred by the criminal justice system (Tseloni, Thompson and Tilley 2018). Documentaries like '999: What's your emergency?' (2018) showcase the real impact of burglary, including the psychological harms. These can include loss of sentimental items, anxiety of being targeted again, feeling their privacy has been invaded. Victims can also be physically affected in the immediate aftermath e.g., shaking, and longer-term feelings of not being safe which can lead to making lifestyle changes e.g., moving out of their home into an over 55 complex.

The Sentencing Council (2015) sets out the range of sentences applied to each type of theft offence. These sentences include imprisonment, community orders and fines. Prevention of theft and burglary involves more than criminal justice agencies e.g., police. Often, the onus is on the public to take responsibility and engage with initiatives and approaches that aim to prevent burglaries (Tseloni, Thompson and Tilley 2018). Situational crime prevention techniques focus on reducing the opportunities for crime, working on the basis that criminal activity is a result of rational choice. Therefore, the environment is manipulated and modified to increase the effort offenders must exert to commit a crime, increase the risks offenders face in completing the crime, reduce the possible rewards obtained from the crime, reduce the temptation to engage in criminal acts and remove the excuses that offenders may use to justify their actions (Newburn 2017). Situational crime prevention techniques could include use of burglar alarms, marking items, installing CCTV and establishing Neighbourhood Watch schemes.

However, this situational crime prevention approach has been criticised as it does not address the causes of crime, whether these be social or psychological (Newburn 2017). Therefore, understanding that burglary aids fulfilment of PHGs is important. Taylor (2016) outlines how adopting a rehabilitative approach to offenders can assist in developing pro-social methods of achieving PHGs, so that burglary is no longer perceived as the only available option. This could also be applied in a proactive, rather than reactive manner, impacting all theft offences. Addressing structural inequalities and the social conditions in which we live, work and age would increase the opportunities available to everyone in fulfilling PHGs in pro-social ways. In turn, increasing population health and well-being whilst reducing criminal activity.

Suggested Further Reading

Mawby, R. I., 2012. *Burglary.* 2nd ed. Oxon: Routledge.
Tseloni, A., Thompson, R., and Tilley, N., 2018. *Reducing burglary.* Switzerland: Springer.

Conclusion

This chapter has identified the continued prejudices apparent in the police and identified that more must be done to address this. Coverage of the penal crisis focussed on the over-representation of the BAME community and their negative experience of prison. As well as the under-representation of female offenders, but equally negative experience and impact. Restorative justice provides hope of an alternative way to respond to crime, reducing reoffending and empowering victims. Exploration of sexual and theft offences highlights the complex causes of crime, acknowledging these are beyond the scope of the criminal justice system to address. The wider health and social care sector can contribute to reducing inequalities, increasing the opportunities available to all, with a focus on prevention and rehabilitation to improve population health, well-being and reduce crime.

Moment of Reflection

It has been identified that the causes of crime are complex and relate to the wider health and social care sector. Although criminal justice responses are required once an offence has been committed, there are calls for a public health approach to crime. This focus on prevention could address the biological, social and psychological factors contributing to criminal behaviour. What strategies, initiatives and programmes can you identify to achieve this?

Summary of Main Points

You should be able to:

- Identify key issues affecting criminal justice agencies
- Provide explanations for criminal behaviour
- Discuss the ways criminal behaviour can be addressed through health, social care and criminal justice services

References

999: What's your emergency?, 2018. [TV] More4, 24 December 2018.

Allely, C.S., and Creaby-Attwood, A., 2016. Sexual offending and autism spectrum disorders. *Journal of Intellectual Disabilities and Offending Behaviour* [online], 7 (1), 35–51. 10.1108/JIDOB-09-2015-0029

Beard, J., 2019. *The prison estate* [online]. London: House of Commons Library, Available at https://commonslibrary.parliament.uk/research-briefings/sn05646/ [Accessed 16 December 2020].

Beard, J., 2017. *Registration and management of sex offenders* [online]. London: House of Commons Library. Available at: https://commonslibrary.parliament.uk/research-briefings/sn05267/ [Accessed 18 January 2021].

Beard, J., 2018. *Transgender prisoners* [online]. London: House of Commons Library. Available at: https://commonslibrary.parliament.uk/research-briefings/cbp-7420/ [Accessed 10 January 2021].

Blagden, N., and Winder, B., 2019. *Helping to rehabilitate sex offenders is controversial – but it can prevent more abuse* [online]. London: The Conversation. Available at: https://theconversation.com/helping-to-rehabilitate-sex-offenders-is-controversial-but-it-can-prevent-more-abuse-111861 [Accessed 8 June 2021].

Brown, J., 2020a. *Policing in the UK* [online]. London: House of Commons Library. Available at: https://commonslibrary.parliament.uk/research-briefings/cbp-8582/ [Accessed 16 December 2020].

Brown, J., 2020b. *Police powers: an introduction* [online]. London: House of Commons Library. Available at: https://commonslibrary.parliament.uk/research-briefings/cbp-8637/ [Accessed 16 December 2020].

Cavadino, M., Dignan, J., Mair, G., and Bennett, J., 2019. *The penal system: an introduction*. 6th ed. London: Sage.

Corston, J., 2007. *The Corston report: a review of women with particular vulnerabilities in the criminal justice system* [online]. London: Home Office. Available at: https://webarchive.nationalarchives.gov.uk/20130206102659/http://www.justice.gov.uk/publications/docs/corston-report-march-2007.pdf [Accessed 8 June 2021].

Craissati, J., 2018. *The rehabilitation of sexual offenders: complexity, risk and resistance*. London: Routledge.

Crewe, B., Hulley, S., and Wright, S., 2017. The gendered pains of life imprisonment. *British Journal of Criminology* [online], 57 (6), 1359–1378. 10.1093/bjc/azw088 [Accessed 8 June 2021].

Criminal Justice and Courts Act 2015 (c. 2) [online]. Available at: https://www.legislation.gov.uk/ukpga/2015/2/contents/enacted [Accessed 17 January 2021].

Crown Prosecution Service, 2019. *Restorative justice* [online]. London: Crown Prosecution Service. Available at: https://www.cps.gov.uk/legal-guidance/restorative-justice [Accessed 16 December 2020].

Crown Prosecution Service, 2020. *Rape and sexual offences: Chapter 5: issues relevant to particular groups of people* [online]. London: Crown Prosecution Service. Available at: https://www.cps.gov.uk/legal-guidance/rape-and-sexual-offences-chapter-5-issues-relevant-particular-groups-people [Accessed 18 January 2021].

Davies, M., 2015. *Davies, Croall and Tyrer's criminal justice*. 5th ed. London: Pearson Education.

Gauke, D., 2018. *Prison reform speech* [online]. London: HM Government. Available at: https://www.gov.uk/government/speeches/prisons-reform-speech [Accessed 10 January 2021].

Gavin, H., 2019. *Criminological and forensic psychology*. 2nd ed. London: Sage.

Goodwill, A.M., Stephens, S., Oziel, S., Yapp, J., and Bowes, N., 2012. Multidimensional latent classification of 'street robbery' offences. *Journal of Investigative Psychology and Offending Profiling* [online], 9 (1), 93–109. 10.1002/jip.1351 [Accessed 8 February 2021].

Gorden, C., Hughes, C., Roberts, D., Astbury-Ward, E., and Dubberley, S., 2017. A literature review of transgender people in prison: an 'invisible' population in England and Wales. *Prison Service Journal* [online], 233, 11–22. Available via: https://www.researchgate.net/publication/327184888_A_Literature_Review_of_Transgender_People_in_Prison_An_'invisible'_population_in_England_and_Wales [Accessed 10 January 2021].

Home Office, 2020a. *Stop and search* [online]. London: Home Office. Available at: https://www.ethnicity-facts-figures.service.gov.uk/crime-justice-and-the-law/policing/stop-and-search/latest [Accessed 17 December 2020].

Home Office, 2020b. *Police workforce* [online]. London: Home Office. Available at: https://assets.publishing.service.gov.uk/government/uploads/system/uploads/attachment_data/file/905169/police-workforce-mar20-hosb2020.pdf [Accessed 18 December 2020].

Javaid, A., 2018. The unheard victims: gender, policing and sexual violence. *Policing and Society* [online], 30 (4), 412–428. 10.1080/10439463.2018.1539484

Jewkes, Y., Jordan, M., Wright, S., and Bendelow, G., 2019. Designing 'healthy' prisons for women: incorporating trauma-informed case and practice (TICP) into prison planning and design. *International Journal of Environmental Research and Public Health* [online], 16 (20), 3818–3833. 10.3390/ijerph16203818 [Accessed 8 June 2021].

JUSTICE, 2019. *Prosecuting sexual offences* [online]. London: JUSTICE. Available at: https://justice.org.uk/wp-content/uploads/2019/06/Prosecuting-Sexual-Offences-Report.pdf [Accessed 2 February 2021].

Lammy, D., 2017. *The Lammy review: an independent review into the treatment of, and outcomes for, Black, Asian and Minority Ethnic individuals in the criminal justice system* [online]. London: GOV.UK. Available at: https://assets.publishing.service.gov.uk/government/uploads/system/uploads/attachment_data/file/643001/lammy-review-final-report.pdf [Accessed 10 January 2021].

McCartan, K.F., Hoggett, J., and Kemshall H., 2018. Risk assessment and management of individuals convicted of a sexual offence in the UK. *Sex Offender Treatment* [online], 13 (1). Available via: http://www.sexual-offender-treatment.org/177.html [Accessed 2 February 2021].

McKee, Z., Mueller-Johnson, K., and Strang, H., 2020. Impact of a training programme on police attitudes towards victims of rape: a randomised controlled trial. *Cambridge Journal of Evidence-Based Policing* [online], 4, 39–55. 10.1007/s41887-020-00044-1 [Accessed 8 June 2021].

Mews, A., Di Bella, L., and Purver, M., 2017. *Impact evaluation of the prison-based core sex offender treatment programme* [online]. London: Ministry of Justice. Available at: Impact evaluation of the prison-based Core Sex Offender Treatment Programme (publishing.service.gov.uk) [Accessed 2 February 2021].

Ministry of Justice, 2018. *Female offender strategy* [online]. London: HM Stationery Office. Available at: https://assets.publishing.service.gov.uk/government/uploads/system/uploads/attachment_data/file/719819/female-offender-strategy.pdf [Accessed 10 January 2021].

Ministry of Justice, 2020a. *Tackling racial disparity in the criminal justice system: 2020 update* [online]. London: Ministry of Justice. Available at: https://assets.publishing.service.gov.uk/government/uploads/system/uploads/attachment_data/file/881317/tackling-racial-disparity-cjs-2020.pdf [Accessed 8 June 2021].

Ministry of Justice, 2020b. *Offender management statistics quarterly: April to June 2020.* [online]. London: Ministry of Justice. Available at: https://www.gov.uk/government/publications/offender-management-statistics-quarterly-april-to-june-2020/offender-management-statistics-quarterly-april-to-june-2020 [Accessed 17 January 2021].

Ministry of Justice, 2021. *Extra funding for organisations that steer women away from crime* [online]. London: Ministry of Justice. Available at: https://www.gov.uk/government/news/extra-funding-for-organisations-that-steer-women-away-from-crime [Accessed 8 June 2021].

Myhill, A., 2019. Renegotiating domestic violence: police attitudes and decisions concerning arrest. *Policing and Society* [online], 29 (1), 52–68. 10.1080/10439463.2017.1356299

Neal, S., 2003. The Scarman report, the Macpherson report and the media: how newspapers respond to race-centred social policy interventions. *Journal of Social Policy* [online], 32 (1), 55–74. 10.1017/S004727940200689X

Newburn, T., 2017. *Criminology* [online]. 3rd ed. London: Routledge. Available via: Criminology – Tim Newburn – Google Books

Office for National Statistics, 2018. *Sexual offending: victimisation and the path through the criminal justice system* [online]. Newport: Office for National Statistics. Available at: https://www.ons.gov.uk/peoplepopulationandcommunity/crimeandjustice/articles/sexualoffendingvictimisationandthepaththroughthecriminaljusticesystem/2018-12-13 [Accessed 17 January 2021].

Office for National Statistics, 2019a. *Restorative justice, year ending March 2011 to year ending March 2019; Crime Survey for England and Wales* [online]. Newport: Office for National Statistics. Available at: https://www.ons.gov.uk/peoplepopulationandcommunity/crimeandjustice/adhocs/010238restorativejusticeyearendingmarch2011toyearendingmarch2019crimesurveyforenglandandwalescsew [Accessed 17 January 2021].

Office for National Statistics, 2019b. *Crime in England and Wales: year ending 2019* [online]. Newport: Office for National Statistics. Available at: https://www.ons.gov.uk/peoplepopulationandcommunity/crimeandjustice/bulletins/crimeinenglandandwales/yearending-june2019#rises-in-some-types-of-property-crime [Accessed 8 February 2021].

Peleg-Koriat, I., and Klar-Chalamish, C., 2020. The #MeToo movement and restorative justice: exploring the views of the public. *Contemporary Justice Review* [online], 23 (3), 239–260. 10.1080/10282580.2020.1783257

Police and Social Responsibility Act 2011 (c.13). [online] Available at: https://www.legislation.gov.uk/ukpga/2011/13/contents/enacted [Accessed 16 December 2020].

Prison Reform Trust, 2017. *Why focus on reducing women's imprisonment?* [online]. London: Prison Reform Trust. Available at: http://www.prisonreformtrust.org.uk/Portals/0/Documents/Women/whywomen.pdf [Accessed 10 January 2021].

Prison Reform Trust, 2021. *The government has met less than half of Female Offender Strategy commitments almost three years on* [online]. London: Prison Reform Trust. Available at: http://www.prisonreformtrust.org.uk/PressPolicy/News/vw/1/ItemID/1011 [Accessed 8 June 2021].

Purshouse, J., 2020. 'Paedophile hunters', criminal procedure and fundamental human rights. *Journal of Law and Society* [online], 47 (3), 384–411. 10.1111/jols.12235

Restorative Justice Council, 2016. *What is restorative justice* [online]. London: Restorative Justice Council: Available at: https://restorativejustice.org.uk/criminal-justice [Accessed 17 January 2021].

Rowe, M., 2017. *Introduction to policing* [online]. 3rd ed. London: Sage.

Sarraf, Z., 2021. Ministers reveal plans to create 500 new places for women in prisons. *The Justice Gap* [online], 25 January. Available at: https://www.thejusticegap.com/ministers-reveal-plans-to-create-500-new-places-for-women-in-prisons/ [Accessed 8 June 2021].

Sentencing Council, 2013. *Sexual offences: definitive guideline* [online]. London: Sentencing Council. Available at: https://www.sentencingcouncil.org.uk/wp-content/uploads/Final_Sexual_Offences_Definitive_Guideline_content_web1.pdf [Accessed 18 January 2021].

Sentencing Council, 2015. *Theft offences: definitive guideline* [online]. London: Sentencing Council. Available at: https://www.sentencingcouncil.org.uk/wp-content/uploads/Theft-offences-definitive-guideline-Web.pdf [Accessed 17 February 2021].

Sex Offences Act 2003 (c.42) [online]. Available at: https://www.legislation.gov.uk/ukpga/2003/42/contents [Accessed 17 January 2021].

Shapland, J., Robinson, G., and Sorsby, A., 2011. *Restorative justice in practice*. London: Routledge.

Shaw, D., 2020. Eleven transgender inmates sexually assaulted in male prisons last year. *BBC News* [online], 21 May. Available at: https://www.bbc.co.uk/news/uk-52748117 [Accessed 10 January 2021].

Sturge, G., 2020. *UK prison population statistics* [online]. London: House of Commons Library. Available at: https://commonslibrary.parliament.uk/research-briefings/sn04334/ [Accessed 10 January 2021].

Taylor, E., 2013 Honour among thieves? How morality and rationality influence the decision-making processes of convicted domestic burglars. *Criminology and Criminal Justice* [online], 14 (4), 487–502. 10.1177/1748895813505232 [Accessed 17 February 2021].

Taylor, E., 2016. 'I should have been a security consultant': The good lives model and re-sidential burglars. *European Journal of Criminology* [online], 14 (4), 434–450. 10.1177/1477370816661743 [Accessed 17 February 2021]

The Survivors Trust, 2019. *The effects of sexual violence* [online]. Rugby: The Survivors Trust. Available at: https://www.thesurvivorstrust.org/the-effects-of-sexual-violence-how-to-support-a-survivor [Accessed 18 January 2021].

Theft Act 1968 (c.60). [online] Available at: https://www.legislation.gov.uk/ukpga/1968/60/contents [Accessed 8 February 2021].

Thomas, T., 2013. Sex crime. In: Hale, C., Hayward, K., Wahidin, A., and Wincup, E., eds. *Criminology* [online]. 3rd ed. Oxford: Oxford University Press, 2013, 210–226. 10.1093/he/9780199691296.003.0010

Tonkin, S., 2016. Father, 42, was 'mistaken for a paedophile by a vigilante gang who chased him through the streets and stabbed him to death then went inside and ordered a pizza'. *Mail Online* [online], 12 April. Available at: https://www.dailymail.co.uk/news/article-3535839/Father-42-killed-lured-vigilante-gang-kicked-punched-stabbed-death-mistakenly-thought-paedophile.html [Accessed 8 June 2021].

Tseloni, A., Thompson, R., and Tilley, N., 2018. *Reducing burglary*. Switzerland: Springer.

Ward, T., and Beech, A., 2016. The integrated theory of sexual offending – revised. In: Boer, D.P., ed. *The Wiley Handbook on the theories, assessment and treatment of sexual offending*. Oxford: Wiley-Blackwell, 2016, 123–137.

Ward, T., Polaschek, D.L.L., and Busch, A.R., 2006. *Theories of sexual offending*. Oxford: Wiley-Blackwell.

Watson, T., 2020. *Valuing victims: a review of police and crime Commissioners' delivery of restorative justice 2018/19* [online]. London: Why me?. Available at: https://why-me.org/wp-content/uploads/2020/03/Why-me-Restorative-Justice-Valuing-Victims-Report-2020.pdf [Accessed 17 January 2021].

Youth Justice and Criminal Evidence Act 1999 (c. 23) [online]. Available at: https://www.legislation.gov.uk/ukpga/1999/23/contents [Accessed 18 January 2021].

Zempi, I., 2020. 'Looking back, I wouldn't join again': the lived experiences of police officers as victims of bias and prejudice by fellow staff within an English police force. *Police Practice and Research* [online], 21 (1), 33–48. 10.1080/15614263.2018.1525381

9 Person-Centred Interventions

*Richard Machin, Dolores Ellidge, and
Verusca Calabria*

The person is at the centre of the delivery of health and social care interventions. Understanding a critical knowledge of the principles and theory of humanistic and existential philosophies that underpin person-centred interventions is essential. Legislation and policy are examined. Working with and valuing service users as equal partners in the decision-making process challenges the intersectional nature of discrimination in health and social care. Reflecting on a case study develops and applies person-centred interventions.

Introduction

Service users are at the centre of the design, planning and delivery of health and social care services, and developing a critical knowledge and understanding of person-centred approaches is essential for health and social care practitioners. This chapter explores how the person-centred approach recognises the assets and preferences of service users and seeks to avoid services dictating the support that they provide. The person-centred approach aims to give more choice and control to the service user and should be underpinned with high-quality advice, guidance and advocacy. Partnership is a key element of person-centred care, both between the professional and the service user and collaboration across services. In this way, the person-centred approach is of critical importance to 'universal services' such as schools, GPs, transport and leisure.

This chapter introduces the paramount importance of working with service users as equal partners in the planning and delivery of services, valuing them as experts in their own right and central to the decision-making process. The benefits and challenges of using the person-centred approach in multi-disciplinary and multi-cultural settings are discussed. This chapter will help the reader to critically reflect on their own person-centred skills and how they can be applied in a wide range of health and social care roles. These include assessment and care planning, coaching and guidance, professional supervision, negotiation and advocacy.

There are three sections to this chapter. The first section explores the origins of person-centred care, it analyses the influence of humanistic and existentialist philosophies, and the role of the anti-psychiatry and service-user movements in democratising patient versus professionals relationships in mental health. The second section sets out the legislation and policy which underpins person-centred care and discusses how person-centred approaches have been assimilated into contemporary Health and Social Care practice. This section explains what is meant by self-directed support, personal budgets, direct payments and independent living. In the third

DOI: 10.4324/9781003079873-11

section, a case study is presented which will help you to apply your learning by considering your approach to assessing the needs of an older service user. After the completion of the case study, an in-depth discussion is provided which will help you to reflect on your understanding. The chapter concludes by critically engaging with the limitations and future of person-centred approaches.

Origins of Person-Centred Approaches to Care

Within health and social care at a global level, putting patients at the centre of care is becoming increasingly central to the design, planning and delivery of care (McCance et al. 2011). In the contemporary landscape of health and social care in the UK, the notion of service users as equal partners in the planning, developing and monitoring of care is embedded in all major policies, including the NHS five-year forward view (2014). Person-centred approaches to care have a long and multifaceted history; the principles and the theories that inform person-centred approaches to care have their origins in humanistic and existentialist philosophies, which emerged from the 1940s onwards in the Western world. Existentialism offers a philosophy of existence, it focuses on the real world, in the everyday life of people and how people experience the world. It is concerned with freedom and responsibility. The fundamental concepts of existentialism are as follows: human beings are unique, and human conduct is intentional and freely chosen action not behaviour; human beings possess free will (Barnard 2017: 37). Actions are not caused, individuals choose to act in certain ways. In this sense, human conduct is active, not passive, as human beings freely initiate a course of action. Jean Paul Sartre (1905–1980) was the main proponent of existentialism as a philosophy of existence, which emerged in the Second World War during a period of great uncertainty. Sartre believed that there is no essence to human nature and that we are responsible for our own actions. Our ideas are the product of experiences of real-life situations. The essence of existential philosophy rests on the notion that the choices and actions define individuals, not any a priory quality of humanity (Sartre 1943, 1948). In one of his most influential works, 'Being and Nothingness', Sartre (1948) argues that the individual's existence is prior to the individual's essence, namely existence precedes essence; this theory seeks to demonstrate that free will exists (Barnard and Sawtell, 2017). Existentialism gives us an understanding of the interaction of individual factors, such as choices, values, actions that are central to person-centred interventions, and sociopolitical factors, such as the oppressions of sexism or racism.

The humanist approach to psychology emerged in the 1950s as a reaction against two major theories, namely Freudian psychoanalysis (Freud 1953) and behaviourism (Commons and Goodheart, 1999). Humanistic psychology centres around building on a client's existing resources. It focuses on the present, and the functioning in the here and now. It is an approach that is reflexive and therapeutic in character. Person-centred approaches to psychology were influenced by existentialism, which put emphasis on personal responsibility by implying choice and acknowledging the phenomenology of the individual, namely free will. The key attributes of humanistic psychology are honesty and genuineness, warmth, honesty and acceptance, and empathic understanding. It centres on the notion that individuals are relational, namely that individuals can only understand themselves in relation to others (DeCarvalho 1991). Abraham Maslow (1908–1970) was a leading proponent of humanistic psychology. Maslow's hierarchy of needs (1943) is a motivational theory of human psychology based on a five-tier model of human needs comprising the following: physiological, safety, belonging and love, social needs or esteem and self-actualisation. All these needs must be met in order for individuals to self-actualise (Moore and Shantall, 2003). Carl Rogers (1902–1987) was another major proponent of the humanistic approach to psychology. Rogers introduced the radical idea that only the client is responsible for their therapeutic direction, thus putting into question the authority of experts. For Roger the role of the therapist is to create conditions for self-exploration, the right conditions to allow clients to accept themselves and achieve personal goals (Schneider 2014). This was to pave the way for the foundations of humanist psychotherapy. Rogers was a proponent of the concept of self-actualisation: putting emphasis on personal growth, becoming the best that we can be within the context of our lives. Rogers' view of mental health focused on the environmental and social causes of suffering, reflecting a wave of progressive thinkers that were part of the 'social turn' in mental health in the post-war period in Europe and North America shifting the focus towards humanistic approaches to mental health to deal with the effects of environmental stresses on well-being, posing a challenge to the dominant medical model of the time (Fussinger, 2011; Kritsotaki et al. 2018). The medical model is based on the assumption that abnormal behaviour is the result of physical problems and should be treated medically such as through medication to reduce symptoms and it is in contrast to the social model of mental health, which rests on the notion that disability is caused by the way society is organised, rather than by a person's impairment or difference. The social model of mental health centres on removing barriers that restrict life choices for disabled people (Repper and Perkins, 2003). For a comprehensive explanation of the social and medical models of disability see Hogan (2019). The following humanist attributes are central to contemporary person-centred counselling: genuine and congruent where the choices relating to care are led by clients not imposed by workers; unconditional positive regard and empathy with service users' views. Unconditional positive regard for clients is at the centre of the person-centred approach, to enable self-exploration and for the client to become fully functioning. An example of this approach is the paraphrasing and the reflection of feelings, standard counselling techniques (Gillon 2007). It is important to note that the second wave of feminism in the 1960s and 1970s strongly supported humanistic values in the provision of therapy by arguing for a humanistic therapeutic practice in which the inherently paternalistic patient/doctor model is replaced by a client/practitioner relationship. The latter is characterised by equality, respect and choice (Bondi 2001). In addition, reflective practice is a central component of person-centred care. Reflective practice acknowledges the phenomenology of individuals; it is epitomised by Schön's seminal notion of the reflective practitioner. The concept of Schön's reflection-in-action and reflection-on-action is fundamental to professional development where responding to uncertainties is necessary (1991: 50–51). Reflective practice acknowledges the complexity of the person-centred interventions in Health and Social Care; it allows health and social care workers to work with uncertainty as a key issue in Health and Social Care and professional practice (Timmins 2015).

Existentialism and humanism influenced major paradigm shifts in mental health from the mid-to-late twentieth century. The anti-psychiatry movement in the 1960s sought radical reform in psychiatry. The movement proposed a critical approach towards traditional theories and practices of psychiatry including the workings of the asylum, and the bio-organic theories of mental illness. Its central tenet was the constitution and removal of institutional power – encompassing the ethos of the larger counter-cultural movements of 1960s (Fussinger 2011, Foot 2015). The movement advocated equality with the patients by removing barriers as part of the therapy and challenged the paternalism of coercive psychiatry in favour of liberty and the autonomy of the individual (Chow and Priebe 2013; Calabria et al., 2021). A notable example of existentialism applied in the clinical setting is R.D. Laing's (1927–1989) radical ideas in psychiatry. Laing was an influential Scottish existential psychotherapist who wrote extensively on mental health and in particular on the experiences of psychosis (Crossley 1998). A proponent of the anti-psychiatry movement, he rejected the biomedical model of mental health by proposing a social approach to understanding and treating mental health problems (Crossley 2006). Unique to Laing's approach was the paramount importance he put on the validity of the lived experiences of his clients – rather than dismissing them as just symptoms of an illness (Laing 1967; Crossley 2001). The survivor movement in Britain was made out of anti-psychiatry thinkers, and various associations and self-governing groups of mental health service users and their allies, such as MIND. It called into question the traditional definitions and diagnoses of mental illness (Foot 2015).

The rise of consumerism in Health and Social Care in the 1980s redefined the role of mental patients as passive to active consumers of services, expressed in some key policy papers at the time (Department of Health 1989). The new ideology of consumerism that dominated the agenda of shaping public services had the unexpected consequences of strengthening the social movement of disenfranchised service users that posed a challenge to the traditional medical elite and allowed for tipping the balance of power in their favour (Rogers and Pilgrim 2001; Calabria 2020: 33–36). The service users' movements that emerged from the 1960s to the 1980s served to propose a social model of mental distress and recommended various reforms from the modernisation to the shutdown of mental hospitals, which gathered momentum in the 1980s (Crossley 2006; Beresford and Branfield 2012; Kritsotaki et al. 2016). In recent years, the emphasis shifted from including the service users as 'subjects' of the research to also actively involving them in the planning, undertaking and evaluating of health and social care research, planning and delivery (Smith et al. 2008; Beresford). This shift towards working *with* rather doing *to* is informed by the recovery model in mental health, an influential paradigm in mental health services in Britain today, based on the individual responsibility and self-management (Slade 2009). The centrality of empathetically working in partnership with service users to reduce inequalities is identified in the QAA benchmark in Social Work (2019) and is embodied in the principles of co-production (Steen and Tuurnas 2018).

As illustrated above, the key tenets of humanistic philosophy and psychology are of key relevance to person-centred care. The implications of adopting person-centred approaches to Health and Social Care rest on the centrality of rights, justice and equality for all. It is of paramount importance for client work in Health and Social Care situations as it challenges 'common-sense' and 'taken-for-granted' assumptions about power and authority, such as the traditional authority of experts by calling for reciprocal ways of working with service users and the public to improve outcomes (Beresford 2000). Ultimately, the key contributions of existentialism and humanism to person-centred approaches to health and social care rest on fundamental principles of freedom and responsibility. These philosophies incorporate the individual/personal and social/collective dimensions of lived experience to the provision of interventions. Importantly, it provides a basis for understanding and challenging oppression, which will be a key theme in the next section of this chapter.

Person-Centred Approaches: Practice and Policy

The opening to this chapter explored the increasing influence of person-centred approaches on Western academic and professional discourse. This section explores how these ideas have been assimilated into Health and Social Care practice and policy. Over the last two decades, the process of implementing the person-centred approach has often been referred to as 'personalisation'. We will explore what personalisation means, and how it is delivered in practice. Personalisation seeks to avoid health and social care professionals and services adopting a 'one size fits all' approach. However, there are undoubted challenges to this way of working; Hart (2014, p. 112) stresses that there is a real risk that personalisation has 'over-promised and under-delivered'.

> *Personalisation means recognising people as individuals who have strengths and preferences and putting them at the centre of their own care and support. The traditional service-led approach has often meant that people have not been able to shape the kind of support they need, or receive the right kind of help*
> (Social Care Institute for Excellence 2012).

As the quote above demonstrates, personalisation is a fundamental, indeed radical, shift from the conventional ways of working with Health and Social Care service users. Personalisation aims to place the service user at the centre of decision-making recognising them as the expert in their needs. It involves giving people more choice and control, focusing on the person rather than processes. If this way of working with people is to be something more than aspirational it requires services to shape their provision in a way that is genuinely enabling. The identification of needs should only be the starting point on the journey; appropriate and high-quality guidance, advice and advocacy must be available to allow the outcomes that service users desire to be fulfilled. Personalisation should not just be of importance to Health and Social Care agencies and professionals; it has a much broader significance. Community-based and user-led organisations should also embrace this approach, and there should be an emphasis on enabling access to what are referred to as 'universal services' such as transport, leisure, housing, employment and education. Collaboration is a key element of personalisation; collaboration between a service user and services is often referred to as co-production and draws on an individual's assets as they work alongside a professional. See Figure 9.1 for an illustration of the key principles of co-production. Collaboration is also important from an organisational perspective as positive, personalised outcomes can only be achieved when agencies work in partnership and resist being subsumed with their own agendas and processes: 'In order to make the best efforts to meet the needs of client groups with complex needs, professionals, organisations and sectors need to work together' (Solomon 2019, p. 391). This requires ethical leadership at all levels of an organisation and an emphasis on the continuing professional development of the workforce. In Higher Education, it is

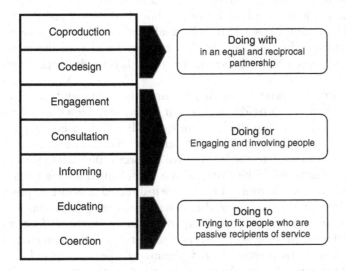

Figure 9.1 Co-production and service-user involvement (National Council of Voluntary Organisations).

important that students are given the time and space to reflect on their own experiences and values-base so that they can develop the awareness and skills required to work in a person-centred way in their future careers (Timmins 2015).

Personalisation is now an integral part of Health and Social Care practice. A long and uneven path has brought us to this point. We have seen the significant impact of the service users' movement and the acknowledgement of the social model of disability. Community Care reforms (notably the National Health Service and Community Care Act 1990), the influence of social work values and lobbying have led to the introduction of a sometimes-disparate range of personalisation-focused policies and legislation. Key policies include the Valuing People Strategy (2001) which introduced person-centred planning for people with learning disabilities, Putting People First (2007) where personal budgets were offered to all people eligible for social care, and the Think Local Act Personal (TLAP) cross-sector partnership (TLAP 2010) encouraging personalised care and prevention across the public, voluntary and private sectors. The NHS Five Year Forward View (2014, p. 4) recognised that 'England is too diverse for a "one size fits all" care model' and promoted personalised and coordinated health services for patients.

Person-centred approaches have also become embedded through legislation. Health and Social Care students should pay particular notice to the Mental Capacity Act (2005) which embodies the key principles of personalisation by enabling people to make their own decisions and the Equality Act (2010) which provides legal protection from discrimination in the workplace and wider society. Of particular importance is the Care Act (2014) which acknowledges that individuals are in the best position to determine their own needs. The Act sets out that a local authority has a duty to ensure well-being when carrying out care and support functions; there is a statutory duty to undertake an assessment for any adult who presents with a care or support need regardless of financial capability (Barnes et al. 2017). An individual should be fully involved in the assessment, access to an advocate should be provided, and the provision of preventative and community-based services should be considered (SCIE). Care Act Statutory guidance emphasises that individuals should not be passive recipients of support services, rather services should be co-produced with the active involvement of the service users who design services to meet their needs (Department of Health, 2014).

Personalisation is a broad approach which promotes the views and needs of service users, but it is hard to provide a clear-cut definition. However, there are some key concepts which are important to understand: self-directed support, personal budgets and direct payments, and independent living. The term self-directed support can be traced back to the 'In Control' project (2003) and refers to the culture and systems which should be fostered in a professional setting to give more choice and control to service users. Effective self-directed support requires mechanisms to be in place to assess, plan and review; it requires professionals at all levels to embed the person-centred approach to working practices. Systems should be in place to allocate funding to the service user; this is often referred to as resource allocation. The terms person-centred planning or person-centred care are often used in professional settings. Again, these refer to the process of integrating personalisation into professional practice, often in services for older people or those with dementia (SCIE 2012).

Putting People First (2007) set out that everyone who is eligible for social care should be able to exercise choice and control through the provision of a personal budget. A personal budget is the amount of money that a local authority will pay towards the social care and support which a service user is assessed as needing. The Care Act (2014) mandates local authorities to give all eligible service users a personal budget. A personal budget can be managed in three different ways. Firstly a local authority managed account, secondly a third party managed account (the third party is sometimes referred to as a broker, typically an organisation such as a care provider) or thirdly a direct payment where the service user is directly given funds, in line with a care plan, to arrange and pay for the support needed.

Independent living is a key aim of personalisation and is influenced by the social model of disability (Beresford 2000). In 2009, the UK adopted the UN Convention on the Rights of Persons with Disabilities (CRPD, 2006); article 19 of the convention 'Living independently and being included in the community' sets out the rights of disabled people to live in the community with equal choices to others. Independent living does not mean living alone, rather it promotes the choice and control of key decisions in life, including those relating to finances, housing, education, employment, education, transport and health (SCIE 2012).

Theory in Practice

This case study activity aims to support you in applying your learning to practice by giving you an opportunity to assess needs and determine your approach to providing a person-centred intervention. A key element of this is for you to complete the activity before progressing to reading the discussion as this will enable you to reflect on your understanding and application of your learning to practice. Your learning from the 'Working with People' chapter will support you to complete this activity.

Introducing Margaret

Margaret is a 70-year-old retired head teacher living in a village with her partner of 40 years. Up until her retirement five years ago she was an active member of the village community in which she worked and had a busy social life. Her plans for retirement life have changed dramatically with her partner becoming increasingly dependent, with very limited mobility, so the couple spend long periods of time together alone and they have very limited contact with Margaret's two sons who do not live in the area. Margaret is increasingly socially isolated as she has not sustained friendships and rarely has contact with anyone outside her partner and their carers.

Margaret is physically healthy with no underlying health conditions but has a tendency to drink alcohol which results in fluctuating levels of personal hygiene, self-care, safety and behaviour. When intoxicated Margaret becomes belligerent which has resulted in her being banned from the village supermarket and local shop due to her verbal abuse of staff. Her supply of alcohol is maintained by manipulation of her sons and neighbours who all think they are the only one buying vodka for her.

Margaret is referred to social services for assessment as her GP is concerned about self-neglect following a home visit and discussion with the partners' carers. Margaret fell whilst drunk resulting in facial bruising and damaged wrist and has refused to go to the hospital despite being knocked out and unable to use her wrist. When the GP visited Margaret was intoxicated and continued to refuse treatment however the GP felt Margaret understood her injuries and the potential risk and was making an informed but ill-advised decision. The GP advised Margaret that she was making a safeguarding referral.

Activity 1   Case study

Reread the case study from the perspective of the Social Worker who will be undertaking a needs assessment with a view of initiating ongoing support for Margaret.

As you read the case study think about the questions below and make notes of your answers:

- What approach would you use and why?
- What skills would you need to use and why these would be beneficial?
- What needs do you identify for Margaret?
- Should anyone else's needs be taken into account and why?

Discussion

Approach

The TLAP collaboration (2018) promotes personalisation as an approach to all interventions and identifies the importance of ensuring all individuals have the opportunity to voice what they want from life and discuss how any support interventions can enable them to achieve their desire. It is essential therefore that the social workers' approach to Margaret is based on partnership empowerment and choice. However, it is also the social workers' responsibility to assess and reduce risk. To achieve this outcome, practitioners need to balance 'what is important for someone' and 'what is important to her' (Sanderson and Lewis 2012, p. 39). This approach will support the social worker to understand the contributing factors to Margaret's situation, which will influence suggestions for interventions and therefore meet Margaret's needs in a manner which is preferable to her. Motivational interviewing, an approach which can support people to look at influencing factors which impact on and promote change (Moss 2017) could support the social worker in delivering a person-centred intervention to Margaret.

Price (2019) suggests that at the point of contact with a practitioner, service users have developed a narrative about their situation or symptoms which may be perceived as implausible to others but are plausible to the individual. This may result in Margaret denying or not recognising the extent of their drinking therefore an approach which supports Margaret to recognise the risks to her health and impact on her partner is essential. Rao et al. (2019) identify that to meet needs, services for elderly substance misusers must be age-appropriate and based in partnership.

Effective communication is key to positive engagement and the development of therapeutic relationships (Kornhaber et al. 2016). Margaret has the potential to be verbally abusive therefore the social worker should use non-verbal communication to reduce or manage any aggression by remaining calm, keeping still and relaxed, maintaining eye contact without staring and speaking slightly slower than usual (Moss 2017).

The concept of 'good enough' in relation to personal hygiene and self-care is important in this situation. An individual's perception of personal hygiene and frequency of bathing and changing clothes varies greatly; therefore it is important to develop an understanding of Margaret's 'norm' to determine whether observed changes in Margaret's physical presentation are detrimental to her well-being and are a result of her alcohol consumption rather than personal preferences.

Assessment of Need

Cargiulo (2007, p. 56) states that 'Alcohol dependence is a maladaptive pattern of alcohol use' which impacts on an individual's decisions regarding alcohol consumption and on their life and behaviour. This may be difficult to identify in elderly women as it is often undiagnosed due to their reduced socialisation and stereotypes of behaviour and drinking held by professionals (Eliason 1998). Developing an understanding of Margaret's pattern of drinking, factors which contribute to her drinking and understanding Margaret's perception of the risks and impacts of her drinking are important elements of assessing Margaret's needs. Part of this assessment of Margaret's alcohol dependency is her desire to make changes to her behaviour.

Alcohol dependency is associated with a broad range of physical and psychological conditions which impact on quality and duration of life (Cargiulo 2007). As a social worker your primary focus is on overall well-being and whilst needing to be aware of the potential for physical ill-health their role would be one of support to access services and with Margaret's consent co-working with other professionals to ensure those needs are assessed and met.

An important part of a social worker's assessment is to determine Margaret's capacity to make informed decisions regarding her drinking and refusing treatment for her injury. The Mental Capacity Act (2005) aims to empower individuals to make decisions about their care and treatment. It is important that the social worker assesses Margaret presuming that she has the capacity to make decisions (Principle 1). The GP has discussed Margaret's injury with her; however the social workers' assessment should determine Margaret's ability to make the decision not to access treatment as well as her understanding of health and well-being risks associated with her intoxication. An individual may be considered incapable of making a decision if they are unable to do one or more of the factors listed below:

- Understand information given to them
- Retain that information long enough to be able to make the decision
- Weigh up the information available to make the decision
- Communicate their decision (SCIE 2017)

If Margaret is able to articulate her understanding of her injury and the risks associated with not seeking treatment, and she continues to decline, the social worker would consider Margaret to have the capacity to make that decision.

Interventions

A partnership approach should be used to determine what interventions Margaret may find beneficial and accessible. Interventions which may be beneficial to Margaret include:

- Brief intervention – this creates an opportunity to talk about a health behaviour such as Margaret's drinking to explore concerns and motivation to change behaviour (Prochaska and DiClementi 1983). This approach will support Margaret to not only understand the risks of her behaviour on herself but to consider the impact on her partner and family which could influence Margaret's motivation and ability to change her behaviour (Scott and Kenner 2015).
- Increased socialisation – how people age is influenced by their lifestyle and environment (Farley, McLafferty and Hendry 2006) therefore increasing isolation and loss of purpose since retirement may be a contributing factor in Margaret's alcohol dependency. Referral to a befriending service such as Age UK may provide support and increase Margaret's confidence to change her behaviour. Evidence suggests that befriending services can support people to realise that 'they had a reason to keep going, they had a purpose in life and, importantly, life was once again worth living' (Cattan, Kime and Bagnall 2011, p. 201).

Activity 2   Reflection

Now you have read the discussion, reflect on your answers in Activity 1. Focus on considering the following:

- How do your ideas compare with the points in the discussion?
- What are the strengths of your answers?
- What are the gaps in your knowledge or understanding and what can you do to resolve these gaps?

Limitations of Personalisation

Practitioners, academics, service users and activists broadly support the aims and ethos of personalisation. However, significant concerns have been raised about the effectiveness of personalisation in practice, particularly as this approach has been delivered in a period of austerity and cuts to public sector services. Beresford (2014) argues that the pace at which personalisation has been introduced means there is a lack of evidence-based scrutiny. He asserts that the formulation of this policy has too often marginalised the views of professionals, and more importantly service users and carers. Personalisation should be about empowerment, but rather than being a genuine grassroots movement, it is argued that a top-down approach has imposed overly bureaucratic systems and unnecessary performance targets (Duffy 2014; Dunning 2011). Furthermore, in practice personalisation can lead to reductions in support for key vulnerable groups and be used as a justification for cuts in services and jobs. Personalisation can place a high degree of responsibility on service users, particularly those who receive direct payments and fund their own care and support (often referred to as 'self-funders'). Self-funders can find that increased purchasing power does not always equate to genuine choice or the provision of appropriate services (Henwood 2014), exposing an inherent contradiction in the ideology of consumerism in Health and Social Care.

There are a number of ethical issues for professionals to navigate when delivering person-centred services. There can be tensions between promoting the independence and choice of service users and safeguarding health and well-being. Professionals may need to manage conflict between the views of a service user and a carer. Effective partnership work is an essential element of person-centred care and professionals must expertly manage not only relationships with service users, but also work collaboratively with other agencies. Budgetary pressures and competing organisational agendas can impede partnership work, although austerity measures can also force agencies to collaborate and deliver joined-up outcomes for service users. Personalisation requires professionals to facilitate access to universal services. However, a decade of austerity has left a 'shrinking state' (Labao et al. 2018), which has led to the fragmentation of services in Health and Social Care. Positive outcomes for service users are harder to achieve with diminished levels of public finance, services and personnel. Increased choice and control for service users must be accompanied by access to support and person-centred care should promote positive professional, caring and familial relationships (Glasby and Needham 2014).

Conclusion

Tracing the history of a person-centred approach supports practitioners to understand the theoretical principles which focus on the individual and their right to acceptance, respect and choice. Using a person-centred approach in practice is reliant on practitioners valuing and respecting an individual's right to be involved in the planning and delivery of their care. It is more than having the knowledge and skills to make an assessment and provide care it requires personal qualities and skills which enable practitioners to advocate and empower service users. However, success of a personalised approach is dependent on more than the values, behaviour and attitudes of practitioners, it involves organisational culture, professional guidance and government policy.

Personalisation continues to evolve and further research in this area is needed (Rousltone 2014). At the start of this chapter, we set out the importance of the service user movement to the development of person-centred care, and research that promotes the service user voice is particularly important. Glasby and Needham (2014, p. 189) see personalisation as an 'evolutionary process' and COVID-19 will have an enduring influence on this process and the delivery of social care. The pandemic has had a disproportionately negative impact on disabled people (ONS, 2020) and widened health, ethnic and gender inequalities (IFS, 2020); person-centred care must respond to these challenges. Professionals engaged with the design, planning and delivery of services must take a critical stance on the person-centred care in the context of the fragmentation of services and the increasing socio-economic and health inequalities emerging in the twentieth century.

References

Abraham, M., 1943. A theory of human motivation. *Psychological Review*, 50 (4), 370–396.

Barnard, A., and Sawtell, H., 2017. Philosophy for professionals. In: Barnard, A., ed. *Developing professional practice in health and social care*. London: Routledge, 2017, 31–59.

Barnes, D., Boland, B., Linhart, K., and Wilson, K., 2017. Personalisation and social care assessment – the Care Act 2014. *BJPsych Bulletin* [online], 41 (3), 176–180. 10.1192/pb.bp.116.053660

Beresford, P., 2000. Service users' knowledge and social work theory: conflict or collaboration?. *The British Journal of Social Work*, 30 (4), 489–503.

Beresford, P., 2014. *Personalisation: Critical and radical debates in social work*. Bristol: Policy Press.

Beresford, P., and Branfield, F., 2012. Building solidarity, ensuring diversity: lessons from service users' and disabled people's movements. In: Barnes, M., and Cotterell, P., eds. *Critical perspectives on user involvement*. Bristol: Bristol University Press, 2012, 33–45.

Bondi, L., and Burman, E., 2001. Women and mental health a feminist review. *Feminist Review*, 68 (1), 6–33.

Calabria, V., 2020. *Oral histories of the Nottinghamshire mental hospitals: exploring memories of giving and receiving care*. PhD thesis, Nottingham Trent University.

Calabria, V., Bailey, D., and Bowpitt, G., 2021. More than bricks and mortar: meaningful care practices in the old state mental hospitals. In: Ellis, R., Kendall S., and Taylor, S.J., eds. *Voices in the history of madness: Patient and practitioner perspectives*. 191–215. London: Palgrave Macmillan.

Care Act 2014 (c. 23) [online]. Available at: https://www.legislation.gov.uk/ukpga/2014/23/contents/enacted

Cargiulo, T., 2007. Understanding the health impact of alcohol dependence. *American Journal of Health-System Pharmacy* [online], 64 (5), 5–11. Available via: https://link.gale.com/apps/doc/A165364076/AONE?u=tou&sid=AONE&xid=163ced36 [Accessed 27 Nov. 2020].

Cattan, M., Kime, N., and Bagnall, A., 2011. The use of telephone befriending in low level support for socially isolated older people – an evaluation. *Health and Social Care in the Community* [online], 19 (2), 198–206. 10.1111/j.1365-2524.2010.00967.x (Accessed 27 November 2020].

Chow, W.S., and Priebe, S., 2013. Understanding psychiatric institutionalization: a conceptual review. *BMC Psychiatry*, 13 (1), 169.

Commons, M.L., and Goodheart, E.A., 1999. The origins of behaviorism. In: Thyer, B.A., ed. *The philosophical legacy of behaviorism.* Dordrecht: Springer, 1999, 9–40.

Convention on the Rights of Persons with Disabilities, 2006. Available at: https://www.un.org/development/desa/disabilities/convention-on-the-rights-of-persons-with-disabilities.html

Crossley, M.L., and Crossley, N., 2001. Patient' voices, social movements and the habitus; how psychiatric survivors 'speak out. *Social Science & Medicine*, 52 (10), 1477–1489.

Crossley, N., 1998. RD Laing and the British anti-psychiatry movement: a socio–historical analysis. *Social science & Medicine*, 47 (7), 877–889.

Crossley, N., 2006. *Contesting psychiatry: Social movements in mental health.* Brighton and Hove: Psychology Press.

DeCarvalho, R.J., 1991. *The founders of humanistic psychology.* Santa Barbara: Praeger Publishers.

Department of Health, 2014. *The Care Act.* London: HMSO.

Department of Health, 1989. *Caring for people: Community care in the next decade and beyond.* London: Department of Health. Available at: https://navigator.health.org.uk/theme/caring-people-community-care-next-decade-and-beyond-white-paper

Duffy, S., 2014. Personalisation was supposed to empower vulnerable citizens. It failed. *The Guardian* [online], 30 January. Available at: https://www.theguardian.com/public-leaders-network/2014/jan/30/personalisation-social-care-support-bureaucracy-service-failure

Dunning, J., 2011. How bureaucracy is derailing personalisation. *Community Care* [online], 24 May. Available at: https://www.communitycare.co.uk/2011/05/24/how-bureaucracy-is-derailing-personalisation/

Eliason, M.J., 1998. Identification of alcohol-related problems in older women. *Journal of Gerontological Nursing*, 24(10), 8–15. Available via: https://search.proquest.com/docview/204186964?rfr_id=info%3Axri%2Fsid%3Aprimo&accountid=14693

Equality Act 2010 (c. 15) [online]. Available at: https://www.legislation.gov.uk/ukpga/2010/15/contents

Farley, A., McLafferty, E., and Hendry, C., 2006. The physiological effects of ageing on the activities of living. *Nursing Standard* [online], 20 (45), 46–52. Available via: https://go.gale.com/ps/i.do?p=AONE&u=tou&id=GALE|A149070713&v=2.1&it=r [Accessed 27 November 2020].

Foot, J., 2015. *The man who closed the asylums: Franco Basaglia and the revolution in mental health care.* London: Verso Books.

Freud, S., 1953. Three essays on the theory of sexuality (1905). In: Freud, S. ed. *The standard edition of the complete psychological works of Sigmund Freud, volume VII (1901–1905): A case of hysteria, three essays on sexuality and other works.* London: Hogarth Press, 1973, 123–246.

Fussinger, C. 2011. 'Therapeutic community', psychiatryas reformers and antipsychiatrists: reconsidering changes in the field of psychiatry after World War II. *History of psychiatry*, 22 (2), 146–163.

Gillon, E., 2007. *Person-centred counselling psychology: An introduction.* London: Sage.

Glasby, J., and Needham, C., 2014. Conclusion: glass half full or glass half empty? In: Needham, C., and Glasby, J., eds. *Debates in personalisation.* Bristol: Policy Press, 185–191.

Hart, V., 2014. A view from social work practice. In: Needham, C., and Glasby, J., eds. *Debates in personalisation.* Bristol: Policy Press, 2014, 111–119.

Henwood, M., 2014. Self-funders: the road from perdition?. In: Needham, C., and Glasby, J., eds. *Debates in personalisation* [online]. Bristol: Policy Press, 2014, 75–87. 10.2307/j.ctt1t892xn.12

Hogan, A.J., 2019. Social and medical models of disability and mental health: evolution and renewal. *CMAJ*, 191 (1), 16–18.

Institute of Fiscal Studies, 2020. Gendered Economic inequalities: a social policy perspective.

Kornhaber, R., Cross, M., Betihavas, V., and Bridgman, H., 2016. The benefits and challenges of academic writing retreats: An integrative review. Higher Education Research & Development, 35 (6), pp. 1210–1227.

Kritsotaki, D., Long, V., and Smith, M., 2016. *Deinstitutionalisation and after: Post-war psychiatry in the western world.* London: Palgrave Macmillan.

Kritsotaki, D., Long, V., and Smith, M., eds., 2018. *Preventing mental illness: Past, present and future.* London: Springer.

Laing, R.D., 1967. *The divided self (London: Tavistock, 1960) and the politics of experience.* New York: Pantheon.

Lobao, L., Gray, M., Cox, K., and Kitson, M., 2018. The shrinking state? Understanding the assault on the public sector. *Cambridge Journal of Regions, Economy and Society* [online], 11 (3), 389–408. 10.1093/cjres/rsy026

McCance, T., McCormack, B., and Dewing, J., 2011. An exploration of person-centredness in practice. *Online Journal of Issues in Nursing* [online], 16 (2), 1. 10.3912/OJIN.Vol16No02 Man01

Mental Capacity Act 2005 (c. 9) [online]. Available at: https://www.legislation.gov.uk/ukpga/2005/9/contents

Moore, C., and Shantall, T., 2003. The self-actualisation theory of Abraham Maslow. In: Rapmund, V., Moore, C., Oosthuizen, P., Shantall, T., van Dyk, A., and Viljoen, H. ed. *Personality theories.* Pretoria, South Africa: University of South Africa, 2011, 119–147.

Moss, B., 2017. *Communication skills in health and social care.* London: Sage.

National Council for Voluntary Organisations, 2019. *Co-production and service-user involvement* [online]. London: National Council for Voluntary Organisations. Available at: https://knowhow.ncvo.org.uk/organisation/collaboration/coproduction-and-service-user-involvement [Accessed 2 July 2021].

National Health Service and Community Care Act 1990 (c. 19) [online]. Available at: https://www.legislation.gov.uk/ukpga/1990/19/contents

Needham, C., and Glasy J., 2014. *Debates in personalisation.* Bristol: Policy Press.

NHS England, 2014. *Five Year forward view* [online]. London: NHS England. Available at: https://www.england.nhs.uk/wp-content/uploads/2014/10/5yfv-web.pdf

NHS England, 2014. *The forward view into action: planning for 2015/16* [online]. London: NHS England. Available at: www.england.nhs.uk/wp-content/uploads/2014/12/forward-view-plning.pdf [Accessed 6 November 2020].

Office for National Statistics, 2020. *Coronavirus and the social impacts on disabled people in Great Britain: September 2020* [online]. Newport: Office for National Statistics. Available at: https://www.ons.gov.uk/peoplepopulationandcommunity/healthandsocialcare/disability/articles/coronavirusandthesocialimpactsondisabledpeopleingreatbritain/march2020tode-cember2021

Price, B. 2019. *Delivering person-centred care in nursing.* London: Sage.

Prochaska, J.O., & DiClemente, C.C., 1983. Stages and processes of self-change of smoking: Toward an integrative model of change. *Journal of Consulting and Clinical Psychology*, 51 (3), 390–395. https://doi.org/10.1037/0022-006X.51.3.390

Quality Assurance Agency, 2019. *Subject benchmark: Social work* [online]. Gloucester: Quality Assurance Agency for Higher Education. Available at: https://www.qaa.ac.uk/docs/qaa/subject-benchmark-statements/subject-benchmark-statement-social-work.pdf?sfvrsn=5c35c881_6 [Accessed 1 November 2020].

Rao, R., Crome, I., Crome, P., and Iliffe, S., 2019. Substance misuse in later life: Challenges for primary care: A review of policy and evidence. *Primary Health Care Research & Development* [online], 20, e117. 10.1017/S1463423618000440

Repper, J., and Perkins, R., 2003. *Social inclusion and recovery: A model for mental health practice.* Oxford: Elsevier Health Sciences.

Rogers, A., & Pilgrim, D., 2001. *Mental health policy in Britain.* London: Palgrave/Macmillan.

Roulstone, A., 2014. Personalisation – plus ca change? In: Beresford, P., ed. *Personalisation: Critical and radical debates in social work*. Bristol: Policy Press, 2014, 47–51.

Sanderson, H., and Lewis, J., 2012. *A practical guide to delivering personalisation: Person-centred approach in Health and Social Care*. London: Jessica Kingsley Publishers.

Sartre, J.-P., 1943. *Being and nothingness: An essay on phenomenological ontology*. New York: Washington Square Press.

Sartre, J-P., 1948. *Existentialism and humanism, translated by Philip Mairet*. Cambridge: Cambridge University Press.

Schneider, K.J., Pierson, J.F., and Bugental, J.F., eds., 2014. *The handbook of humanistic psychology: Theory, research, and practice*. London: Sage Publications.

Schön, D.A., 1991. *The reflective turn: Case studies in and on educational practice*. New York: Teachers College Press.

Scott, S., and Kanner, K., 2015. Brief alcohol interventions [online]. In: Neuberger, J., and DiMartini, A., eds. *Alcohol abuse and liver disease*. New Jersey: Wiley-Blackwell, 2015, 147–154. Available at: 10.1002/9781118887318.ch16

Slade, M., 2009. *Personal recovery and mental illness: A guide for mental health professionals*. Cambridge: Cambridge University Press.

Smith, E., Ross, F., Donovan, S., Manthorpe, J., Brearley, S., Sitzia, J., and Beresford, P., 2008. Service user involvement in nursing, midwifery and health visiting research: a review of evidence and practice. *International Journal of Nursing Studies*, 45 (2), 298–315.

Social Care Institute for Excellence [SCIE], 2012. *Personalisation: a rough guide* [online]. London: Social Care Institute for Excellence. Available at: Personalisation: Rough guide – SCIE.

Social Care Institute for Excellence [SCIE], 2017. *Mental capacity act (MCA): Assessing capacity* [online]. London: Social Care Institute for Excellence. Available at: https://www.scie.org.uk/mca/practice/assessing-capacity [Accessed 27 November 2020].

Solomon, M., 2019. Becoming comfortable with chaos: making collaborative multi-agency working work. *Emotional and Behavioural Difficulties*, 24 (4), 391–404.

Steen, T., & Tuurnas, S. (2018). The roles of the professional in co-production and co-creation processes. In Co-production and co-creation (pp. 80–92). Routledge.

Taylor, A.L., 2012. Best practice in substance misuse. *Archives of Disease in Childhood Education and Practice Edition*, 97(4), 143.

Think Local Act Personal, 2010. *Think local act personal: Next steps for transforming adult social care* [online]. London: Think Local Act Personal. Available at: https://www.thinklocalactpersonal.org.uk/Browse/ThinkLocalActPersonal/

Timmins, F., 2015. *A–Z of reflective practice*. London: Palgrave Macmillan.

United Nations Convention on the Rights of Persons with Disabilities [CRPD], 2006. *United nations convention on the rights of persons with disabilities* [online]. New York: United Nations. Available at: https://www.un.org/disabilities/documents/convention/convention_accessible_pdf.pdf

Valuing People Strategy, 2001. *Valuing people: A new strategy for learning disability for the 21st century* [online]. London: Department of Health. Available at: https://assets.publishing.service.gov.uk/government/uploads/system/uploads/attachment_data/file/250877/5086.pdf

10 Valuing Research in Health and Social Care

Louise Griffiths, Verusca Calabria, and Melanie Bailey

By the end of the chapter, you should be able to:

- Evaluate underpinning values and ethics in health and social care research
- Analyse and evaluate research and other forms of evidence
- Explain how theory, policy and research underpin practice in a range of health and social care settings across informal, voluntary, public and private sectors
- Understand the key principles required for developing a research proposal

Introduction

Research is becoming increasingly important in the current world in which we all live. Whilst research for many is aligned to scientific laboratory research it takes many different forms, such as the testing of hypotheses under controlled environments to social research conducted within communities. Indeed, whilst the remit of research is broad, there is a need for continued high-quality research in order to reduce the inequalities which are currently present within our communities. Research can aid in the reduction of the ever-growing health-related inequalities, which are evident and increasing at a rapid pace between countries and between communities in the UK and elsewhere. For instance, as a result of COVID-19, health inequalities between countries are set to increase especially for mothers and children within the poorest countries who are experiencing indirect implications of the pandemic on their health, which can result in adverse long-term impacts (International Child Health Group and the Royal College of Paediatrics and Child Health 2021).

What Is Research?

Research is the examination of human behaviour, individually, in groups, cultures or organisations. In the academic world, social research is conducted by students and academics to extend knowledge on areas of interest (Henn et al. 2009). The purpose of research is to develop new insights and theories to help understand the processes behind behaviours and theories to bring about positive change in an attempt to reduce inequalities. For example, research might be conducted on the impact of COVID-19 on students' education from disadvantaged backgrounds (Drane et al., 2020). Furthermore, it is important to consider how the lockdown enforced by the

DOI: 10.4324/9781003079873-12

UK government in 2020 and 2021 research informed these measures to reduce the transmission of the coronavirus. Once you start to study research and think about daily decisions you start to notice that research informs decisions ranging from medical procedures to implementing policy changes.

Research Paradigms

Epistemology and Theories of Knowledge

Epistemology considers the theory of knowledge and has two contrasting schools of thought, interpretivism and positivism.

Interpretivism

Weber (1949) contended that in order to increase social knowledge, the cause-and-effect model should be rejected and that we should seek the views of those who are being researched and that participants should provide accounts of their own worlds, namely, to focus on the phenomenology of events. This is an approach embraced in structured, semi and unstructured qualitative methods such as participant observations/interviews/focus groups (Denzin and Lincoln 2011).

Positivism

The term 'positivism' was founded by Auguste Comte in the late 1800s. This approach uses a range of scientific methods to reveal the dynamics of society and individuals (Corry et al. 2018). Research conducted following the positivist paradigm uses quantitative research and statistical analysis. This paradigm has a strong emphasis on reliability, validity and objectivity. The positivist approach does not focus on the lived experiences of individuals or the researchers (McGregor and Murnane, 2010). The quantitative methods which could be used include surveys, experiments, observations.

Research Evaluations for Critical Literature Reviews

An important part of research is to explore and assess what research has already been conducted on your research topic. This is conducted for several reasons, which include assessing the merit of previous research, exploring the depth and breadth of the research, providing justifications for the focus of new research projects. This exploration of previous research is a **literature review** and is the starting point of new research projects.

The early days of a research project involve detailed planning and conducting an expansive review of previous research. This involves using search terms which relate to the topic you are researching and returning to the literature several times to conduct subsequent searches. During these initial literature searches whilst planning your research project, your aim is to identify gaps in knowledge, assess whether a limited amount of research has previously been conducted on your potential research topic and whether the previous research you have identified is outdated.

Example: Research on women in prison

Imagine that you are conducting literature searches of all the academic articles/ books on research with male prisoners. Once an expansive search of the literature has been conducted you can say that you have found a 'gap in knowledge'. Indeed, if most of the previous research is on male prisoners by focusing a new research project on women in prison you have found a 'gap' and will be adding a significant contribution to knowledge, in other words providing original insights that have not yet been provided by academics.

When assessing previous research it is important to develop a research strategy, namely the key ideas and concepts that you need to research, once these have been identified you can write down your **keywords** relating to your research topic which you will need to use to search the literature. During the initial searches of the literature, these search terms will likely be **broad terms** such as mental health. However, these keywords can be refined further during subsequent searches of the literature as you develop your final research topic to a particular mental health problem such as anxiety. When conducting your searches, it is important to remember that whilst books and websites provide some useful information, journal articles often provide more up-to-date information. In addition, journal articles include citations and a reference list which can help you to find additional articles on your research topic.

Health and Social Care Literature Reviews

A literature review in Health and Social Care involves exploring the findings of previous research and how this information relates to your research question/s (Aveyard 2019). A literature review shows how your research fits in with what has gone before and puts it into context. It is an analysis of existing research, which is relevant to your topic and shows how it relates to your investigation. It also explains and justifies how your investigation may answer questions or gaps in this area of research.

There are two types of literature reviews to consider in your Health and Social Care studies, a traditional (or narrative) literature review or a systematic review. A systematic review is a summary of the literature that uses explicit and systematic methods to identify, appraise and summarise the literature according to predetermined criteria. If this description (of the methods) is not present, it is not possible to make a thorough evaluation of the quality of the review. Whilst a traditional (or narrative) literature review critiques and summarises a body of literature (Aveyard 2019).

Organising and Evaluating Your Sources

Creating a mind map can help provide an overview of your reading and connections between ideas. In addition, group your reading notes into topics or themes by using highlighters to identify which topic each article, chapter, report, etc. fits into. Be selective – ask yourself 'why am I including this?' You don't have to refer to everything you read in the same depth as in your literature review. Prioritise the recent research and avoid using older studies that were relevant in the past but are now out of date, their methods surpassed by more accurate methods.

Writing Your Literature Review

Introduction

- Explains the context of your research area and the main topics being investigated
- Highlights the relevant issues or debates
- Includes signposting for the reader – explains the sequence of topics covered and the scope of the research (Aveyard 2019)
- Outlines the aims and objectives of your research

Main body

- An analysis of the literature by themes or topics that bears on the aims and objectives on your research
- Linked together in a coherent, logical structure
- Shows how your research builds on previous research and provides justification for what, why and how you are going to do it (Aveyard 2019)

Conclusion

- Summarises the **current state** of the research in your field as analysed in the main body
- Identifies any **gaps or problems** with the existing research
- Explains **how your research** will address these gaps or build on the existing research

(Aveyard 2019)

Critical Analysis

Once you have identified the literature to include within your review, you will need to compare and contrast the different views from the literature in relation to your themes. This is where you become critical with what you are reading. If you agree with the findings or viewpoint of the article, provide the reasons for your decision. If you do not agree also justify this. There are a number of reasons why you may agree or disagree with the findings within the literature. For example, the research may have been conducted a long time ago and new research contradicts this school of thought. Alternatively, there may be perceived limitations with the methods used within the study e.g. small scale. Indeed, here you will assess the strengths of previous research in relation to your research question/s (Aveyard 2019).

As you progress with your literature review, explain in turn how each theme relates to your research question/objectives, whilst assessing the findings within each theme. It is key to ensure you are not being descriptive and just repeating the findings but that you are discussing any limitations of previous research that has been conducted, which in turn supports the aims of your research project.

Research Design

The design of your research project involves a number of important decisions which should be considered in relation to your chosen research topic and aligned with what you want to achieve from your research. In addition, other considerations may play a role when deciding on your research design, such as previous research knowledge, funding, the time schedule and previous research which has already been conducted on your topic. The decision initially may not be solely focused on the methods but rather on what you are wanting to explore (Bell 2018). Once you have considered these factors you will need to decide on whether your research design will be quantitative, qualitative or a mixed methods approach.

Mixed Methods

Mixed methods design stands for the use of both qualitative and quantitative data collection to answer your research question. Mixed Methods methodology has become very popular in the social sciences world. This design is used to give a stronger understanding between the connections of the quantitative and qualitative sets of data (Shorten and Smith 2017). If the researcher selects this design, they have a good grasp of both the quantitative and qualitative design. A table that summarises the key elements of qualitative and quantitative research methods can be found in Hesse-Biber and Levy (2017, p. 12).

There are three mixed-method designs:

> Convergent Design – the researcher's aim is to collect both the quantitative and qualitative data, analyse the two sets of data simultaneously and then amalgamate them together (Creswell 2015, p. 37).

> Explanatory Sequential Design – the researcher collects the quantitative data first and collects the qualitative to help explain the findings of the quantitative data (Creswell 2015, p. 38). It provides a richer in-depth overall picture of the findings.

> Exploratory Sequential Design – the researcher initially explores the problem area using qualitative data and analysis. From this analysis an intervention or tool is developed, and the third stage of this design is a quantitative study then takes place of the new intervention or tool (Creswell 2015, p. 39).

Quantitative Methodology

What Is Quantitative Research?

Quantitative research is the adoption of natural scientific experiment module for research methods (Henn et al. 2009), which is associated with the positivist school of thought. The focus is on collecting data in a standardised approach using a range of variables to test existing theories by testing hypotheses and searches for causal relationships between variables. The research decisions with this approach are made before the research is conducted.

An example of quantitative data which we have all come to recognise since COVID-19 emerged at the start of 2020 is the 'R number'. This statistical number is not just linked to COVID-19 but to all infectious diseases. The reproductive number is an epidemiologic metric used to describe the transmissibility of an infectious agent (Diekmann et al. 2013). In this example the infectious agent is COVID-19. How the 'R number' is calculated is based on a variety of factors; infectious period; contact rate; mode of transmission (Sanche et al. 2020). Once the reproductive number is above 1 this shows that the infectious disease is likely to continue spreading. If the reproductive number is below 1 the transmission of the infectious disease is likely to die out in the selected population (Liu et al. 2020).

A final example of the use of quantitative data in the public health domain is the Index of Multiple Deprivation. This official measure ranks every small area in England from 1 to 32,844. The number 1 is classed as the most deprived area and 32,844 as the least deprived area. The Index of Multiple Deprivation scores help distribute funding and focus on programmes in areas which are the most deprived. The most current IMD was produced in 2019 (Ministry of Housing, Communities and Local Government 2019).

Quantitative Methods

Quantitative Approach

When considering the most appropriate approach for your research project you may assess the reliability of the approach and associated methods. Quantitative research is deemed to be high on reliability as this refers to the ability of the data to produce similar results on all occasions (Bell 2018).

Experiments

This quantitative method is conducted within controlled environment of a laboratory or field setting where manipulating a controlled environment can be implemented to explore the cause-and-effect relationships between variables, with the independent variable (cause) and the dependent as (effect) (Punch 2013).

The researcher manipulates certain controlled conditions in order to identify if the independent variable (cause) has an impact on the dependent variable (effect) to explain 'cause and effect' relationships. Experimental enquiry offers the researcher considerable control by effecting change and observing the research participants' subsequent behaviour (the effect) (Henn et al. 2009, p. 142). Researchers will often have two groups when conducting an experiment. For instance, on a new treatment for cancer the experimental group would receive the new treatment, whilst the control group would not. The only difference should be that the experimental group are exposed to the treatment.

Some challenges of experimental research include:

> Internal validity (factors which affect true measurement of variables). Factors to consider that might affect the integrity of experimental research are factors outside the control of the researcher despite careful planning, such as mortality, historical events, variations in the measurement process and testing.

External validity examines the extent of how much the research findings can be related and generalised to the whole population outside of the experimental controls (Taylor 2013). There are three ways which could affect the external validity, therefore making the findings gathered not as generalised as first thought. These are the participants, time and the environment. If you can get a representative sample, conduct the experiment at different times of the day and conduct the research in varied environments this would allow your findings to be generalised to the real world.

'The Hawthorn Effect'

In experimental research, the researcher needs to be aware of 'The Hawthorne Effect'. This is when the participant may change their behaviour once being asked about it or if they are aware of being observed when conducting that behaviour (Breakwell 2012). An example related to COVID-19 is if someone asks whether you follow the 2-meter guidelines inside a supermarket before you enter; you may be more aware of keeping that 2 meters distance than you have done previously. The Hawthorne effect could have an impact on the generalisation of the results to the population.

Sample Surveys

Surveys are another type of quantitative design. Surveys generally collect large-scale data, which is beneficial in terms of the reliability and validity of the collected data. Surveys can be distributed to a large geographic diverse sample (Kumar 2019). An example would be the Census which in England and Wales takes place every 10 years. The most recent census was conducted in 2021.

There are several ways that surveys can be delivered including postal surveys, face-to-face surveys, telephone surveys and online surveys. All forms of delivery of surveys have their benefits and their limitations. The most common delivery is a face-to-face survey, this is when the interviewer is present and writes down the answers. The survey may be conducted at a specific location or interviewers might catch the participant when they are doing a certain activity (Stopher 2012). A strength of this form of data collection is that it minimises nonresponse or partial response. Having an interviewer there can also help to clarify questions (Dialsingh 2008).

Online surveys have increased since the pandemic in 2020 due to reduced amount of face-to-face contact. The 2021 Census recommended that the survey be completed online instead of postal method. Strengths using online surveys include being able to prevent the participant to move on to the next question if they have not answered the previous questionnaire meaning a complete set of data (Breakwell 2012). A critique would be that not everyone has access to online systems and therefore we would be ignoring a group of the population (Kumar 2019). Conducting a telephone survey is also another form of collecting information without direct contact. An advantage for conducting a telephone survey is that the interviewer can reach more participants than when interviewing face-to-face. A limitation of using such a survey is that the sample may not be representative of the population. Some people may not own a telephone, for example, those who are homeless (Block and Erskine 2012).

A Critique of Sample Surveys

A perceived limitation of a sample survey is measurement validity, namely whether the survey provides a true picture of what is being measured (Punch 2013). Can

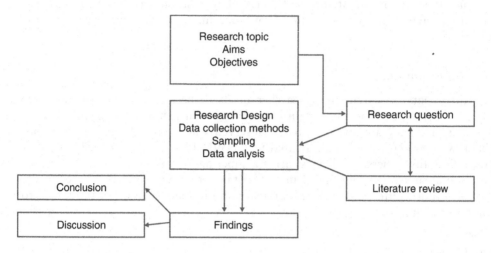

Figure 10.1 Good qualitative research follows the process above.

human behaviour be understood by posing a series of structured questions? Indeed, surveys can be seen to lack depth and context (Punch 2013). Critics of quantitative research claim that survey-based research offers limited insights into understanding people's behaviours and attitudes (Henn et al. 2009).

Qualitative Research Design Process

Ethnography

Ethnography involves study through observation of institutions, cultures and customs (Henn et al. 2009), which inquires systematically about the world people see, to develop theories about the social world. This type of qualitative method is used when researchers want to see the world in a different way from the point of view of the participants under investigation, researchers join in with the everyday life and activities of those being studied. This method is often used when researchers wish to discover something new or different than has already been noted (Punch 2013).

Ethnography has benefits and limitations to consider before selecting this qualitative method, some benefits are that questions will not be perceived as intrusive and a true reflection can be obtained if the researcher is accepted by the group (Punch 2013). However, reactivity (behaviours are modified) may occur if the group are not accepting of the researcher (Punch 2013). Further strengths and limitations of this method can be located in Punch 2013.

Collaborative Research Designs in Health and Social Care

This section of the chapter introduces two collaborative research methods, oral history and participatory-action research, which are becoming recognised in mainstream social sciences and are being increasingly used in research within health and social care for their emancipatory qualities.

Participatory Action Research

Participatory action research (PAR) involves researchers and participants working together to understand a problematic situation and change it for the better. It is a research approach that emphasises the active participation of research subjects, who usually occupy a passive role in traditional research. PAR can be viewed as an alternative form of research practice that seeks to place participants in a position of influencing research findings (Kemmis et al. 2014). The main tenet of PAR is to bring about practical change through iterative and reflexive practice (Reason and Bradbury, 2001). It calls for the active participation of research participants in the planning, the action and reflection of a research project. Doing PAR research involves working with participants instead of doing research on them (Slade et al. 2017). Within the PAR research cycle both researcher and the research participants stay partners throughout the process. This is achieved through stakeholders' authentic involvement and the exercise of personal agency in order to challenge the conventional imbalance of power in research (Calabria and Bailey 2021). Participants are encouraged to become active in all aspects of the research cycle, see Figure 10.2.

PAR calls into question the validity of the knowledge produced by researchers as privileged to the knowledge produced by participants. The goal is to uncover different kinds of realities from those limited by conventional inquiry that privileges the knowledge of experts (Kemmis et al. 2014). It is a methodology that is oriented towards social action by involving stakeholders who have the most to gain from the outcomes of the research, in order to bring about changes in knowledge, policy and practice. With its emphasis on grassroots empowerment, it is particularly suitable for conducting research with marginalised communities. PAR is an applied and cyclical research process that invites all interested stakeholders, who have a vested interest in knowledge constructed about them, to produce action towards social change.

The importance of harnessing the active involvement of service users in mental health research has become an important feature of the discussions and planning related to current approaches to prevention, care and treatment in mental health. It fits in with the current health policy agendas that call for the design of services in partnership with service users (Mental Health Taskforce 2016). PAR makes valuable theoretical and practical contributions when undertaking research in health and social care. It is part of a growing trend of action-oriented research in health and social care in the UK for its empowering and inclusive features such as the

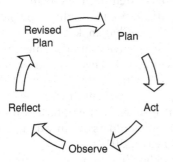

Figure 10.2 The action research cycle (Kemmis and McTaggart, 1982).

participatory research on the impact of the modernisation of mental health day services carried out with service users with enduring mental health problems (Bryant 2011); participatory oral history research that revealed important aspects of inpatient care in the now-closed mental hospitals, overlooked during the transition to community care (Calabria et al. 2021), and participatory arts-based research with teenage mothers to challenge negative assumptions made about them and provide alternative understandings of teenage pregnancy and young parenthood (Brady and Brown, 2013).

There are limitations to the PAR methodology. Firstly, although the method may bring about some practical change at the local level, it does now necessarily challenge structural inequalities; working collaboratively with research participants does not necessarily bring about change at the local or national level (Russo 2012). Secondly, Cook and Kothari (2001) coined the term 'tyranny of participation' in PAR, namely participants may not want to be involved in all stages or may be unable to do so despite the imperative to do so. Overall, researchers committed to PAR methodology need to embrace the necessary long-term commitment, and manage expectations of what can be achieved. There are also possible social, practical, emotional implications of conducting participatory research, which call for a reflective approach of the positionality of the researcher (Calabria 2019). In addition, there are important ethical issues to be addressed when conducting PAR research with vulnerable groups. Safeguards are required to explain roles and promote openness in research relationships; strategies include self-awareness, research logs, supervision and encouraging a reflexive approach on the part of the researcher that help foster authenticity in research relationships (Atkinson 2005).

Oral History Methodology

Oral history is the recording of people's memories and past life experiences in the form of an audio or video recording; oral history interviewing entails the researcher and participants spend extended time engaged in the process of storytelling and listening. This methodology is particularly suitable to investigate how given populations experienced historical events (Hesse-Biber and Leavy, 2017). Oral history relies on first-person testimony and memory to arrive at a more comprehensive or different understanding of past events, experienced both individually and collectively. Crucially, oral history produces a unique source of history for future research in which the oral history interview becomes the primary instrument in researching the past (Perks and Thomson 2015). It has often been associated with both grassroots and progressive politics, the democratic desire to amplify the voices of marginalised and oppressed groups (Freund, 2013). What makes oral history different is that it allows a window into the realm of subjectivity and the emergence of a multiple realities about a given situation (Portelli 2015). This method of data collection is inherently participatory as it relies on the active collaboration of the participants in sharing their unique perspectives about a past event or experience in the context of the individual's life. Like PAR, oral history puts emphasis on developing mutual and reciprocal relationships with stakeholders in an attempt to democratise the research process (Hesse-Biber and Leavy, 2010).

The main critique of oral history lies in the unreliability of memory such as omissions and misremembering. However, since the social turn in the Humanities and

Social Sciences, there has been a shift away from positivistic interpretations of events to embrace the social production of knowledge (Thomson 2007). The unique strength of oral history lies in understanding the personal and collecting meanings attached to past events and the purposes these serves (Portelli 2015). The potential of this method, in the context of health and social care research, centres around the emerge of multiple realities about given past events and how this knowledge by experience can help redress inequalities.

Oral history both as a research method and a subject of research in its own right has the potential to decolonise not only academic curricula but also to broaden perspectives in research by including the voices of black and ethnic minority groups, usually denied a voice in the public discourse. In addition, oral history is becoming an emerging practice to improve public policy in the twenty-first century. Hoffman (2017) refers to the 'hidden gold' of oral history, namely the wealth of local knowledge and expertise of otherwise disenfranchised groups, which can be utilised to improve public policy. Hoffman advocates sharing findings from oral histories with decision-makers to influence change at the policy level. Example of how oral history has been used to improve outcomes and reduce inequalities in health and social care is Rickard's 'Oral History of Prostitution' in the UK project (2003). The project took a sex positive perspective on prostitution by recording the oral histories of sex workers. Rickard facilitated practical change by responding to the stakeholders' concerns that emerged from the interviews with the aid of the oral histories for educational and political purposes. Moreover, research on the impact of recording the oral histories of people with life-limiting illnesses in palliative care has demonstrated the tangible benefits in providing a validating and dignified social activity (Winslow and Smith, 2019). In addition, Calabria's oral histories of former staff and patients of the now-closed mental hospitals demonstrated the importance of the therapeutic environment of the mental hospital, as well as the relationships fostered within it, for patients' recovery (Calabria et al. 2021; Calabria 2022).

Qualitative Data Collection Tools

Semi-Structured Interviews

Semi-structured interviews are particularly suitable method of gathering data about individual experiences; it allows flexibility to further investigate any emerging insights and the achievement of detailed narratives from each participant (Henn et al. 2009). By choosing to interview your participants, you will be able to control the pace and direction of the interview. Conducting qualitative interviews enables the researcher to explore further areas of interest which may be identified by your participants, a technique referred to as grounded theory (Charmaz 2014). The strengths of weakness of conducting research remotely are considered later in this chapter.

Some benefits of semi-structured interviews include the ability of the researcher to build rapport with participants which can lead to increased levels of disclosure and information on the research topic (Denzins and Lincoln, 2011). Whilst some limitations of semi-structured interviews are that you will be unable to generalise because of the depth and detail obtained from participants (Denzins and Lincoln, 2011), the interviews can be distressing for the participant/researcher if discussing a particularly sensitive topic (Charmaz 2014). For further benefits and limitations of semi-structured interviewing please see Denzin and Lincoln (2011).

Focus Groups

Focus groups represent a group discussion which is guided or unguided by the researcher. Most manuals of qualitative research advise setting up small focus groups in order to effectively manage data collection.

There are benefits and limitations of focus groups which should be carefully considered when deciding if this method is most appropriate for your research project. Indeed, focus groups enable the participants to build on each other's responses with the group interactions representing a vital element of the research and the collection of data (Krueger and Casey, 2014). Whilst some difficulties may arise trying to arrange a mutually agreeable date and time for the focus group to be conducted (Krueger 2007), the control of the focus group should not lie with the researcher, but with the participants (Getrich et al., 2016). Further strengths and limitations of this method can be located in (Denzin and Lincoln, 2011).

Observations

Observations is a method of data collection that offers fresh insights into the research, which lead to new directions (Charmaz 2014). When considering observations as a research method it is important to select whether these will be unstructured, structured or participant observations. Unstructured observations may be selected by researchers who have some ideas but may not know the exact part of the research topic they want to explore, whilst structured observations involve selecting a focus (Bell 2018). Participant observations involve the researcher becoming involved in the daily lives of those under research. Punch (2016) explored the use of research observations to explore the social role of police in Amsterdam, findings indicated that the police modified their behaviour, which is called Reactivity. Reactivity has been found to undermine the researcher's ability to record accurate details.

Observations have associated benefits and limitations. Some benefits are that observations enable fresh insights and directions for research (Charmaz 2014) with participants disclosing behaviours that they may not discuss during interviews (Punch 2016). Whilst some limitations include the involvement of the research within the observed behaviour and the ability to make accurate notes (Punch 2016). Further strengths and limitations of this method can be located in Punch 2016.

Activity 1   Equality and Opportunity Research

1   Explore the likelihood of the UK having a black/ethnic minority prime minister.
2   What qualitative or quantitative methods would be most appropriate to use for a research project which investigates equality and opportunity (in relation to becoming a prime minister)?

Please refer to the table of key differences between qualitative and quantitative research methods in Hesse-Biber and Levy, 2017, p. 12.

Sampling

The main aim of qualitative research is to understand the participants involved in the research as opposed to providing a representative sample (Punch 2016). Some of the key sampling strategies employed when using a qualitative approach to your research project include snowball sampling which relies on the researcher establishing a significant contact to identify other participants; theoretical sampling, a form of sampling which uses the findings from the earlier stages of data collection to guide the sampling of participants from specific areas (Charmaz 2014). In addition, other popular qualitative sampling strategies include Purposive sampling which involves the selection of participants through a known criterion (Punch 2016). For further qualitative sampling strategies and information please see Creswell et al. (2007).

Remote Research

The recent COVID-19 pandemic has reconceptualised how research is conducted in health and social care. Research is being carried out remotely to reduce the chances of transmission. This shift has important implications on the doing of qualitative research. There are some clear advantages to conducting fieldwork online such as the ability to automate transcription of usually lengthy interviews, and the ability to conduct research in multiple countries concurrently (Archibald et al. 2019). Some of the common pitfalls are the difficulty of establishing rapport with research participants, issues of data security, and structural inequalities impeding participation such as participants' lack of access to a personal computer and internet connection. Conducting research remotely is likely to become a defining feature of the twenty-first century. Moreover, qualitative researchers who take a participatory approach to sensitive research in health and social care would discourage conducting online interviews for it is difficult to gauge the effect an interview can have on participants in online environments, making it difficult to protect participants from harm, central ethical consideration aspects of user-led research. However, there are also many advantages of conducting remote interviews; these include the ability to involve participants from wider geographical areas and reducing costs and time involved in this kind of research (Dodds 2020). Your university research ethics committee will have put in place guidance that you must adhere to when doing remote research interviews.

Evidence-Based Practice

Evidence-Based Practice in Health and Social Care is the interlinking of research and practice by being able to explain the rationale behind the care you may provide as future practitioners, this is done by using the most up-to-date evidence (research), see Aveyard and Sharp (2017). There are three elements to Evidence-Based Practice which are considered when deciding on a care plan for a service user. The latest research is explored whilst also considering the expertise/experience of the professional alongside the preferences of the service user.

Example of Evidence-based Practice

A social work student undertakes a placement with disadvantaged families, one of the families has a five-year-old with behavioural problems.

Rationale – research evidence suggests parenting groups can help parents to manage the behaviour of the child and reduce anxiety for the parents (Barlow et al. 2016). Whilst also considering the expert opinions of the student's placement supervisor and the preferences of the parents and the family, who are advised to attend parenting skills workshops in their local community.

Ethical Considerations in Health and Social Care Research

Ethics govern the protecting of participants versus the freedom to conduct research (Punch 2016). Ethical dilemmas can be presented whilst the research is being conducted, which may not have previously been considered within the research planning. These ethical concerns have been termed by Bryan et al. (2016) as 'in the moment' challenges for ethics, which are also a consideration when planning your research project and represent an important element when planning research proposals. Such ethical considerations identify the unpredictable nature of the research environment.

All research must take into account ethical considerations. Whilst some research projects are more sensitive than others, requiring additional ethical considerations, basic ethical considerations are present for all research projects. Ensuring participants are fully informed about the research topic and voluntarily agree to be part of your project is central to all research projects and is referred to as gaining *'informed consent'*. Furthermore, not sharing the information with others outside of the research (*confidentiality*) and ensuring individuals are not identified within your research (*anonymity)* are central to all research projects, regardless of the topic (Hesse-Biber and Leavy, 2017).

A good starting point when considering the ethical considerations of your research is to consider various stakeholders within your research, such as who your participants will be, guidance from your supervisor for your research project, the ethics board at your university and any potential examiners or markers (Punch 2016).

A key ethical responsibility that you hold as a researcher is to ensure your research does not cause harm to yourself or the participants as part of the research process, by adhering to ethical principles. Researchers need to combine the following ethical guidelines whilst also contributing knowledge on the research topic. The ethical considerations of a research project are central and should be considered in the early stages of the research project planning.

Ethics Application

The importance of ethics is demonstrated with each university having an ethics application process and an ethics board who considers proposed research projects. In addition, this ethics application can also be combined with ethical applications if the research is taking place in an external organisation e.g. NHS.

Research Location

When planning your research, it is essential to consider the location where you plan to conduct the research and collect your data. For example, when conducting face-to-face interviews, consider using a private space at the research site. Alternatively, you could justify for the interviews to be conducted remotely.

Ethical Responsibilities to Research Participants

When planning your research project, it is important to consider the ethical responsibilities to your research participants, which include the following:

Voluntary Informed Consent	Research participants should have the full description of the research and be fully informed what their individual participation will involve.
Deception	Participants should not be deceived unless it can be ethically justified.
Right to Withdraw	Participants should always have an opportunity to withdraw from the research and the information they provided will not be used as part of the research.
Children, Vulnerable Young People and Vulnerable Adults	All participants should have the capacity to consent, parental consent should be sought for under 18s.
Incentives	Incentives can be used as part of research but may be more appropriate for some research projects than others.
Detriment Arising from Participation in Research	Participants may be distressed as part of your research and this needs to be considered with further support contacts provided.
Anonymity	Participants should not be identifiable in the research e.g. participants 1, 2, etc. should replace their names.
Confidentiality	The information provided as part of the research should be kept secure (password-protected computer files/ locked cupboards) with only the researchers and project supervisors having access.

To deepen your understanding of ethical considerations please explore the Stanford Prison Research by Zimbardo et al. (1971).

Data Analysis Approaches

When designing your research project, it is important to consider how you will analyse the data that you collect. The data analysis approach that you select for your research project must align to your methodology. For example, if you have selected a qualitative methodology, you should analyse your data using a qualitative data analysis approach.

Quantitative Data Analysis

Descriptive vs Inferential Statistics

Descriptive statistics consist of a range of measures used to describe and explain the results from a specific dataset. Whilst inferential statistics consist of a group of statistical tests designed to calculate a level of confidence that a random probability sample is representative of a population – these tests result in a measure of statistical significance (Punch 2013).

Analysing Quantitative Data Sets

There are a variety of tools you need to analyse quantitative data, which include graphical and tabular demonstration of data. The analysis of quantitative data explores the relationship between two variables to assess the statistical significance of variables which can produce correlations between variables (Punch 2013). For example, we might correlate two variables of substance misuse and homelessness to assess if misusing substances leads to homelessness.

Statistical Analysis of More Complex Datasets

When analysing quantitative data special software packages are available to assess the significance between variables these include the Statistical Package Social Sciences (SPSS). When analysing quantitative data, you will be measuring the *reliability* which refers to the effectiveness of data collection instruments for taking accurate and consistent measures (Bell 2018). In addition, you will be assessing the *significance* between variables. How do we know whether the correlation between variables is statistically significant? Using SPSS, several tests can be conducted on the data. There are numerous statistical tests for association (examples include Phi, Pearson's r, Spearman's rho, Lamda, Gamma). These indicators offer evidence of the strength of a relationship between two variables, the lower the P-level the more significant the relationship, $P = .05$ (Punch 2013). Indeed, these tests determine whether the results of a sample group can be applied to the wider population (Henn et al. 2008).

Qualitative Data Analysis

Once you have decided on a qualitative approach and therefore a qualitative type of analysis, you will need to select the form of analysis which best fits your research and your prior knowledge. One form of qualitative analysis which is appropriate for undergraduate and master's level is Interpretative Phenomenological Analysis (IPA), which identifies themes from within the data. Indeed, IPA explores personal perspectives to investigate how participants make sense of their social world as opposed to in relation to a particular event. An undergraduate student conducted a qualitative research project exploring the impact of exercise on student anxiety using IPA to analyse the interview transcripts (answers provided by the participants) to identify themes.

Narrative Analysis considers the lived experiences of participants and how they use language to convey meaning, *Grounded theory* presents a form of thematic analysis, which looks to identify themes within the data to develop explanations and theory (Glaser and Strauss, 2017). *Analytic Induction* involves examining social phenomena using case studies to explore similarities which contributes to the generation of new ideas and concepts (Punch 2013). *Discourse Analysis* considers the language of the participants within social contexts, 'discourse' relates to exploring ideas from people at points in time to explore their knowledge in relation to other groups of people. Please see (Creswell et al. 2007) for further information.

Conclusion

This chapter has illustrated the vital role research plays to raise awareness of existing inequalities, whilst also providing evidence to reduce such inequalities within communities in the UK and between countries. Research is an integral part of all welfare decisions made by the UK Government, without which such decisions would become problematic. This chapter has shown that research is paramount for the health and social care sector by aligning current priorities such as conducting qualitative remote research and COVID-19 quantitative research. In addition, this chapter has provided detailed guidance on completing a research proposal within the Health and Social Care Sector by enabling the development of evaluative skills to research which will further seek to reduce inequalities through the encouragement of further research. Crucially, students in health and social care must gain a sound understanding of research designs, methods and ethical principles before embarking on research projects in health and social care.

References

Archibald, M., Ambagtsheer, R.C., Casey, M.G., and Lawless, M., 2019. Using Zoom videoconferencing for qualitative data collection: perceptions and experiences of researchers and participants. *International Journal of Qualitative Methods* [online], 18, 1–8. 10.1177% 2F1609406919874596

Atkinson, D., 2005. Research as social work: participatory research in learning disability. *British Journal of Social Work*, 35 (4), 425–434.

Aveyard, H., and Sharp, P., 2017. *A beginners guide to evidence based practice in health and social care*. Maidenhead, UK: McGraw-Hill Education.

Aveyard, H., 2019. *Doing a literature review in health and social care: a practical guide*. 4th ed. London: Open University Press.

Barlow, J., Bergman, H., Kornør, H., Wei, Y., and Bennett, C., 2016. Group-based parent training programmes for improving emotional and behavioural adjustment in young children. *Cochrane Database of Systematic Reviews*, (8).

Bell, J., and Waters, S., 2018. *Doing your research project*. 7th ed. London: Open University Press.

Block, E.S., and Erskine, L., 2012. Interviewing by telephone: specific considerations, opportunities and challenges. *International Journal of Qualitative Methods*, 11 (4), 428–445.

Brady, G., and Brown, G., 2013. Rewarding but let's talk about the challenges: using arts based methods in research with young mothers. *Methodological Innovations* [online], 8 (1), 99–112. 10.4256/mio.2013.007

Breakwell, G.M., 2012. *Research methods in psychology*. London: SAGE Publications.

Bryan, V., Sanders, S., and Kaplan, L., 2016. *The helping professional's guide to ethics: a new perspective*. Chicago: Lyceum Books.

Bryant, W., Tibbs, A., and Clark, J., 2011. Visualising a safe space: the perspective of people using mental health day services. *Disability & Society*, 26 (5), 611–628.

Calabria, V., 2019. Self-reflexivity in oral history based research: the role of positionality and emotions. In: Bray, P., ed. *Voices of illness: Negotiating meaning and identity*. Brill Publishing, 2019, 271–292.

Calabria, V., 2022. With care in the community, everything goes: using participatory oral history to re-examine the provision of care in the old state mental hospitals. *Oral History Journal*, 50 (1), 93–103.

Calabria, V., and Bailey D., 2021. Participatory Action Research and Oral History as natural allies in mental health research. *Qualitative Research Journal (Sage)* 10.1177/14687941211 039963 [Accessed 10 January 2022].

Charmaz, K., 2014. *Constructing grounded theory*. London: SAGE Publications.

Cooke, B., and Kothari, U. eds., 2001. *Participation: the new tyranny?*. London: Zed books.

Corry, M., Porter, S., and Mckenna, H., 2018. The redundancy of positivism as a paradigm for nursing research. *Nursing Philosophy*, 20 (1), e12230.

Creswell, J.W., 2015. *A concise introduction to mixed methods research*. Los Angeles: SAGE Publications, 37–39.

Creswell, J.W., Hanson, W.E., Clark Plano, V.L., and Morales, A., 2007. Qualitative research designs: selection and implementation. *The Counseling Psychologist*, 35 (2), 236–264.

Denzin, N.K., and Lincoln, Y.S. eds., 2011. *The Sage handbook of qualitative research*. London: SAGE.

Dialsingh, I., 2008. Face-to-Face Interviewing. In: Lavrakas, P.J., ed. *Encyclopedia of survey research methods*. Thousand Oaks: SAGE Publications, 2008, 276–261.

Diekmann, O., Heesterbeek, H., and Britton, T., 2013. *Mathematical tools for understanding infectious disease dynamics* [eBook]. Princeton: Princeton University Press. 10.2307/j.cttq9530.

Dodds, S., and Hess, A.C., 2020. Adapting research methodology during COVID-19: lessons for transformative service research. *Journal of Service Management*, 32 (2), 203–217.

Drane, C., Vernon, L., and O'Shea, S. 2020. The impact of 'learning at home' on the educational outcomes of vulnerable children in Australia during the COVID-19 pandemic. Literature Review Prepared by the National Centre for Student Equity in Higher Education. Curtin University, Australia.

Drane, C.F., Vernon, L., and O'Shea, S., 2021. Vulnerable learners in the age of COVID-19: a scoping review. *The Australian Educational Researcher*, 48 (4), 585–604.

Freund, A., 2013. Toward an Ethics of silence? Negotiating off-the-record events and identity in oral history. In: Sheftel, A., and Zembrzycki, S., eds. *Oral history off the record*. New York: Palgrave Macmillan, 2013, 223–238.

Getrich, C.M., Bennett, A.M., Sussman, A.L., Solares, A., and Helitzer, D.L., 2016. Viewing focus groups through a critical incident lens. *Qualitative Health Research*, 26 (6), 750–762.

Glaser, B.G., and Strauss, A.L., 2017. *The discovery of grounded theory: strategies for qualitative research*. Oxfordshire: Routledge.

Henn, M., Weinstein, M., and Foard, N., 2008. *A critical introduction to social research*. London: SAGE Publications.

Hesse-Biber, S.N., and Leavy, P., 2017. *The practice of qualitative research*. London: SAGE Publications.

Hoffman, M., 2017. *Practicing oral history to improve public policies and programs*. Oxfordshire: Routledge.

International Child Health Group, International Child Health Group and Royal College of Paediatrics & Child Health, 2021. Impact of the COVID-19 pandemic on global child health: joint statement of the International Child Health Group and the Royal College of Paediatrics and Child Health. *Archives of Disease in Childhood*, 106 (2), 115–116.

Kemmis, S., and McTaggart, R. 1982. The action research planner. Victoria, Deakin.

Kemmis, S., McTaggart, R., and Nixon, R., 2014. Introducing critical participatory action research. In: Kemmis, S., McTaggart, R., and Nixon, R. *The action research planner*. London: Springer, 2014, 1–31.

Krueger, R., 2007. Problems, challenges and headaches with focus group interviewing and strategies for responding. In: *Workshop presented at the American Evaluation Association annual conference, Baltimore, Maryland*.

Krueger, R.A., and Casey, M.A., 2014. *Focus groups: a practical guide for applied research.* London: SAGE Publications.

Kumar, R., 2019. *Research methodology: a step-by-step guide for beginners.* London: SAGE Publications Ltd. Available via: https://app.talis.com/ntu/player#/modules/5f68843802ad9425 f0b5a469/resources/5f688fa402ad9425f0b5a4d4 [Accessed 10 January 2022].

Liu, Y., Gayle, A.A., Wilder-Smith, A., and Rocklöv, J., 2020. The reproductive number of COVID-19 is higher compared to SARS coronavirus. *Journal of Travel Medicine,* 27 (2), 1–4.

McGregor, S.L.T., and Murnane, J.A., 2010. Paradigm, methodology and method: intellectual integrity in consumer scholarship. *International Journal of Consumer Studies,* 34 (4), 419–427.

Mental Health Taskforce, 2016. *The five-year forward view for mental health* [online]. London: Department of Health. Available at: https://www.england.nhs.uk/wp-content/ uploads/2016/02/Mental-Health-Taskforce-FYFV-final.pdf

Ministry of Housing, Community and Local Government, 2019. *The English indices of deprivation 2019* [online]. London: Ministry of Housing, Community and Local Government. Available at: https://assets.publishing.service.gov.uk/government/uploads/system/uploads/ attachment_data/file/835115/IoD2019_Statistical_Release.pdf [Accessed 10 January 2022].

Office for National Statistics, 2021. *About the census* [online]. London: Census. Available at: https://census.gov.uk/about-the-census [Accessed 10 January 2022].

Perks, R., and Thomson, A., 2015. *The oral history reader.* Oxfordshire: Routledge.

Portelli, A., 2015. What makes oral history different. In: Perks, R., and Thomson, A., eds. *The oral history reader.* Oxfordshire: Routledge, 2015, 48–58.

Punch, K., 2013. *Introduction to social research: quantitative and qualitative approaches.* London: SAGE Publications. Available at: https://app.talis.com/ntu/player#/modules/5f68843802ad9425 f0b5a469/resources/5f68c60902ad9425f0b5a653 [Accessed 10 January 2022].

Punch, K., 2016. *Developing effective research proposals.* London: SAGE Publications.

Reason, P., and Bradbury, H., 2001. *Handbook of action research: participative inquiry and practice.* London: SAGE Publications.

Rickard, W., 2003. Collaborating with sex workers in oral history. *Oral History Review,* 30 (1), 47–59.

Russo, J., 2012. Survivor-controlled research: a new foundation for thinking about psychiatry and mental health. *Forum Qualitative Sozialforschung/Forum: Qualitative Social Research,* 13 (1).

Sanche, S., Lin, Y.T., Xu, C., Romero-Severson, E., Hengartner, N., and Ke, R., 2020. High contagiousness and rapid spread of severe acute respiratory syndrome coronavirus 2. *Emerging Infectious Diseases,* 26 (7), 1470–1477.

Shorten, A., and Smith, J., 2017. Mixed methods research: expanding the evidence base. *Evidence-Based Nursing,* 20 (3), 74–75.

Slade, M., Oades, L., and Jarden, A., 2017. *Wellbeing, recovery and mental health.* Cambridge: Cambridge University Press.

Smith, J.A., and Osborn, M., 2015. Interpretative phenomenological analysis as a useful methodology for research on the lived experience of pain. *British Journal of Pain,* 9 (1), 41–42.

Stopher, P., 2012. *Collecting, managing, and assessing data using sample surveys.* Cambridge: Cambridge University Press.

Taylor, C.S., 2013. *Validity and validation* [online]. Oxford: Oxford University Press. Available via: https://ebookcentral.proquest.com/lib/ntuuk/reader.action?docID=1480995 [Accessed 10 January 2022].

Thomson, A., 2007. Four paradigm transformations in oral history. *The Oral History Review,* 34 (1), 49–70.

Weber, M., 1949. "Objectivity" in social science and social policy. The methodology of the social sciences. New York: Routledge. pp. 49–112.

Winslow, M., and Smith, S., 2019. The development of oral history with users of palliative care services in the UK. *Sociological Problems,* 51 (1), 26–37.

Zimbardo, P.G., Haney, C., Banks, W.C., and Jaffe, D., 1971. *The Stanford prison experiment.* Zimbardo, Incorporated.

11 Managing Health and Social Care

Amy Allen

Chapter aims:

- Explore 'good practice' in the management of people working in health and social care
- Review a range of challenges facing managers of health and social care services in an ever-changing industry
- Analyse the impact of recent social, fiscal and political changes on a range of health and social care services

Introduction

The health and social care sector is one of UK's biggest employers. In 2020, the adult social care sector alone employed 1.52 million people (Skills for Care 2020). A vast majority of these were employed by independent organisations. Meanwhile, the NHS employs approximately 1.33 million people in hospitals and community health services (NHS Digital 2020). This sector is a subject of constant debate in the media, with it's triumphs and failings attracting much attention. It is also at the mercy of political shift, with regular changes in policy, funding and structuring presenting frequent challenges. These factors make the management of health and care services a challenging occupation; but it is also a vital one. This chapter seeks to explore the challenges faced by the managers of health and care services in modern Britain.

This chapter is split into two distinct sections. The first section focuses on three key responsibilities of those managing health and care settings which are: managing the disclosure of poor practice, supervision and managing stress and preventing burnout. Whilst managers have a highly varied range of responsibilities, the three responsibilities covered here are seen as uniquely important when managing staff providing care to vulnerable individuals but are also difficult to implement and can present challenging dilemmas. It is well known that good management of poor practice disclosures is vital to ensuring high quality care and avoiding abuse or harm. However, high-profile cases in recent years have shown that concerns from staff about the poor practice of their peers often go unreported or are not responded to appropriately, allowing harmful or undignified care to go on unchecked. This section seeks to explore the reasons for this and proposes strategies for improvement.

Supervision in the caring professions has a specific meaning and purpose, distinct from the usage of the term in other industries. Supervision as a regular, supportive professional discussion between a caregiver and their supervisor is explored in this

DOI: 10.4324/9781003079873-13

chapter. The importance of supervision for maintaining both care quality and employee health are discussed. The third responsibility covered in section one is reducing stress and burnout. Working in the caring professions can be highly taxing on the individual for a number of reasons. Anti-social hours and shift patterns can be both physically exhausting and also present challenges to maintaining a healthy work-life balance. The emotional impact of caring for others in distress, alongside the challenges faced by working in an underfunded and over subscribed service can add further strain. As a result, incidences of stress and burnout are disproportionately high amongst health and care professionals. This section explores the reasons for this in more depth and discusses possible solutions for prospective managers.

The second section of this chapter uses five current issues to explore the wider political, economic and sociological context in which care services operate. These are wider challenges which, whilst out of the direct control of managers, have a significant impact on the way services are managed. The five current issues discussed are: staffing shortages, funding, commissioning, consumer expectations, and service level targets. The discussion of each of these challenges aims to make links between decisions made at national level and their impact on front line practice in health and care services.

Section 1: Good Practice in Management

Managing the Disclosure of Poor Practice

Management style and workplace culture can have a significant impact on professional behaviour. A supportive, accepting and open culture can encourage individuals to ask questions, inspire change and ensure high quality care as a result (André et al. 2014; Schein 2015). However, if employees are not encouraged to voice their opinion and to ask questions when they are struggling, poor practice can go on unchallenged. If an employee worries that they will be ignored or even punished in some way for challenging poor practice, they are much less likely to come forward with their concerns. In the wake of recent, high-profile malpractice cases in the caring industries, there has been a renewed interest in whistleblowing and the reasons why professionals do not disclose. For example, whilst there were a small number of professionals guilty of directly abusing residents at Winterborne view, there were many more staff working in the setting who observed this criminal behaviour and did not report it. Other professional from agencies who worked closely with the setting also failed to raise concerns about the quality of care given in the setting. Following the publication of the Francis Report (2013) and The NHS Five Year Forward View (2014), training programmes for care staff have sought to re-emphasise the importance of whistleblowing and settings have taken action to encourage staff to report any concerns.

It is important for managers to understand the potential barriers which prevent staff from reporting concerns. The desire to be accepted by the team and avoid ostracization can be a strong motivator not to disclose concerns about the behaviour of colleagues (Ion et al. 2015). Levett-Jones and Lathlean (2009) found that the relationship with supervisors or senior members of the team exerted a strong influence. Some student nurses conformed to incorrect clinical practices to avoid 'rocking the boat' and cited the threat of alienation as a key factor. Several students cited the fear negative consequences as significant in deciding whether to voice concerns. Such studies highlight the importance of a trusting and mutually respectful relationship between junior staff and their managers. A manager must encourage their supervisees to ask questions about how care is being provided and to challenge things they feel are being done wrong. There must also be processes in place to protect and support those who report poor practice.

Managers have a key role in ensuring staff feel safe and supported to raise concerns about care quality. Strategies such as having an 'open door policy' can encourage employees to 'pop in' to see a manager on an adhoc basis as and when they have concerns, rather than delaying doing so until a formal meeting can be arranged. Managers should also encourage a culture of professional discussion, ensuring colleagues feel they can ask questions and receive feedback on their practice within their team without fear of reprisals.

Supervision

Although the term 'supervision' is used to describe a wide range of managerial roles, it has a specific meaning and purpose in health and social care. Cassedy (2010) defines supervision in clinical settings as *"A regular and formal agreement to engage in a professional working relationship, facilitated by the supervisor to support the supervisee to reflect on practice, with the aim of developing quality care, accountability, personal competence and learning."*

Because of the emotionally taxing nature of work in the caring professions and the importance of professional judgement in decision making, it is vital that employees have a 'safe space' to discuss work-related issues with someone who understands. Supervision in the caring industries usually consists of a regular meeting between two professionals where one can discuss dilemmas, unusual cases or workplace stressors in a confidential and supportive space. Generally, the supervisor will be a more experienced or senior member of the team. For supervision to be effective, the relationship between the supervisor and supervisee is important. The supervisee needs to trust that the supervisor will maintain confidentiality and be non-judgemental, otherwise they will not feel comfortable opening up about their work-based concerns. For example, a social worker may have had to make a difficult decision about whether a home setting was safe or not. Although they followed the guidance and carried out their professional duties appropriately, they may have doubts about the decision they made. They may find themselves worrying about the welfare of the family in their own time and wondering 'what if ...'. The social worker would discuss this with their supervisor at their next session. The supervisor would invite the supervisee to explain the case, talk about their feelings, discuss how they made the decision, reassure them that they did the right thing or even support them in taking steps to change the decision if needed. The supervisor may also have additional knowledge or experience which they can share with the supervisee to help them to feel more confident in the decision they made. By discussing the case in this way, the supervisee will hopefully feel more comfortable with the decision they made, reducing the emotional impact of their work and promoting professional wellbeing (Bourn and Hafford-Letchfield 2011).

Different professional bodies have differing guidelines for how regularly supervision should take place, but it is important that supervision sessions are clearly scheduled times where the supervisor and supervisee can meet in private and with clear purpose. Often, in a busy care setting, supervision meetings can be postponed or cancelled due to issues with staffing levels. It is also common for supervision meetings to be 'hijacked' by discussions about other day-to-day matters, rather than being used for their true purpose (Lambley and Marrable 2013). In emotionally taxing professions, it is vital that managers protect supervision time to support the welfare of their employees and prevent emotional burnout.

Reducing Stress and Preventing Burnout

Wall et al. (1997) found that NHS employees were significantly more likely to suffer from minor psychiatric disorders (e.g. depression) than the general public. Factors such as shift work, handing emotionally challenging situations, and making vital decisions under pressure, make working in health and social care demanding for individual workers which can be detrimental to their physical and psychological wellbeing. However, when the intense nature of the work itself is combined with the pressures of working in an overstretched or struggling system, it can become a stressful occupation. In 2018, 8.7% of staff leaving employment in the NHS cited a lack of work-life balance as their reason for resigning. This figure had increased from 3,689 to 10,257 per year between 2010 and 2018 (NHS Digital 2019). These figures may be indicative of the significant changes in the management and working conditions within the NHS during this period. The term 'burnout' describes a breaking point in the wellbeing of an employee, a point at which they no longer feel able or willing to continue in their current role. Maslach (2003) defined job burnout using three dimensions: exhaustion, cynicism, and a sense of inefficacy. Burnout is particularly prevalent in the caring and human services professions and is the result of continued emotional and interpersonal stress experienced in the workplace. Bowers et al. (2011) found that good quality leadership led to effective teamwork which significantly lowered burnout levels amongst staff in UK psychiatric wards, showing that managers have a vital role in helping to reduce stress and avoid burnout. Job dissatisfaction and alienation, resulting from changes to the nature of caring roles may also be associated with burnout (Iliffe and Manthorpe 2019). The restructuring of teams, increases in paperwork, focus on quantitative targets and increased reliance on technology has reduced the amount of meaningful face-to-face time many caring professionals spend with service users. Over time, this erosion of the interpersonal dimension of the role may lead to dissatisfaction with the job, causing stress and increasing the likelihood of burnout or resignation.

The Covid-19 pandemic has added to the pressure experienced by staff in the industry. A mixed methods study by Gemine et al. (2021) found that being in a role directly involved in managing the Covid-19 pandemic, feeling unable to rest during breaks and having concerns about PPE supply, were linked to significantly higher levels of stress and risk of burnout. Whilst the added workload and pressure of the pandemic itself could not have been avoided, ensuring that staff felt able to rest during breaks without interruption could have helped reduce stress and increase productivity in the workforce. It is important that managers encourage staff to take breaks, even during busy periods, and that they ensure these breaks are not interrupted. Measures which can help with this may include providing a 'break room' or similar space away from the workstation, having a 'no meetings at lunchtime' policy, and encouraging staff to disconnect from their work emails outside of working hours. Whilst individual managers have a key role in reducing stress and avoiding burnout within their team, wider policy changes and interventions are clearly needed to tackle this endemic issue. Industry wide initiatives such as workload reviews, counselling support for workers, and flexible working arrangements need to be explored if we hope to make significant improvements.

Section 2: External Factors Influencing the Management of Services in Recent Years

Funding the NHS

The UK has a national health system (the NHS), a publicly funded organisation providing care to all for free at the point of access. This means that all citizens are entitled to healthcare without needing to pay for their care directly or through personal medical insurance. Services are funded by the contributions of taxpayers. We have various types of taxes in the UK, which are either collected directly from households, individuals, and companies (e.g. income tax) or indirectly (e.g. value added tax on products or services). Individuals in the UK also pay National Insurance contributions during their working life which fund a variety of services. The majority of revenue from taxation is managed by the central government who use it to provide services nationally. We also have taxes raised by local government (e.g. council tax) which fund some services within the specific region where they were raised (Baggott 2004). The UK was the first in the world to have a fully publicly funded health care system, though may other countries now have similar systems. Examples include: Egypt, Hong Kong, Sri Lanka, Sweden and Cuba. Other countries have healthcare systems which are predominantly government funded, though citizens have to pay a contribution either through regular insurance payments or one-off payments for certain services (Britnell 2015).

An alternative to having a publicly funded health care system is to have a private system in which individuals must pay for their care either through private medical insurance or by paying for their treatment directly. For example, the USA has a predominantly private health care system meaning that whilst some basic health care is provided free of charge to the most vulnerable, the majority of citizens must pay for private health insurance. The cost of health insurance can be high, and the quality of cover varies greatly depending on how much you pay, with many having additional costs. It is common for Americans to have to pay top-up charges for individual treatments or find that certain types of care are not covered by their insurance leaving them with difficult choices to make. For example, if you need a life-saving surgery that is not covered by your insurance, you may have to pay hundreds of thousands of dollars to have it. Unexpected medical bills are a common cause of bankruptcy in the USA (Britnell 2015).

Whilst the NHS is held in high esteem by many, there is much debate about whether such a system continues to be viable in the modern era. The cost of funding the NHS is continuously rising, and it needs an influx of money to support modernisation. Under the current system, it is difficult to see how such money could be raised without significant increases in taxation. In the near future we could see a move towards more of a hybrid public-private healthcare system where the majority is funded by taxation but individuals also make top-up contributions too. We already pay prescription charges in England which make a contribution towards the true cost of our medication, we could see similar charges being introduced. For example, a charge of £10 for GP consultations would raise an additional £1.2 billion for the NHS annually (Warner and O'Sullivan 2014). Countries such as France and Australia have introduced similar measures in recent years. It could be argued that these measures would reduce waste as it would deter individuals from missing appointments. However, such changes would undoubtably be met with significant resistance both from the public and left-wing political parties and raise concerns about equal access to health care for all.

Commissioning Healthcare Services

The term commissioning refers to the planning, funding and monitoring of a service. The health and care industry consists of a wide range of public sector, private sector and third sector organisations, each with their own priorities, methods of governance and ways of working. In this section we will explore how the NHS is funded to explore what effect this has on the planning, provision and management of healthcare services.

Whilst the NHS is overseen at national level by the Minister for Health and Social Care and NHS England, it is divided into 211 smaller Clinical Commissioning Groups (CCGs) with relative autonomy over their own budget for a specific area. These CCGs came into being as a result of the Health and Social Care Act (2012) which bought in a range of reforms to improve the efficiency and quality of health and care services in the UK. Essentially, each CCG is allocated a budget to spend on providing health care services in their area. The benefit of this is that each CCG can examine the health needs of their area and provide services to meet these localised needs. Each CCG still has to comply with national standards governing the range and type of healthcare they must provide. However, they have flexibility in the way they do this in their area. For example, a CCG in a rural area with lots of remote villages and an ageing population may decide that air ambulances, district nursing and geriatric services are a priority. By contrast, an urban CCG covering a city with a younger population may prioritise services such as 24-hour walk-in centres. Critics of this system argue that this can result in a 'Postcode-lottery' where individuals are entitled to different types of care dependent on where they live.

Each CCG also has control over who provides their services. For example, if a CCG needs to commission 1,000 hours of counselling sessions in an area they can invite local providers to tender for the contract to deliver this. So, if there is a local private counselling practice which could provide this, they can put in a bid to the CCG for the contract. The CCG may receive bids from a range of providers, including charities and private organisations. The CCG will carefully consider each bid and choose the provider which is most suitable to provide the service and the best price. This process of commissioning services is effectively a marketplace for care provision. One benefit of this system is that it can save money as providers are competing with each other for the CCG contract, this encourages them to lower their prices to ensure their bid is most attractive. Private companies are often able to operate more efficiently than large public sector organisations and so can offer services at a cheaper rate. However, this process of providing services as cheaply as possible can result in a reduction in the quality of care provided. It has also been criticised as it results in large amounts of public sector money being spent with private sector contractors (Dowd 2019; Hurley 2021). Many people feel that public sector money should not be given to private sectors organisations who make a profit from it.

Consumer Expectations

At its inception in 1948, the purpose of the NHS was to provide medical care to all, free at the point of delivery. This was a radical idea with many critics doubtful that it was possible. Many questioned the cost as well as the social impact of free health care – would it make people more careless with their health? Over the last seven decades, the NHS has become a prized institution which many Britons feel proud to be part of. However, it is still the subject of much criticism. The cost of the NHS has risen consistently since 1948 as medical science has developed. Many conditions which were incurable 70 years ago now have cures. The development of surgical technology, genetic sciences and pharmacological advances have undoubtably increased the overall health and life expectance of the nation. However, such treatments are expensive. Our expectations of what the NHS should provide have also changed over time. Aneurin Bevan's proposal for a National Health System in the 1940s did not include the holistic and preventative care we expect today. Prompt access to vaccination programmes, health screening initiatives, preventative medicine, community based mental health care, contraceptive provision, and social care costs are examples of things which would not have been expected by NHS service users in 1948. A modern, holistic care system comes with a modern price tag. In the financial year 2020/2021 the Department of Health and Social Care's total budget was £149.8bn (plus £51.9bn of additional Covid-19 funding) (The King's Fund 2022). This is by far the biggest departmental budget and represents a significant proportion of the government's total spending. Such significant expenditure requires scrutiny to ensure that taxpayer money is being spent in the taxpayer's best interests.

Modern consumers are accustomed to private companies asking for feedback on their service and expect them to respond to complaints appropriately. Similarly, service users often view themselves as customers or consumers of NHS services, with expectations about the quality of care they should receive (Hunt et al. 2015). These consumer expectations can be seen as a challenge or an opportunity by managers of services. Whilst unrealistic expectations can be hard to manage, feedback is a rich source of information leading to significant improvements in service quality (Adams 2011). The views of service users can be invaluable in helping care providers understand what it feels like to use the service and often propose creative solutions to issues which may not have been previously considered.

Health and social care providers gather service user feedback in a variety of ways, including:

- Focus groups
- Suggestion boxes
- A dedicated feedback or complaints email address
- Online questionnaires
- Resident's committee meetings

One key tool used by the NHS to gain feedback is the 'Friends and Family Test' (NHS 2020). This is a simple two question survey which patients are asked to complete after an appointment or being discharged. It asks the patient how likely they are to recommend the service to friends or family on a six-point scale from 'extremely likely' to 'extremely unlikely'. It then asks them to explain why they scored their experience the way they did. The overall score received by the service is published on the NHS website for the service. Many providers also collate the written responses and create a display showing what has been implemented in response to any issues raised.

In modern health and social care, managers must be aware of the expectations the community has of their service. It is vital that they involve service users in helping to improve service quality. Complaints must be responded to promptly, ensuring that the service user understands the actions taken in relation to their complaint.

Service Level Targets

With a huge proportion of the government's budget being spent on health and social care, it is important that service providers are held accountable for the quality of the service they provide. One method used to ensure this is to set service level targets. These are targets which are used to measure how well a service is performing in relation to key performance indicators, for example waiting times, resource utilisation, or MRSA infection rates. In 1999, the Performance Assessment Framework (PAF) was introduced which set out a range of quality indicators against which NHS services would be measured. Services were inspected and audited regularly and given a star rating based on how well they were performing. It was hoped that this system would improve services and hold individual providers accountable for quality. However, the use of such targets was heavily criticised. Many managers felt that the targets were unachievable with the budget and resources they had available and that the system actually demotivated staff as they felt they were being blamed for failing to reach targets over which they had little control. Such targets are also criticised for being overly reductionist and quantitative, rather than measuring the quality of care holistically (Bardsley in Walshe & Smith 2016, pp. 390–416).

The content and parameters of these targets is constantly debated, with such frameworks under regular review to try to develop a fair and representative set of measures. In recent years, the CCG Improvement and Assessment Framework 2018/19 was implemented, and then replaced again by the NHS Oversight Framework 2019/20 (NHS England 2021). For managers of services, these frequent changes to the measures against which they are assessed can be a source of great stress. These issues are often compounded when there are political changes. For example, the appointment of a new Minister for Health and Social Care often foreshadows significant changes to the priorities or structure of the NHS, which has a cascade effect through the sector. New policies or initiatives at national level must eventually be implemented at local level by service managers. An example which has attracted much media attention in recent years is the four-hour waiting time target for Accident and Emergency (A&E) services. In 2004, the government announced that it aimed for 98% of patients attending A&E departments in

England would be seen within four hours of arriving. In the years following this announcement, providers of A&E services experienced intense pressure to meet this target. Many were expected to reduce waiting times without being allocated additional funds or resources to do so which seemed an impossible task. This target was criticised for putting pressure on hospitals to admit or discharge patients quickly as the four-hour point loomed to ensure they hit the target. Such practices are a wasteful use of resources and can result in harm to patients (Eatock, Cooke and Young 2017). This example shows how targets can in fact be harmful to care quality, rather than improve it as intended.

Conclusion

This chapter has introduced a range of challenges currently faced by managers of health and care services. In discussing managers' key responsibilities, it is clear that the role of 'manager' in health and social care is different to similar roles in other industries. Managers of care services play a key role in ensuring the quality of care provided and in safeguarding the wellbeing of their staff. Managers of services are also subjected to a wide range of external pressures which impact on the way a service is run.

Whilst this chapter has explored several challenges faced by managers of health and care services in 21st century Britain, there are many more to come. With the development of communication technologies, artificial intelligence and robotics, it is likely that managers of services will soon be faced with difficult decisions about how to integrate technological advancements into their services. The Covid-19 pandemic has shown that care can be provided effectively at a distance, using video calling to triage care or provide consultations for issues which do not need direct physical contact for diagnosis. Therapeutic interventions such as counselling therapies have also been delivered successfully using video calling. Multiagency teams have learned quickly to work together effectively without physical meetings. Vaccines have been developed by sharing knowledge across vast distances using online communication to accelerate research. This raises questions about the value of face-to-face encounters. Managers may need to weigh the cost of retaining office and consultation spaces against the value of a face-to-face encounter. Do service users gain the same feeling of care quality via a screen? Does an employee truly feel supported by a manager whom they have never met in person? Such debates are likely to be ongoing in years to come.

The Covid-19 Pandemic also shone a light on the endemic issues with staffing numbers within health and care services. Understaffed providers struggled to deliver care safely with significant levels of staff illness and the additional workload which social distancing, quarantine and screening procedures imposed. Urgent intervention is needed to ensure that the current staffing and skills shortage within the health and social care industry does not present a significant risk to care quality and care provision (The King's Fund 2018). It is likely there will also be intense debate about the viability of maintaining an NHS which is free to all at the point of delivery in the modern world. In short, whilst this chapter has discussed some of the current challenges faced by managers in the industry, it is clear that there are turbulent times ahead and services will need to adapt rapidly to change.

Moment of reflection

After reading this chapter, take time to reflect upon or discuss the following questions:

- To what extent is the wellbeing of a professional the responsibility of their manager?
- What impact can good management have on the quality of service provision?
- What makes a good manager: a professional who has 'risen through the ranks' or someone with qualifications and experience in management?

Key Terms

- Whistleblowing
- Supervision
- Stress
- Burnout
- Privatisation
- Commissioning
- Consumer expectations
- Clinical Commissioning Groups
- Service Level Targets

References

Adams, S.A., 2011. Sourcing the crowd for health services improvement: The reflexive patient and "share-your-experience" websites. *Social Science & Medicine (1982)*, 72 (7).

André, B., Sjøvold, E., Rannestad, T., and Ringdal, G.I., 2014. The impact of work culture on quality of care in nursing homes - A review study. *Scandinavian Journal of Caring Sciences*, 28 (3).

Baggott, R., 2004. *Health and Health Care in Britain*. 3rd ed. London: Palgrave.

Bardsley, M., 2016. Measuring and managing healthcare performance. In: Walshe, K., and Smith, J., eds. *Healthcare management*. London: Mcgraw Hill, 2016, pp. 390–416.

Bourn, D., and Hafford-Letchfield, T., 2011. The role of social work professional supervision in conditions of uncertainty. *The International Journal of Knowledge, Culture and Change Management*, 10 (9), 41–56.

Bowers, L., Nijman, H., Simpson, A., and Jones, J., 2011. The relationship between leadership, teamworking, structure, burnout and attitude to patients on acute psychiatric wards. *Social psychiatry and Psychiatric Epidemiology*, 46 (2), 143–148.

Britnell, M., 2015. In *Search of the Perfect Health System*. London: Palgrave.

Cassedy, P., 2010. *First steps in clinical supervision*. Maidenhead: Open University Press.

Dowd, A., 2019. NHS is spending more on private providers despite government pledges. *BMJ* [online], 336. DOI: 10.1136/bmj.l4812

Eatock, J., Cooke, M., and Young, T., 2017. Performing or not performing: What's in a target?. *Future Health Journal*, 4 (3), 167.

Francis, R., 2013. *Report of the Mid Staffordshire NHS Foundation Trust: Public Inquiry Executive summary* [online]. London: House of Commons. Available at: https://assets. publishing.service.gov.uk/government/uploads/system/uploads/attachment_data/file/ 279124/0947.pdf [Accessed 12 March 2022].

Gemine, R., Davies, G.R., Tarrant, S., Davies, R.M., James, M., and Lewis, K., 2021. Factors associated with work-related burnout in NHS staff during COVID-19: A cross-sectional mixed methods study. *BMJ Open* [online], 11 (1), e042591. DOI: 10.1136/bmjopen-2020-042591

Hunt, D., Koteyko, N., Gunter, B., 2015. UK policy on social networking sites and online health: From informed patient to informed consumer? *Digital Health*, 1, 2055207615592513

Hurley, R., 2021. Covid-19: Billions spent on private contacts should have gone to public services, says people's inquiry. *BMJ*, 374.

Iliffe, S., and Manthorpe, J., 2019. The unexpected return of alienation: Job dissatisfaction, 'burnout' and work estrangement in the NHS. *Renewal: a Journal of Labour Politics* [online], 27 (4), 50–60.

Ion, R., Smith, K., Nimmo, S., Rice, and McMillan, M., 2015. Factors influencing student nurse decisions to report poor practice witnessed while on placement. *Nurse Education Today*, 35 (7), 900–905.

Lambley, S., and Marrable, T., 2013. *Practice enquiry into supervision in a variety of adult care settings where there are health and social care practitioners working together* [online]. London: Social Care Institute for Excellence. Available at: https://www.scie.org.uk/ publications/guides/guide50/#:~:text=Practice%20enquiry%20into%20supervision%20in, of%20settings%20including%20integrated%20settings [Accessed 12 March 2022].

Levett-Jones, R., and Lathlean, M., 2009. 'Don't Rock the Boat': Nursing students' experiences of conformity and compliance. *Nurse Education Today*, 29 (3), 342–349.

Maslach, C., 2003. Job burnout: new directions in research and intervention. *Current Directions in Psychological Science*, 12 (5), 189–192.

NHS Digital, 2019. *Leavers from the NHS by age and reason for leaving 2010–2019* [online]. London: NHS Digital website. Available at: https://digital.nhs.uk/data-and-information/ find-data-and-publications/supplementary-information/2019-supplementary-information-files/leavers-and-joiners/leavers-from-the-nhs-by-age-and-reason-for-leavingrom the NHS by age and reason for leaving 2010–2019 AH3120 - NHS Digital [Accessed 16 March 2021].

NHS Digital, 2020. *NHS workforce statistics July 2020* [online]. London: NHS digital. Available at: https://digital.nhs.uk/data-and-information/publications/statistical/nhs-workforce-statistics/july-2020. [Accessed 1 April 2021].

NHS England, 2021. *NHS oversight and assessment* [online]. London: NHS England. Available at: www.england.nhs.uk/commissioning/regulation/ccg-assess/ [Accessed: 01 April 2021].

NHS, 2020. *Friends and Family Test (FFT)* [online]. London: NHS England. Available at: https://www.nhs.uk/using-the-nhs/about-the-nhs/friends-and-family-test-fft/ [Accessed 16 March 2021].

Schein, E.H., 2015. Whistle blowing: A message to leaders and managers comment on 'cultures of silence and cultures of voice: The Role of Whistleblowing in Healthcare Organizations'. *International Journal of Health Policy and Management*, 5 (4), 265.

Skills for Care, 2020. *The Size and Structure of the Adult Social Care Sector and Workforce in England* [online]. Leeds: Skills for Care. Available at: Size and structure infographic 202 https://www.skillsforcare.org.uk/adult-social-care-workforce-data/Workforce-intelligence/documents/Size-of-the-adult-social-care-sector/Size-and-structure-infographic-2020.pdf 0 (skillsforcare.org.uk) [Accessed 16 March 2021].

The King's Fund, 2018. *The healthcare workforce in England: Make or Break?* [online]. London: The Kings Fund. Available at: https://www.kingsfund.org.uk/sites/default/files/2018-11/The%20health%20care%20workforce%20in%20England.pdf [Accessed 19 March 2021].

The King's Fund, 2022. *The NHS budget and how it has changed* [online]. London: The Kings Fund. Available at: https://www.kingsfund.org.uk/projects/nhs-in-a-nutshell/nhs-budget?gclid=CjwKCAiAprGRBhBgEiwANJEY7KxhJh1grFLp0tSDvsn8cKYwrRc7a8VXKKhq_keKWsWa_EDZ3bxutRoC3skQAvD_BwE [Accessed 12 March 2022].

Wall, T.D., Bolden, R.I., Borrill, C.S., Carter, A.J., Golya, D.A., Hardy, G.E., Haynes, C.E., Rick, J.E., Shapiro, D.A., and West, M.A., 1997. Minor psychiatric disorder in NHS trust staff: Occupational and gender differences. *British Journal of Psychiatry*, 171 (6), 519–523.

Warner, N., and O'Sullivan, J., 2014. *Solving the NHS Care and Cash Crisis: Routes to Health and Care Renewal*. London: Reform. Available at: https://www.bl.uk/collection-items/solving-the-nhs-care-and-cash-crisis-routes-to-health-and-care-renewal# [Accessed 18 March 2021].

Part III

12 Young People and Social Care

Aslihan Niscanci

Chapter Aims:

- Explore the impact of individual, familial and social factors that generate young people's social care needs
- Review and explain major policies and legislation regulating social care as it relates to young people
- Explore the impact of social, economic, and political forces on young people's social care and related public services
- Explore the impact of young people, who face increasing economic and social challenges, on society
- Highlight the increasing role of new technologies and new media on young people's social care
- Discuss the approaches and best practices to direct work and interventions with young people in need/with challenging behaviours
- Introduce approaches in social care service delivery systems and social policies which relate to young people

Introduction

Young people may need assistance and care for reasons including, but not limited to, abuse or neglect, health and mental health issues, drug and alcohol use, disabilities, sexual exploitation, immigration status, anti-social behaviours, harmful sexual behaviours, and being young carers. Social care aims to meet one or more of these needs. Service and intervention models are offered to young people and their families within the context of the existing policies, legislation, and service delivery systems. Numerous complex, dynamic and interrelated structural issues like poverty, unemployment, racism, discrimination surround these service systems and social care experiences of young people and their families. In this chapter, social care provided to young people with different needs and conditions is discussed with reference to relevant legislation and surrounding social forces. As commonly used and overarching frameworks, developmental-ecological perspective and strengths-based approach are elaborated for working with young people in social care. Examples of best practices are also presented under each subtitle with a focus on young people with disabilities and chronic health conditions, Refugees and Asylum Seekers, and young offenders. Thus, the chapter aims to help the readers critically evaluate a variety of theories,

DOI: 10.4324/9781003079873-15

models, approaches, and interventions targeting young people across a range of social care and institutional settings.

In legal documents, anyone under the age of 18 is defined as a child. The United Nations defines "youth" as persons between 15 and 24. The definition of youth or young people is more ambiguous and depending on the cultural context, the age range may change (United Nations, n.d.). For the purposes of this chapter, the definition of young people includes both children, teenagers, and even young adults.

Policy Context

In the UK, the main responsibility for the social care of children and young people is on the statutory sector, which provides services established by the law. Safeguarding children is the responsibility of the local authorities (UK Parliament 2021). Under the organisational scheme of the local authorities, the Director of Children's Services coordinates and provides social services such as assessing the needs of the young people and providing support. This support includes family support in the form of daycare for children under five, parenting support, family support work, practice home help and access to children's centre (NHS 2020). Voluntary and private sectors also provide social care services to children, young people and their families.

According to National Statistics, 3% of the 12 million children in England (400,000) are in the social care system at any one time and more than 80,000 of these children are children in care (Ofsted 2021). Within the social care system, 3,402 providers serve the children and young people's social care sector. These settings are (Ofsted 2021):

- Children's homes:

  - Secure children's homes
  - Residential special schools registered as children's homes
  - Short-break-only children's homes
  - Children's homes

- Independent fostering agencies
- Residential family centres
- Residential holiday scheme for disabled children
- Adoption support agencies
- Voluntary adoption agencies
- Secure training centres
- Boarding schools
- Residential special schools
- Further education colleges with residential accommodation

As of 31 March 2021, the number of providers in each setting is shared by Ofsted (2021): Table 12.1.

Table 12.1 The number of social care setting providers which serve children and young people as of 31 March 2021 (Ofsted 2021)

Setting	Number
Children's homes of all types	2,706
Independent fostering agencies	317
Residential family centres	59
Residential holiday schemes for disabled children	18
Adoption support agencies	38
Voluntary adoption agencies	37
Secure training centres	2
Boarding schools	60
Residential special schools	126
Further education colleges with residential accommodation	39

Safety, Risk and Safeguarding

Safeguarding is at the centre of young people's social care and is related to their protection from any kind of risk, harm, and threat to their wellbeing. The threat to young people's wellbeing can take the forms of "sexual, physical and emotional abuse; neglect; domestic abuse, including controlling or coercive behaviour; exploitation by criminal gangs and organised crime groups; trafficking; online abuse; sexual exploitation and the influences of extremism leading to radicalisation" (Department for Education 2018: p. 9). The government defines safeguarding as "preventing harm to children's health or development, ensuring children grow up with the provision of safe and effective care, and taking action to enable all children and young people to have the best outcomes" (Department for Education 2018: p. 9). This means that any social care activity that serves children and young people's wellbeing safeguards them directly or indirectly. Child protection is part of the safeguarding process and refers to the activity that is undertaken to protect specific children who are suffering, or are likely to suffer, significant harm (Department for Education 2018: p. 106).

The main issues related to safeguarding are abuse, neglect, and child sexual exploitation. Child abuse may be in the form of emotional abuse, physical abuse, sexual abuse, and neglect. Offences relating to modern slavery, human trafficking, female genital mutilation, child sexual exploitation, and witnessing domestic violence or abuse are categorised under child abuse. It is not easy to give an accurate estimate of the prevalence of child maltreatment. However, the rate of looked after children gives an idea of the prevalence of abuse and neglect. In 2019, there were 49,570 looked after children due to the risk of abuse or neglect in England (Office for National Statistics 2020a).

In the UK, local authorities have the duty of safeguarding children under 18, young people with disabilities, and looked after young people even when they are over 18. The Children Act 1989 and the Children Act 2004 are the main legal documents that bind the practitioners. Section 17 of the Children Act 1989 gives the local authorities the duty of safeguarding children in their area. After a "child in need" assessment, the family may receive support to safeguard the child's welfare. Under Section 17, the child is considered "in need" if:

- They need local authority services to achieve or maintain a reasonable standard of health or development
- They need local authority services to prevent significant or further harm to health or development
- They are disabled (The Children Act, 1989)

Based on this definition, different groups of children can be defined as "in need" such as disabled children, young carers, or asylum-seeking children. If there is a risk of suffering from significant harm, Section 47 of the Children Act 1989 holds local authorities responsible for investigating the child's situation if there is suffering or risk of suffering from significant harm. Consequently, the local authorities may take the child under their care. If the child is under local authority's care or is provided with accommodation for more than 24 hours, they are considered "looked after child" (The Children Act 1989).

Organisations need to follow best practices in safeguarding and use guidelines such as the NICE guidelines, Child Protection Evidence, and Child Protection Companion (Turney et al. 2018). They should work in collaboration and follow "Working together to Safeguard Children" (Department for Education 2018), which regulates the procedures of inter-agency working for the safeguarding of children. Being child-centred, which means keeping the child in focus when making decisions about their lives and working in partnership with them and their families (Department for Education 2018: p. 9), and putting children's needs first are fundamental to child safeguarding. In the midst of complex risks and safeguarding needs of today's society, high quality assessments should also be holistic, strengths-based, ecological, collaborative, rights-based, and evidence-informed (Department for Education 2018).

Safeguarding cannot be limited to the family environment and risks go beyond young people's home environment. Considering the multi-layered nature of risks of abuse and harm, contextual safeguarding (CS) was proposed as a practice model (Firmin 2020). Contextual safeguarding draws attention to the interplay of the environments surrounding the child. It is acknowledged that harm occurs within the context of individual choice-environmental constraints interaction and ways of creating safe environments may differ for each young person (Firmin and Lloyd 2020). In today's rapidly changing societies, the internet and social media, which can pose risks for young people, should also be part of the risk assessment procedures. We are facing new risks of harm such as cyberbullying, which is more complex than traditional bullying and may pose greater emotional and social risks (Ansari 2020). In England and Wales, 70% of children reported that they were emotionally affected by online bullying and it mostly happened at school (Office for National Statistics 2020b). Extremism, which young people are often exposed to via the internet environment, is another risk. Research shows that social media is one of the factors that may lead to young people's radicalisation (Alava, Frau-Meigs, and Hassan 2017) and precautions should be taken to protect young people.

Child welfare involvement in children's lives for safeguarding purposes is not independent of structural factors. Recent and eye-opening research (Bywaters 2020) clearly showed that children from low socioeconomic status families and economically deprived neighbourhoods had a higher likelihood of being involved in child protection services in the UK. Consequently, we can confidently argue that child protection is not limited to safeguarding services but also includes advocacy for social justice.

Young People with Disabilities and Chronic Health Conditions

A child is defined as disabled "if he is blind, deaf or dumb or suffers from mental disorder of any kind or is substantially and permanently handicapped by illness, injury or congenital deformity or such other disability as may be prescribed" (The Children Act 1989). Some young people may have two or more disabilities, or a disability and a mental health condition, which require high levels of support on a daily basis. This group is called "young people with complex needs" (YPCNs). A child is defined to have "complex needs" when they are diagnosed with an illness, disability, cognitive impairment, behavioural or social communication disorders, learning disability or sensory impairment which requires additional daily support (NHS National Institute for Health and Care Excellence 2019). Complex needs may come from birth or emerge after an illness or injury. In this sense, it is reasonable to say that 'complex needs' is a narrower category under disability. 8% of children in the UK are disabled (Department for Work and Pensions 2019). The number of disabled children with complex needs is rising, which is attributed to technological advances and the survival of preterm babies (Council for Disabled Children and the True Colours Trust 2017). While the number of disabled children and young people with complex and life-limiting conditions (aged 0–19) was 49,300 in 2004, it reached 73,000 in 2017 (Council for Disabled Children and the True Colours Trust 2017). This trend means that the social care needs of this population have been and will be increasing along with health and education needs.

Disabled children are defined as children "in need" by Section 17 of The Children Act 1989. As of 2020, 12.6% of all 389,260 children in need has a disability recorded in England (UK Government Statistics 2020). To meet the ongoing health, mental health, care, education needs of children and young people with a long-term condition, every child or young person is registered and monitored by the local NHS services and local authorities. Education, health and care (EHC) need assessments are implemented by social care teams, disabled children's teams, and special education needs and disability teams within local authorities (Council for Disabled Children 2016). Voluntary sector organisations such as charities are also involved in service provisions in many cases. Needless to say, collaboration and coordination between these teams are very crucial for effective practice.

Along with their ongoing care needs, children and young people may need specialised social care for reasons such as abuse, neglect, or family difficulties (Council for Disabled Children and the True Colours Trust 2017). Research shows that disabled children and young people are more vulnerable to maltreatment than their non-disabled peers and they are overrepresented in the looked-after population (The Children's Society 2009). These statistics underline the importance of raising awareness on the possibility of maltreatment in practice with this population and several legislative pieces and service plans mention this underestimated risk (Department for Education 2018; Department of Health 2004). Standard 8 of the National Service Framework for Children, Young People and Maternity Services 2004 regulates the legal responsibilities to ensure that all disabled children are safeguarded (The Children's Society 2009).

The disability movement played a pivotal role in addressing disabled individuals' needs properly. The grass-roots disability rights movement from the 1960s onwards heavily criticised the deficit-oriented, medical model of disability and brought about the social model, which indicates that it is the social, not the individual that leads to exclusion of individuals with disabilities (Barnes 2012). This critical perspective permeated into the service provision frameworks/approaches targeting disabled young people. Hence, creating the least restrictive environment and challenging all forms of disability-related exclusion, discrimination and oppression should be the goal of practice and policies. Not doing so would be in contrast with the gains that the disability rights movement achieved as a result of decades of struggle and advocacy. Disability and health issues are often not the only form of oppression disabled children and young people face. Young people may be at the intersections of differences and different forms of oppression. Therefore, other categories of discrimination such as class, race, ethnicity, gender or immigration status should be given due consideration in practice with children and young people with disabilities. Anti-oppressive practice (Dominelli 2002) and intersectionality can be guiding principles.

While addressing young people's issues, too much focus on the challenges they face put us at the risk of ignoring their strengths and potential. Several legislative gains aimed at transforming the social domain. The Disabled Person's Act 1986, the Disability Discrimination Act 1995 and the Disability Discrimination Act 2005 were issued to address individuals' rights to information access, employment, and all service provisions including education and transportation (Larkin 2009). Despite these efforts, discrimination is still rife and legislation could not fully ensure disability rights.

Despite commonalities, each young person's experiences and needs are unique. Moreover, having a disability or complex needs is not their primary defining characteristic. A person-centred approach should be adopted to taylor individual needs. In line with The Children and Families Act 2014, children and families should be regarded as the central partners in the design and delivery of health and social care services and their needs and wishes should be at the centre of planning for their care (Reeder and Morris 2018).

Lastly, the health and social care needs of children and young people with disabilities or complex needs require a joint, integrated, and inter-agency approach. Multi-level, coordinated, continuous, negotiated, with the least intrusive and most effective services are suggested as the principles to provide care across systems to children and young people with complex needs (Ungar et al. 2014).

Social Care with Refugees and Asylum Seekers

An asylum seeker is a person who fled from their country of origin and crosses international borders for reasons of safety and applies for refugee status under Article 1 of the 1951 Genova Convention. An asylum seeker receives the refugee status after their application is assessed and the status is given by the government under the 1951 Genova Convention based on a well-founded fear of persecution if they returned home due to race, religion, nationality, political opinion or membership of a particular group (UNHCR 1951). The UK received 31,752 asylum applications in the year ending in September 2020 (Refugee Council 2020). Amongst asylum seekers and refugees, there are young people with different social care needs and the complex interplay of social care needs and their immigration status may complicate assessment and intervention. Some of these young people are unaccompanied children seeking asylum (UCSAs), which means that they have no responsible adult to care for them. There are two aspects worth discussing here: (1) The issues young people face due to their asylum seeker or refugee status, (2) Young people's specific needs due to their status.

In the UK, asylum seekers are provided housing and financial support via UK Visas and Immigration (UKVI) and Asylum Support (Previously National Asylum Support Service/NASS), while they wait for the government's asylum decision. As part of this scheme, children and young people are eligible for free state school and health care (UK Government 2020). Asylum seekers do not have the right to work. This means that asylum-seeking young people's carers, either parents or relatives, cannot work due to their immigration status.

When asylum-seeking or refugee children and young people have social care needs, the same legislation regulating social care for children and young people in general applies. For example, when they are "in need", Section 20 of the Children Act 1989 is applied and local authorities have the responsibility of safeguarding the young person and meeting the accommodation needs within their areas. In cases including child trafficking, Section 31 of the Children Act 1989 may be more appropriate. Unaccompanied asylum-seeking children (UASCs) are defined as "in need" and entitled to the full assessment and support of their needs by the local authorities. According to The Nationality, Immigration and Asylum Act 2002, local authorities and voluntary organisations are reimbursed for the support they have provided for UASCs. The Children (Leaving Care) Act 2000 also applies to refugee young people and the local authorities provide support to them while they are leaving care after age 18. The UK government gave protection to 41,000 children between 2010 and 2020 and received 2,795 asylum applications from unaccompanied children in 2020, which is 10% of all applications (Refugee Council 2020). It is very important to support UASCs with access to immigration-related advice at the initial phase of the social care planning process because immigration status-related issues may affect young people's rights and entitlements when they move to independence (Children's Legal Centre 2020).

Young people with asylum seeker or refugee status frequently have challenging experiences before, during and after their migration. Research shows that refugee young people either themselves were subject to inhumane treatment or watched their family members being tortured, raped, or murdered (Hek 2005). In addition, it is hard to deny the challenges refugee children and youth face in the UK including poor quality of services (Kohli 2006), adaptation issues, poverty, disconnect from education, health and mental health care access, parent disconnect from education, intergenerational conflict, racism, discrimination, social exclusion, and anti-immigrant discourses and policies (Hek 2005). In the case of unaccompanied refugee young people, highly supportive living arrangements such as foster care is reported to lead to better youth wellbeing outcomes (Rip et al. 2020). In order to consider past and future trauma risks, trauma-informed care principles are recommended in the organisation of all services (Ostrander, Melville, and Berthold 2017). The stabilisation, adaptation and integration needs of young people (Cairns 2013) with traumatic backgrounds should be met in all social care settings. Adopting a child-centred, holistic, inclusive, and needs-based approach and focusing on education, employability, and trauma recovery are suggested depending on the unique experiences of the young person (Ramsay 2020). On the other hand, social care professionals should not underestimate the power of the individual, family, and community-level protective factors in the lives of refugee youth, hence should not ignore their coping skills (Ní Raghallaigh and Gilligan 2010), such as resilience. Stable settlement and social support are the key protective factors for their psychological wellbeing (Fazel et al. 2012). While it is hard to make generalisations, some of the protective factors for refugees in different countries are recorded as strong cultural and family values, bilingualism, valuing education, two-parent families, strong community bonds and better physical health. In practice settings, providing support for present issues is suggested to give hope about the future and increase their present quality of life before handling past issues (Hek 2005). Lastly, social care practitioners should be aware that young people's home environments may display different sociocultural characteristics. It is crucial for them to reflect upon their skills of navigating within the diverse cultural world and work on their cultural competency.

Violence, Crime and Social Care

When young people under 18 commit a criminal offence, they are called "young offenders" (Ministry of Justice 2012) and they become part of the "youth justice system". Youth violence is recognised as a global public health problem by World Health Organisation and globally homicide is the fourth leading cause of death in people aged 10–29 years (WHO 2020). While youth offence rates differ from one country to another and within each country, UK statistics show that there were 49,100 proven offences committed by children in the year ending March 2020 (Ministry of Justice 2021). 31% of all proven offences were violence against the person and sexual offences accounted for 2%, which is the smallest proportion of all offences (Ministry of Justice 2021). While the overwhelming majority of youth violent crime offences are individual offences, 27,000 children identify as gang members (Children's Commissioner 2019). Furthermore, 313,000 children aged 10–17 know someone who is a street gang member (Children's Commissioner 2019).

Two institutions are important for youth offending in the UK: (1) Youth Offending Teams (YOTs) under local authorities, and (2) Youth detention accommodations. In YOTs, 10–18-year-old youth are supervised upon court decision or when they are at risk for an offence. YOTs are multi-agency teams and have been effective on the dramatic decrease in youth reoffending in recent years (Youth Justice Board 2015). When a child is charged with an offence, they attain "looked after" status and are remanded into local authority accommodation or Youth Detention Accommodation. Local authorities implement the care plan and support the child's family. In England and Wales, three are three types of youth detention accommodations:

- Young Offenders Institution (YOI): These institutions are for boys aged 15–17 and young adult men aged 18–21. There are five YOIs in England and Wales.
- Secure Training Centre (STC): These centres are for people aged up to 17. They give 30 hours of education and training a week, following a school day timetable.
- Secure Children's Home (SCH): They are run by local councils and are for people aged 10 to 14.

When a child or person under 18 is remanded or sentenced to custody, the Youth Custody Service (YCS) decides where to place them. Youth offending teams (YOTs) provide information to the YCS's Placement Team about the needs, risks and circumstances of each young person (HM Prison & Probation Service 2020). Over decades, changes occurred in how youth violence and young offenders are viewed and treated. In the first half of the twentieth century, there has been a shift from a punitive approach to a welfare approach in youth justice in the whole world (Trépanier and Rousseaux, 2018). Till the Criminal Justice Act 1991, welfare, care and treatment dominated the youth justice field in England and Wales (Brown 2005). The 1969 Children and Young Persons Act was the legislative expression of this welfare model (Bell, Hodgson, and Pragnell 1999). With the new Labour government in the UK in the 1990s, individuals and communities were targeted in the interventions as they were seen as the root cause of the youth crime problem (France, Bottrell, and Armstrong 2012). In this era, control, surveillance, management, and punishment replaced the welfare model to a great extent. Within this context, increasing emphasis was given to youth anti-social behaviour and "offender management" (Smith and Gray, 2019). From the 1990s onwards, social care agencies have been part of crime reduction strategies in the UK as a key government strategy (Williams 2009) and crime reduction and prevention became part of the obligations of local authorities in the UK (France, Bottrell, and Armstrong 2012).

There are intricate connections between social care and youth violence at institutional and sociological levels. Strikingly, children in care or with a history of care are overrepresented in the youth justice system and children in care are six times more likely to be cautioned or convicted of a crime than other young people (Prison Reform Trust 2016). Care leavers are reported to re-offend at greater rates and at higher levels of seriousness (McFarlane 2008). It is not being in care itself that increases the risk of violence and crime for young people, but the very conditions that led to their involvement in social care do (Youth Justice Board 2015). In other words, the reasons for being in care are often one of the risk factors for youth offending. Most of the risk factors for youth offending, such as problems at home, parental conflict, broken families, poor parental supervision, harsh discipline, abuse/neglect/domestic violence trauma, living in inner-city areas, poverty, homelessness, unstable accommodation, learning disabilities, are the very risk factors for youth offending. It is important for social care practitioners to be aware of the individual and environmental factors that influence youth violence. The individual-level factors include physiological, cognitive, and psychological level factors. Early maltreatment, attachment issues, and mental health problems are particularly important in understanding violent youth behaviour (Seifert and Ray 2012). The environmental level factors (Seifert and Ray 2012) include 1) family stressors such as violence in the household, parental substance use or mental health problems; (2) school stressors such as lack of academic success, school conflict and school suspension without treatment; (3) community stressors such as poverty, community violence, and availability of drugs and firearms; (4) media stressors such as violent TV and violent and anti-social video games. Being involved in social care and violence are often the result of similar factors, which are in a complex interplay with each other.

It is reasonable to say that all preventive and rehabilitative measures in youth social care also serve towards tackling youth violence and crime. Involvement in social care may precede involvement in the youth justice system or vice versa. Regardless, when the health, education and social care needs of young people are not properly met, the offending behaviour worsens (Luton 2012). Therefore, social care plays a vital role in both the prevention and rehabilitation of young people involved in violence and crime. In this case, social care practitioners should work in collaboration with and sometimes within youth offending teams, which implement youth crime prevention programmes and are multidisciplinary in nature. Social care practitioners should be aware of the risks of crime and make referrals to youth offending teams as necessary. Violence risk assessment, which includes comprehensive information from multiple sources on the young person's and their family's history (Seifert and Ray 2012), needs to be part of social care assessments. More specific assessment tools such as the Juvenile Sex Offender Assessment Protocol can be used when harmful sexual behaviours are involved (Turney et al. 2018).

The experiences of young people during care may also pose risks for offending behaviour. The following factors were identified to increase the likelihood of offending for young people in care: (1) Complex unmet emotional needs of looked-after children, (2) Multiple placement breakdowns for teenagers leading to greater instability, (3) Young people placed in high crime and high deprivation areas (Youth Justice Board 2015). Young people in foster care or adoption are less likely to be involved in the youth justice system compared to young people in residential care.

It is important to find a language that does not stigmatise children in need of social care while discussing the relationship between social care and youth offending. The root causes of youth criminal behaviour need to be addressed and work is implemented across multiple systems of the individual, family, school, community, and social welfare policies. Different from a control paradigm, which focuses on controlling the "deviant" behaviour preventing its reoccurrence, social care perspective underlines the circumstances that lead children and young people towards crime and draws attention to the social and political ecology as a contextual understanding of youth offending.

Prevention and early intervention at individual, family, and community levels are at the core of the social care approach to youth crime. Interventions which target young people with problematic behaviours and interventions that include therapeutic approaches such as skills training are shown to be effective prevention strategies (Ross et al. 2011). The evidence-based intervention strategies that focus on the individual, family, school, or community should be incorporated into social care practices to protect at-risk youth from violence and crime. Research shows that control and coercion-based techniques that invoke fear are ineffective in preventing youth crime and anti-social behaviour (Ross et al. 2011). This finding once more underlines the crucial role of social care in preventing and rehabilitating youth violence. Due to the high prevalence of traumatic experiences of the young people involved, youth offending teams should adopt a trauma-informed practice as suggested by the British Association of Social Workers (BASW 2017). In order to keep children and young people safe, a child-centred approach addressing the age-specific needs of the child is suggested (Youth Justice Board 2015).

It is also important to know the evidence-based practice models and the widely used concepts in the youth justice field. The following intervention modalities are commonly used as individual and family-focused intervention models: Multi-systemic therapy (MST), Functional Family Therapy (FFT), Multidimensional Treatment Foster Care (MTFC), Persistent Young Offender Projects (PYOP), Intensive Supervision and Support Programmes (ISSP), and Intensive Family Interventions

(Ross et al. 2011). In England and Wales, the preliminary evidence suggests that they are effective (Ross et al. 2011).

Some approaches and models guide and shape youth justice practice and policy areas. The following are some of the most common examples:

Children First, Offenders Second (CFOS)

Also known as the positive youth justice model, the wellbeing of children are prioritised irrespective of their criminal behaviour in this model (Smith and Gray, 2019). The model challenges the stigmatisation of young people and punitive measures.

Youth Restorative Justice

Implemented by Youth Justice Board and together with YOTs, the model brings the offender and the victim together for communication. The offender hears the effects of their crime on the victim, who in turn has a voice. It aims to divert young people from the criminal justice system in their minor offences and antisocial behaviour and reduces reoffending rates (Restorative Justice Council 2015).

Positive Behaviour Framework

The model uses behavioural strategies to develop positive relationships between staff and young people within the youth custody service (Ministry of Justice and HM Prison and Probation Service 2019).

Government's Serious Violence Strategy

This strategy was published in 2018 as a response to an increase in gang involvement and criminal exploitation (Children's Commissioner 2019). Six pots of funding were announced to support issues facing disadvantaged young people.

The complexity of young peoples' experiences is not confined to protected groups. Housing, caring, the perils of social media, ideological manipulation, and cross-cutting themes of intersectional oppressions contextualise and situate young peoples' experiences in a complex web of overlapping networks from cyberbullying to extremism.

Perspectives in Social Care for Young People

Three perspectives or approaches are pivotal in understanding and contextualising young people's social care needs: (1) Developmental-ecological perspective, (2) Strengths-based approach (SBA), (3) Trauma-informed care. While these are not the only perspectives guiding social care for young people, they need to be prioritised in guiding services.

The developmental-ecological perspective considers both the environmental systems and developmental issues to understand the young person (Derksen 2010). From a developmental point of view, young people are in the midst of rapid biological and psychological changes, including an active search for their identities. They are also surrounded by interacting systems including, but not limited to, family, school, social care agencies, social policies, cultural and political settings.

A strengths-based approach (SBA) is a holistic and multidisciplinary approach that replaces a deficit and pathology-focused view with one emphasising young people's competencies and resources in social care services provision (Sabalauskas, Ortolani and McCall 2014). While young people's needs and difficulties are assessed, their resources are not ignored. The resources include personal, community, and social resources that empower young people. According to SBA, all services need to be rights-based and youth-centred. Young people are considered as the experts and in charge of their own lives as supported by the Mental Capacity Act (Social Care Institute of Excellence 2018). They should be treated with respect and dignity, as promoted by the national (Health and Social Care Act 2008) and international law (UN Convention on the Rights of the Child 1989). In addition, young people's participation in all decision-making processes related to their lives is the essential principle.

Trauma-informed care (TIC), with its micro and macro practice implications, has been highly recommended for use in agencies working with clients with trauma histories. What is astonishing about TIC is its simultaneous focus on both past traumas as well as the future trauma risks of the clients and staff members providing services. TIC needs to be an integral part of social care for young people considering the prevalence of trauma in their lives. When put into practice, TIC has the power of transforming the staff-client relationships, service delivery systems, organisational procedures, communities, and policies along with the principles of safety, trustworthiness and transparency, peer support, collaboration and mutuality, and empowerment. TIC has emerged out of increasing awareness of the prevalence and implications of childhood trauma in presenting issues in social care. Adverse Childhood Experiences (ACEs) of traumatic, harmful or stressful events and experiences have significant and long-lasting effects. Operationalising trauma-informed care and practice are unresolved with the direction, practice and organisational delivery of the big idea to the everyday practice still presenting a challenge. There is a need to develop a common definition that can be operationalized across different systems to address the implementation of TIC versus trauma-specific interventions. Social care for and with young people has work to do.

Conclusion

Young people may need social care, assistance and support for a range of complex and overlapping reasons. As elaborated in the chapter, often times, individual, familial and social factors lead to young people's social care needs. Service and intervention models are offered to young people and their families within the context of the existing policies, legislation, and service delivery systems. Different professions and service sectors play a role in supporting and safeguarding vulnerable children. Numerous complex, dynamic and interrelated structural issues like poverty, unemployment, racism, discrimination surround these service systems and social care experiences of young people and their families. The chapter presented issues of young people with disabilities and chronic health conditions, Refugees and Asylum Seekers, and young offenders. The readers are expected to develop a critical understanding of a variety of models, approaches, and interventions used in social care practice settings. The chapter also expects to support practitioners in planning and developing intervention strategies with a range of young people with complex and multiple challenges. Upon the dynamic and complex nature of the factors influencing young people in social care, the readers will probably reflect on their own personal value base as well. Therefore, the content hopefully contributed to the readers' competence in reflection and the self-awareness necessary to support personal and professional development.

Activity: Frank's Case

The aim of this activity is to show the importance of hearing the children's voice in social care and of assessing the case with a holistic perspective. The reader will look at Frank's case from different parties' perspectives and see the ways different professional groups see and handle cases.

Background Details

Frank is a fourteen-year-old young person, who loves sport and street dancing. Frank is a Child in Care (CIC) and is one of five siblings. He suffered chronic neglect and abuse before entering care from seven years of age. Frank was placed in Foster Care along with his youngest two siblings. When he was eight years of age, Frank was diagnosed with a Growth Hormone Deficiency 2. This is a medical condition caused by problems occurring in the pituitary gland. Following diagnosis, Frank was started on Growth Hormone Therapy.

Agencies involved:

- Children's Social Care (CSC)
- Police
- Local Clinical Commissioning Group (CCG) on behalf of NHSE for Primary Care
- Community Foundation Trust
- School 1
- School 2
- Acute Hospital
- Young Offending Service
- Virtual School
- Educational Psychology

Read the details on Frank's experiences with the police, schools/Virtual Head, foster carers, GP and offer medical staff, and CAMHS (Child and Adolescent Mental Health Service). Then, answer the following questions:

What do you think is going on?

What thoughts do you have on Frank's behaviour and what might you do to help him?

Do you think enough attempts are being made to listen to Frank?

Read the following Script and Assess Frank's Experiences with the Police

Two weeks after moving into the new placement Frank assaulted another pupil in school 1 by slapping and grabbing the pupil around the back of the neck and pulled the pupil towards a window and banged his head three times on the window causing bruising. Frank received an exclusion from School 1 for five days due to behaviour.

Following the assault at School 1, Frank was interviewed under caution by the Police and charged with assaulting a pupil. Frank received support from the Youth Offending Team during this time and engaged well in his sessions although it was noted that they did struggle with some of the concepts covered. Frank also had anger management one-to-one work. The Virtual School also had regular involvement with Frank during his period and weekly sessions were undertaken with them in School 1 to develop strategies for developing positive behaviour.

By the autumn of Frank's 12th year hey had moved to School 2 near to the Foster placement, Frank had settled well and was making good progress. Also, in autumn of the 12th year, Frank disclosed to the Foster Carers that an older sibling had tried to sexually assault him on numerous occasions and that his Mother had made him watch pornography and would hit Frank with a rolling pin. A Section 47 investigation was undertaken; and the younger siblings were also spoken to but made no disclosures.

Frank underwent two ABE (Achieving Best Evidence) interviews and his Mother was voluntarily interviewed by the Police but was released without charge. Frank's older sibling was arrested and interviewed during the investigation process also. After consideration, the decision was made by the Police that there was not a realistic chance of a prosecution. This was because Frank had significantly changed the story from the first interview and it was also of concern that Frank's medical notes, when reviewed, had noted the history of behavioural concerns and more notably "concerns regarding compulsive lying". This led the Police to believe that here would be no realistic chance of a prosecution as Frank would not have been a credible witness.

Read the Following Script and Assess Frank's Experiences with the School

In his eleventh year Frank was being seen by the therapist from the CAMHS. It was noted that Frank had been showing confrontational behaviour which had been getting worse since starting Secondary School. Frank was observed to be more comfortable in one-to-one situations and struggled with unstructured times throughout the day. Of particular concern was that the challenging behaviour observed in School was also developing in the foster placement. The therapist noted that the Foster Carers could at times view Frank in a negative context, but they were struggling with Frank's behaviours which were described as impulsive with Frank's mood changing quickly. Frank was also struggling with managing his emotions.

In January 2015 Frank was excluded by School 1 for three days due to persistent disruptive behaviour and defiance in lessons. School 1 had emailed the Social Worker with details of the incident which caused the exclusion and indicated that a drama/dance route for education would be sought when Frank returned to School.

The following week a meeting was held at the school regarding the exclusion. The Virtual School Head Teacher, Social Worker and the Head of Year met to discuss recent events. Frank's behaviour was not improving and the recent incidences in lessons were escalating. The Virtual School agreed to provide a behaviour support worker who could observe and support Frank and give staff strategies to help with classroom behaviour.

Two weeks after moving into the new placement Frank assaulted another pupil in school 1 by slapping and grabbing the pupil around the back of the neck and pulled the pupil towards a window and banged his head three times on the window causing bruising. Frank received an exclusion from School 1 for five days due to behaviour.

Following the assault at School 1, Frank was interviewed under caution by the Police and charged with assaulting a pupil. Frank received support from the Youth Offending Team during this time and engaged well in his sessions although it was noted that they did struggle with some of the concepts covered. Frank also had anger management one-to-one work. The Virtual School also had regular involvement with Frank during his period and weekly sessions were undertaken with them in School 1 to develop strategies for developing positive behaviour.

At age 14 Frank attended the medical bay in School 2 first thing feeling unwell. The Foster Carer was contacted, and Frank was sent home. Frank also presented at the sick bay on the 22nd day and 23rd day again feeling unwell. On the first occasion it was suggested that Frank try his lesson and come back if he still felt unwell. Frank was given an ice pack to cool his neck. On the second occasion the Foster Father was contacted and suggested that Frank should be encouraged to stay in class.

Assess Frank's Experiences with the Foster Carers

When aged 13 years and nine months Frank and the siblings attended the Endocrine Clinic for the routine six monthly reviews. The Consultant Paediatrician in attendance noted that Frank was compliant with the Growth Hormone treatment. The Growth Hormone dose was increased by 1.2 mg and the endocrine plan was updated to reflect annual blood tests to measure hormones and a repeat bone density scan was to take place in his 15th year.

The next week following the clinic appointment Frank was attended at the medical bay in school 2; Frank had fallen over on the school field after feeling dizzy and landed on the side of his face. Frank felt okay and wanted to go to his street dance lesson. The school nurse ensured that the dance teacher was informed of the incident and also informed the Foster Carers.

Seventeen days following the dizzy spell in school 2, Frank presented at A&E following a fainting episode in church, Frank also had abdominal pain and had fainted for a few seconds after feeling clammy. History which was given at

A&E included loss of consciousness for a few minutes, pale in colour and com plaining of right sided abdominal pain. Frank also had reduced eating and drinking for a few days. Medical investigations were undertaken, which included clinical observations, blood pressure, abdominal scan and urine tests; results of which all came back as within normal range. Frank was discharged home after being given pain relief and the episode was recorded as a vasovagal episode which is also known as a fainting episode. The results of the abdominal scan were received and there was no abdominal or pelvic abnormalities detected.

During this time feedback from Frank's school (2) during the PEP (Personal Education Plan) meeting continued to be very positive. Frank was engaged and working well. His behaviour and effort in lessons was described as excellent. Frank was keen to do well and was working towards becoming a prefect. In contrast, the Foster Carers had started to report some changes in Frank's behaviour which they were attributing to puberty and the impact of recent contact with the Mother. This contact had included his siblings, and all had struggled since his had taken place. The Foster Carers advised their Supervising Social Worker (SSW) hat hey felt that Frank was pulling away from them. Frank's Foster Carer advised Children Services that Frank was stealing money from them. The Foster Carers view was that Frank was stealing the money to buy junk food, this was on the basis that Frank was not eating with the family.

The Foster Carer contacted the GP at the beginning of the 2nd week of June for a telephone consultation. The Foster Carer advised the GP that Frank was complaining of 'not feeling well' and was experiencing cramps in his stomach. Moreover, that Frank was complaining of being dizzy, nauseous and generally unwell. The Foster Carer advised GP that Frank was 'faking' his symptoms and that Frank had started being sick when told to get ready for school. Frank was said to be screaming and crying when asked to get into the car. The Foster Carer believed that the current issues all began after the younger siblings had contact with Frank's mother; Frank had also disclosed abuse by his older sibling. The Foster Carers continued to identify a range of problems that they were experiencing with Frank including stealing money, getting up at night to eat food and having controlling behaviours. The GP was advised that the Social Worker was aware of these concerns. The GP concluded the telephone consultation and arranged for Frank to be brought to the surgery.

Assess Frank's Experiences the GP or other Medical Staff

In mid-June Frank was brought into the doctor's surgery accompanied by his Foster Carer. Frank was seen by the GP who had undertaken the telephone consultation with the Foster Carer. Initial problem was diagnosed as hyper-ventilation. Frank was on crutches and his leg was still in a plaster cast from a recent fracture. Frank was complaining of episodes of pain which spread across the lower ribs and into his chest. Frank also had experienced dizziness and tingly fingers and tingling around the mouth. Frank was observed to be breathing fast. The GP observed a quiet and meek looking child who appeared to be downcast and only smiled occasionally.

The GP attributed the tingling and dizzy sensations down to the fact that Frank was hyperventilating and that the symptoms were likely to be psychological in origin. Frank was offered mental health support but was not keen to access his; contact details for mental health support were given to Frank, and the Foster Carer was advised that this would be discussed with Frank's Social Worker. The GP noted that now Frank was growing up he was more aware of being a CIC. The GP noted that the Foster Carer lacked an empathetic approach. This is noted in the records but not acted upon by GP.

On the 3rd day of July Frank presented at with his Foster Carer, complaining of feeling unwell and was experiencing dizziness and vomiting. The Foster Carer's voice was heard during the consultation; informing the Doctors that Frank was fabricating his illness. Frank had not been attending school and was reported to be vomiting every morning and refusing to eat breakfast. The history taken by the Doctor identified that Frank had a history of depression and had made allegations of sexual abuse against Mother and older sibling. The Foster Carer reported that Frank had been staying in his room for three days refusing to leave. Frank had experienced mood changes and was awaiting an appointment with 'a counsellor'. This reference was likely in respect of the new referral that GP had made to CAMHS.

Frank was spoken to and denied making himself sick; advising hat he was unhappy but could not elaborate why. Clinical observations were carried out and Frank's blood pressure was noted to be elevated during three reviews 144/99, 152/103, 150/109. The Children's Early Warning Tool (CEWT) assessed Frank as Amber. The Early Warning Score is a guide used by medical services to quickly determine the degree of illness of a patient. The assessment at Amber required Frank to be reviewed within twenty,' minutes by a Senior Doctor. The review took place and Frank was diagnosed with regular vomiting and following pain relief and assessment by the crisis team was discharged home. Frank was clear with the practitioner that they felt physically unwell but that everything else was fine.

Continuing challenges in terms of Frank's behaviour led to the placement with his foster carers breaking down and ultimately Frank was placed in report foster care. On the 17th day of July the Respite Foster Carer contacted the GP. The Respite Foster Carer expressed concern that Frank was still being sick and advised that this was not self-induced. Frank was observed to vomit approximately an hour after food, he was also noted to hiccup and when sick observed to be bringing up bile and this was noted to be worse in the morning. The Respite Foster Carer advised the GP that she had been told that Frank's problems stemmed from trauma and that Frank was receiving psychological support from CAMHS but the Respite Foster Carer wondered if there was an acid reflux issue as she had given Frank antacids and these had helped marginally. The GP arranged to see Frank three days later for review.

On the 20th day of July the Respite Foster Carer and Frank presented at the GP surgery and were seen by the same Doctor whom had seen Frank during his previous presentation. Frank advised the GP hat "I feel sick, my eyes go blurry and I see two things, I go dizzy. Frank disclosed that they had been having headaches since month nine of his 13th year".

The Respite Foster Carer advised the GP that Frank was having episodes of vomiting and preferred to lie down. His sleep at night was observed to be poor. The Respite Foster Carer stated that Frank was taking what was happening in his stride. Frank was not currently in School 2. On examination the GP noted that Frank was limping and that his right foot appeared to have a loss of proprioception and Frank had an unsteady wide gait using his arms to balance and preferred to hold onto someone. A full assessment was undertaken. Frank's pupils were equal and reactive, nystagmus to right and diplopia (double vision) looking left. Neurological symptoms at that time were obvious and the GP made an urgent referral to the Acute Hospital for an urgent paediatric assessment that same day.

Assess Frank's Experiences with CAMHS (Child and Adolescent Mental Health Service) Professional

In his eleventh year Frank was being seen by the therapist from the CAMHS. It was noted that Frank had been showing confrontational behaviour which had been getting worse since starting Secondary School. Frank was observed to be more comfortable in one-to-one situations and struggled with unstructured times throughout the day. Of particular concern was that the challenging behaviour observed in School was also developing in the placement. The therapist noted that the Foster Carers could at times view Frank in a negative context, but they were struggling with Frank's behaviours which were described as impulsive with Frank's mood changing quickly. Frank was also struggling with managing his emotions.

During the months following his 13th birthday and following Frank being informed that the Police were to take no further action in respect of the allegations regarding the older sibling, there were some minor changes noted in Frank's behaviour in School 1. Frank was observed to be argumentative and at times defiant. In a five-week period Frank had five behaviour logs completed for disruptive behaviour in school. Around this same time period Frank and the younger siblings were discharged from CAMHS.

When Frank was 14 years of age a new referral was received by CAMHS. The referral stated that the Foster Carer was concerned for Frank's wellbeing. Information contained in the referral indicated that Frank was faking being ill. The referral was accepted by CAMHS. Also, at the end of June the Foster Carer again contacted the GP for a telephone consultation. The Foster Carer was concerned about Frank; the Foster Carer stated that Frank had not contacted CAMHS. Frank was refusing to go to school and would sit naked refusing to dress. When in school 2 the Foster Carer stated she was being contacted as Frank had vomited and needed to be brought home. Frank had attended contact with Mother the previous day and the Foster Carer advised the GP that Frank had asked for the contact to finish early; this was something Frank had never done before. The Foster Carer was concerned that Frank was becoming depressed. GP gave the Foster Carer the number for the CAMHS and advised the Foster Carer to ring that day, in addition GP referred Frank for a fast-track assessment and intervention. There was telephone contact between the Social Worker and the CAMHS practitioner that week. The records indicated that the

Social Worker was concerned as Frank had emotionally withdrawn from the Foster Carers. Frank was still being physically sick and stating he was unwell. There was also telephone contact between the Foster Carer and CAMHS on the same day, it was noted that the Foster Carer was indicating that there was a correlation between the symptoms Frank was experiencing and the trauma experienced in his childhood. Following the consultation an appointment letter was sent.

Frank was seen by CAMHS and a full assessment was undertaken. The assessment indicated that there was a complex picture of physical health issues which sat alongside offer emotional and relational issues. During the consultation it was observed that the relationship between Frank and the Foster Carer appeared to be deterioration further. This same day Frank was given a diagnosis of psychosomatic disorder.

What Happened in the End?

Frank and the Respite Foster Carer attended the Accident and Emergency Department at the local hospital. Clinical tests were undertaken, Frank's blood pressure was elevated 135/92 and pulse rate was 102. An MRI brain scan was undertaken, and a mass was seen on the MRI indicating a Brain Tumour. Paediatric Consultant and Paediatric Registrar discussed the results with the Respite Foster Carer and Frank.

Frank was informed that they were going to be transferred to a Paediatric Specialist Hospital for further treatment and Frank asked that his biological Mother to be present if they had to go to another hospital; his was agreed. Frank's previous Foster Carer was also informed about the diagnosis and attended the hospital. On the 21st day of July Frank underwent surgery to remove part of the tumour. Following the surgery,

Frank required intensive care treatment and was transferred to a ward after two days. Frank subsequently received both radiotherapy and chemotherapy but sadly died some months later in a children's hospice.

Indicative Reading

Bragg, S., and Kehily, M.J., (2013). *Children and young people's cultural worlds*. London: The Policy Press.

Burton, M., Pavord, E., and Williams, B., (2014). *An Introduction to Child and Adolescence Mental Health*. London: Sage Publishing.

A valuable introduction to children and young people and the risks and protective factors in relation to their mental health. Helpful edited chapters review child development, safeguarding, mental health promotion strategies, communication, interventions, group work and ethics and values.

References

Fleming, J., and Boeck, T., (2017). *Involving Children and Young People in Health and Social Care Research*. London: Routledge.

Participation and strategies for engaging children and young people with a focus on research but an absence of presenting issues and problems

Gitterman, A., (ed.) (2014). *Handbook of Social Work Practice with Vulnerable and Resilient Populations.* Columbia University Press.

Horwath, J., and Platt, D. (eds.) (2019). *The child's world: The essential guide to assessing vulnerable children, young People and their families.* Jessica Kingsley Publishers.

Horton, J., and Piyer, M. (eds.) (2017). *Children, Young People and Care.* Routledge.

Jackson, S., (2013). *Pathways Through Education for Young People in Care: Ideas from Research and Practice.* London BAAF.

Larkin, M., (2009). *Vulnerable groups in health and social care.* London: Sage. Broad overview of working with people in health and social care. Strategies, interventions and programmes less well developed.

References

Alava, S., Frau-Meigs, D., and Hassan, G., 2017. *Youth and extremism on social media: mapping the research* [online]. Paris: UNESCO. Available at: https://unesdoc.unesco.org/ark:/48223/pf0000260382 [Accessed 5 November 2021].

Ansari, N. S., 2020. Cyberbullying: concepts, theories, and correlates informing evidence-based best practices for prevention. *Aggression and Violent Behavior,* 50, 1–9.

Barnes, C., 2012. Understanding the social model of disability: past, present and future.

BASW, 2017. *The work of youth offending teams to protect the public* [online]. Birmingham: BASW. Available at: https://www.basw.co.uk/system/files/resources/basw_112231-5_0.pdf [Accessed 10 August 2021].

Bell, A., Hodgson, M., and Pragnell, S., 1999. Diverting children and young people from crime and the criminal justice system. In: Goldson, B., ed. *Youth Justice: Contemporary Policy and Practice.* Oxford: Routledge, 1999, pp. 91–109.

Brown, S., 2005. *Understanding youth and crime: Listening to youth?.* Berkshire: McGraw-Hill Education (UK).

Bullement, A., Meng, Y., Cooper, M., Lee, D., Harding, T.L., O'Regan, C., & Aguiar-Ibanez, R. (2019). A review and validation of overall survival extrapolation in health technology assessments of cancer immunotherapy by the National Institute for Health and Care Excellence: how did the initial best estimate compare to trial data subsequently made available?. *Journal of Medical Economics,* 22 (3), 205–214.

Burton, M., Pavord, E., and Williams, B., 2014. *An introduction to child and adolescent mental health.* London: Sage Publishing.

Bywaters, P., 2020. *The child welfare inequalities project: final report.* Huddersfield: Child Welfare Inequalities Project. Available at: https://pure.hud.ac.uk/ws/files/21398145/CWIP_Final_Report.pdf [Accessed 13 August 2021].

Cairns, K., 2013. The effects of trauma on children's learning. In: Jackson, S., ed. *Pathways through education for young people in care: Ideas from research and practice.* Cardiff: British Association for Adoption and Fostering, 2013. pp. 134–163.

Children's Commissioner, 2019. *Keeping kids safe* [online]. London: Children's Commissioner. Available at: https://cscp.org.uk/wp-content/uploads/2018/04/Childrens-Commissioner-Report-Keeping-kids-safe-gang-violence-and-CCE.pdf 12 September 2021. [Accessed 8 July 2021].

Children's Legal Centre, 2020. *Migrant Children's Project Factsheet: Children in care with immigration issues* [online]. London: Children's Legal Centre. Available at: https://www.

childrenslegalcentre.com/wp-content/uploads/2020/02/Children-in-care-with-immigration-issues.January.2020.pdf [Accessed 8 July 2021].

Council for Disabled Children, 2016. *Identifying the social care needs of disabled children and young people and those with SEN as part of Education, Health and Care Needs Assessments [online]*. London: Council for Disabled Children. Available at: https://councilfordisabledchildren.org.uk/sites/default/files/field/attachemnt/Identifying%20the%20social%20care%20needs_0.pdf [Accessed 14 January 2021].

Council for Disabled Children, 2017. *Understanding the needs of disabled children with complex needs or life-limiting conditions* [online]. London: Council for Disabled Children the True Colours Trust. Available at: https://councilfordisabledchildren.org.uk/sites/default/files/field/attachemnt/Data%20Report.pdf. [Accessed 13 January 2021].

Department for Education, 2018. *Working together to safeguard children: a guide to interagency working to safeguard and promote the welfare of children* [online]. London: Department for Education. Available at: https://assets.publishing.service.gov.uk/government/uploads/system/uploads/attachment_data/file/942454/Working_together_to_safeguard_children_inter_agency_guidance.pdf [Accessed 13 January 2021].

Department for Work and Pensions, 2019. *Family resources survey 2018/19* [online]. London: Department for Work and Pensions. Available at: https://assets.publishing.service.gov.uk/government/uploads/system/uploads/attachment_data/file/874507/family-resources-survey-2018-19.pdf [Accessed 14 January 2021].

Department of Health, 2004. *National service framework for children, young people and maternity services* [online]. London: Department of Health. Standard 8. Available at: https://assets.publishing.service.gov.uk/government/uploads/system/uploads/attachment_data/file/199952/National_Service_Framework_for_Children_Young_People_and_Maternity_Services_-_Core_Standards.pdf [Accessed 15 January 2021].

Derksen, T., 2010. The Influence of ecological theory in child and youth care: A review of the Literature. *International journal of child, youth and family studies* [online], 1 (3–4), 326–339. DOI: 10.18357/ijcyfs13/420102091

Dominelli, L., 2002. *Anti-oppressive social work theory and practice*. Basingstoke, Hampshire: Palgrave Macmillan.

Fazel, M., Reed, R. V., Panter-Brick, C., and Stein, A., 2012. Mental health of displaced and refugee children resettled in high-income countries: risk and protective factors. *The Lancet*, 379 (9812), 266–282.

Firmin, C., 2020. *Contextual safeguarding and child protection: Rewriting the rules*. Oxford: Taylor & Francis.

Firmin, C., and Lloyd, J., 2020. *Contextual safeguarding: a 2020 update on the operational, strategic and conceptual framework*. Bedford: University of Bedfordshire.

France, A., Bottrell, D., and Armstrong, D., 2012. *A political ecology of youth and crime*. New York: Springer Publishing.

Hek, R., 2005. *The experiences and needs of refugee and asylum seeking children in the UK: A literature review*. Birmingham: University of Birmingham.

HM Prison & Probation Service, 2020. *Placing young people in custody: guide for youth justice practitioners* [online]. London: HM Prison & Probation Service. Available at https://www.gov.uk/guidance/placing-young-people-in-custody-guide-for-youth-justice-practitioners

Kohli, R. K., 2006. The comfort of strangers: social work practice with unaccompanied asylum-seeking children and young people in the UK. *Child & Family Social Work*, 11 (1), 1–10.

Larkin, M., 2009. *Vulnerable groups in health and social care*. London: Sage Publishing.

McFarlane, K., 2008. From care to crime – children in state care and the development of criminality. In: Cunneen, C., and Salter, M., eds., *Proceedings of the 2nd Australian & New Zealand Critical Criminology Conference, Sydney, 19-20 June 2008* [online]. New South Wales: The Crime and Justice research Network, 2009, pp. 207–221. Available via: https://papers.ssrn.com/sol3/papers.cfm?abstract_id=1333994

Ministry of Justice and HM Prison and Probation Service, 2019. *Building bridges: a positive behaviour framework for the children and young people secure estate* [online]. London: GOV.UK. Available at: https://www.gov.uk/government/publications/building-bridges-a-positive-behaviour-framework-for-the-children-and-young-people-secure-estate [Accessed 20 January 2021].

Ministry of Justice, 2012. *Offenders young people. Juvenile offenders* [online]. London: Ministry of Justice. Available at: https://www.justice.gov.uk/offenders/types-of-offender/juveniles [Accessed 14 July 2021].

Ministry of Justice, 2021. *Youth Justice Statistics 2019/20* [online]. London: GOV.UK. Available at: https://assets.publishing.service.gov.uk/government/uploads/system/uploads/attachment_data/file/956621/youth-justice-statistics-2019-2020.pdf [Accessed 20 January 2021].

NHS, 2020. *Children and young people's services* [online]. London: NHS. Available at: https://www.nhs.uk/conditions/social-care-and-support-guide/caring-for-children-and-young-people/children-and-young-peoples-services/ [Accessed 13 January 2021].

Ní Raghallaigh, M., and Gilligan, R., 2010. Active survival in the lives of unaccompanied minors: coping strategies, resilience, and the relevance of religion. *Child & Family Social Work*, 15 (2), 226–237.

Office for National Statistics, 2020a. *Child abuse extent and nature, England and Wales: year ending March 2019* [online]. Newport, UK: Office for National Statistics. Available at: https://www.ons.gov.uk/peoplepopulationandcommunity/crimeandjustice/articles/childabuseextentandnatureenglandandwales/yearendingmarch2019 [Accessed 5 January 2022].

Office for National Statistics, 2020b. *Online Bullying in England and Wales: year ending March 2020* [online]. Newport, UK: Office for National Statistics. Available at: https://www.ons.gov.uk/peoplepopulationandcommunity/crimeandjustice/bulletins/onlinebullyinginenglandandwales/yearendingmarch2020 [Accessed 5 January 2022].

Ofsted, 2021. *Main findings: children's social care in England* [online]. London: GOV.UK. Available at https://www.gov.uk/government/statistics/childrens-social-care-data-in-england-2021/main-findings-childrens-social-care-in-england-2021 [Accessed 4 January 2022].

Ostrander, J., Melville, A., and Berthold, S. M., 2017. Working with refugees in the United States: Trauma-informed and structurally competent social work approaches. *Advances in Social Work* [online], 18(1), 66–79. DOI: 10.18060/21282

Prison Reform Trust, 2016. *In care, out of trouble* [online]. London: Prison Reform Trust. Available at: http://www.prisonreformtrust.org.uk/Portals/0/Documents/In%20care%20out%20of%20trouble%20summary.pdf [Accessed 10 November 2021].

Ramsay, A., 2020. *Social work with unaccompanied asylum-seeking children in Scotland* [online]. Glasgow: Iriss. Available at: https://www.iriss.org.uk/resources/insights/social-work-unaccompanied-asylum-seeking-children-scotland [Accessed 11 November 2021].

Reeder, J., and Morris, J., 2018. The importance of the therapeutic relationship when providing information to parents of children with long-term disabilities: The views and experiences of UK paediatric therapists. *Journal of Child Health Care*, 22 (3), 371–381.

Refugee Council, 2020. *Top facts from the latest statistics on refugees and people seeking asylum* [online]. London: Refugee Council. Available at: https://www.refugeecouncil.org.uk/information/refugee-asylum-facts/top-10-facts-about-refugees-and-people-seeking-asylum/ [Accessed 11 November 2021].

Rip, J., Zijlstra, E., Post, W., Kalverboer, M., and Knorth, E. J., 2020. 'It can never be as perfect as home': An explorative study into the fostering experiences of unaccompanied refugee children, their foster carers and social workers. *Children and Youth Services Review*, 112, 104924.

Ross, A., Duckworth, K., Smith, D. J., Wyness, G., and Schoon, I., 2011. *Prevention and Reduction: A review of strategies for intervening early to prevent or reduce youth crime and anti-social behaviour* [online]. London: Centre for Analysis of Youth Transitions. Available at: https://assets.publishing.service.gov.uk/government/uploads/system/uploads/attachment_data/file/182548/DFE-RR111.pdf

Sabalauskas, K. L., Ortolani, C. L., and McCall, M. J., 2014. Moving from pathology to possibility: integrating strengths-based interventions in child welfare provision. *Child Care in Practice* [online]. 20 (1), 120–134. DOI: 10.1080/13575279.2013.847053

Seifert, K., and Ray, K., 2012. *Youth violence: Theory, prevention, and intervention.* New York: Springer Publishing.

Smith, R., and Gray, P., 2019. The changing shape of youth justice: Models of practice. *Criminology & Criminal Justice*, 19 (5), 554–571.

Social Care Institute of Excellence, 2018. *Strengths-based social care for children, young people and their families* [online]. London: SCIE. Available at: https://www.scie.org.uk/strengths-based-approaches/young-people [Accessed 24 August 2021].

The Children's Society, 2009. *Safeguarding disabled children: Practice guidance* [online]. London: Department for Children, Schools and Families. Available at: https://assets.publishing.service.gov.uk/government/uploads/system/uploads/attachment_data/file/190544/00374-2009DOM-EN.pdf [Accessed 24 August 2021].

Trépanier, J., and Rousseaux, X., 2018. *Youth and Justice in Western States, 1815–1950.* London: Palgrave Macmillan.

Turney, D., Taylor, J., Shemmings, D., Shemmings, Y., Bentovim, A., Smeaton, E., Tait, A., Wosu, H., Ruch, G., and Tarleton, B., 2018. *The child's world: the essential guide to assessing vulnerable children, young people and their families.* Exeter: Jessica Kingsley Publishers.

UK Government Statistics, 2020. 'B2 children in need by recorded disability' from 'characteristics of children in need'. London: GOV.UK. Available at: https://explore-education-statistics.service.gov.uk/data-tables/permalink/db5f3740-990b-477b-8106-2cd6fe74edd4.

UK Parliament, 2021. *Children's social care services in England* [online]. London: UK Parliament. Available at https://commonslibrary.parliament.uk/research-briefings/cbp-8543/ [Accessed 17 May 2022].

Ungar, M., Liebenberg, L., and Ikeda, J., 2014. Young people with complex needs: Designing coordinated interventions to promote resilience across child welfare, juvenile corrections, mental health and education services. *British Journal of Social Work*, 44 (3), 675–693.

UNHCR, 1951. *Convention and protocol relating to the status of refugees* [online]. Geneva: UNHCR: The UN Refugee Agency UK. Available at: https://www.unhcr.org/3b66c2aa10.html

United Nations Department of Economic and Social Affairs, [n.d.]. *Definition of Youth* [online]. Geneva: United Nations. Available at: https://www.un.org/esa/socdev/documents/youth/fact-sheets/youth-definition.pdf [Accessed 16 May 2022].

WHO, 2020. *Youth violence* [online]. Geneva: World Health Organisation. Available at: https://www.who.int/news-room/fact-sheets/detail/youth-violence [Accessed 13 November 2021].

Williams, I., 2009. Offender health and social care: a review of the evidence on inter-agency collaboration. *Health & Social Care in the Community*, 17(6), 573–580.

Youth Justice Board, 2015. *Keeping children in care out of trouble: an independent review chaired by Lord Laming* [online]. London: Youth Justice Board. Available at: https://assets.publishing.service.gov.uk/government/uploads/system/uploads/attachment_data/file/543582/YJB_response_Laming_Review_keeping_children_in_care_out_of_custody.pdf [Accessed 24 August 2021].

13 Engaging Vulnerable Groups

Chris Towers

This chapter discusses the importance of vulnerability, and the constructionist and structural aspects of vulnerable populations. Safeguarding and personalisation are explored in the decision-making process. The practice issues and experience of vulnerability is considered.

The aims of this chapter:

- To define vulnerability
- To discuss why this theme is so important to students of health and social care
- To reflect on issues of vulnerability as the term applies to groups and individuals who receive services
- To consider practice issues with vulnerable service users

Introduction: Defining the Term

This challenging and reflective chapter explores the concept of vulnerability and how it can be viewed in relation to the delivery of health and social care. We start however with some reflections on its meaning, within different contexts. The term vulnerability has wide usage in health and social care but whilst widely used it is rarely defined. Virokanaas et al. (2018) says that there are critiques of the term but curiously little in the way of definition and they argue that instead of talking of vulnerable groups it would be more helpful to talk of vulnerable situations. It is argued that people are not vulnerable per se, that it is the social environment that makes one vulnerable. Vulnerability can be situational, or indeed geographical for time and place can shape its meaning. It can also mark out service users deemed eligible for services. One could be vulnerable by lack of access to services. Vulnerability means many things and it is important to define the term and indeed if one works with people who are vulnerable one needs to be aware of effective ways of working with people and whether they are comfortable with seeing themselves as vulnerable or not.

Vulnerability needs to be deconstructed in such a way that one sees the term in a rounded sense with all sorts of meanings and connotations. Consider this depiction of someone I observed whilst in Singapore in 2019.

I focused on the women by the river as she seemed incongruous with the glittery city skyline of Singapore. Her apparent poverty contrasted with opulence far away, down the river. Vulnerability can be perceived in a variety of such ways, seen by sight,

DOI: 10.4324/9781003079873-16

or at least interpreted as such. As a lecturer of health and social care I have observed many students engaging with the term in many ways. One student once observed, in class that creativity allowed her to 'see the world in different ways'. This remark made an impact on me, it was so refreshing to hear a student describe something that has so many- negatives connotations in such positive and affirming ways. Given this, it may now be pertinent to consider the various ways one can understand this term. The term vulnerability has original meanings related to that of being physically attached but at the same time having the ability 'to wound' (Merriam Webster dictionary 2020) with it deriving from the Latin noun 'vulnus'.

The Social Construction of Vulnerability

One may argue that dictionary definitions are not sufficient to understand what this term means from different perspectives. We may have different ways of seeing or knowing vulnerability and how we see people in relation to say risk may tell us something of how we see humans. Vulnerability can be understood in very visceral, physical ways, like when observing the woman by the river in Figure 13.1, but it is

---

Walking by the Kallang River one morning I saw her, she was far from the thriving, bustling city and she caught my eye. What is your understanding of her in this poem I wrote of her, is she vulnerable? If so, how?

By the Kallang River

I saw her as I wandered by
the Kallang River,
far from the opaque
endless shopping malls
of plenitude.

She scavenged voraciously,
with forked fingers,
plucking and picking,
at scraps from the
waste bins.

Shovelling empties of
Coca-Cola bottles into bags
with a voracity
of hungry birds,
pecking and poking.
I could see skyscrapers
with glories and stories
of a country transformed.
Eating opulence.

Meanwhile she devoured the
garbage,
like a cynonmolgus monkey,
feeding on the left behinds
of a feast.

Figure 13.1 Moment of reflection.

important to acknowledge the social aspects. It is seen from different angles and partly down to perception. The idea put forward by Birkmann and Welles (2014) is that these phenomena or these concepts of risk and vulnerability are defined and then named or understood in various ways. Vulnerability is multi-faceted and dynamic (Birkmann and Welle, 2014). Policy makers and practitioners will see it in different ways. Such ideas draw from social constructionist approaches. These is a theory used to develop knowledge of or understand the world in some way. This approach can accept there is such an objective thing called 'vulnerability' but at the same time it can be socially defined (Berger and Luckmann, 1991) and that people in groups and individuals play their part in defining it. There is an objective but also a subjective reality (Segre 2016) with power dimensions (Burr 1995), in other words the powerful or those with power can define others in ways they decide. These theories or approach would say that vulnerability can be defined by society or by people agreeing on what it means to be vulnerable and at the same time what it is to be strong or invulnerable.

Cuts Both Ways

Vulnerability is something of a paradox, it can mean strength and weakness at the same time and this needs remembering for service users of health and social care can be both strong and weak, can be wounded, figuratively and literally of course, but can also wound others.

If we examine words close to vulnerability, synonyms (like) we can cite the following terms:

1   Accessible
2   Defenceless
3   Exposed
4   Sensitive
5   Susceptible
6   Unsafe
7   Weak

Falling in Love With Vulnerability

These words (above) have many associations and meanings and we can say that people could be considered vulnerable through all their lives. It could be argued that being vulnerable is the default state of being human although claiming universal understandings are not an easy claim to make for there can be many cultural and ethnic variations of meanings and language can play its part in shifting meaning. Maybe 'we' are all vulnerable in the sense that we are mortal, and the term applies in a physical and mental health context to describe many different states of mind.

The term is also not simply applicable to just health and social care. Falling in love can place someone in a position of being vulnerable argues Emma Seppala (2012) in the magazine 'psychology today'. She says that when we make ourselves vulnerable we reveal aspects of ourselves to others and we do that she says to connect with them. It is in that sense a positive. But at the same time the term may also be a distraction and unhelpful. It could be seen to ignore the social, economic, and political contexts of our lives that induce or encourage vulnerability and is not therefore regarded as default but something to be explained in wider contexts.

Structural Aspects of Vulnerability

There are psychological and socio-political interpretations of vulnerability. The body and the mind are potentially or indelibly susceptible. But there are wider interpretations of a more sociological nature and these looks to concepts of 'structure and 'agency'. Social structures such as the family or social policy or indeed many aspects of the law give shape to society (Erola et al. 2016). Vulnerability can relate to the way resources are distributed or how power, wealth and opportunity are configured. It is possible to talk about vulnerable groups. For Larkin (2009) vulnerable groups are often those that face social exclusion from those resources, and they tend to be in disadvantaged neighbourhoods. Their problems are often 'linked', such as lack of work leading to lack of income for example, or poor health outcomes. They may have problems accessing services. These social structures will shape or can shape a life whilst at the same time they are potentially balanced or at least partly offset by the issue of agency. With agency the individual is able to direct their own life, that they can enact some form of behavioural change (Frohlic and Potvin 2010). If we consider such an issue in relation to a contemporary issue such as the covid 19 pandemic we can see how interventions by government such as social distancing or mask wearing will shape our own lives and impact upon our vulnerability, maybe protecting us from risk or restricting our freedom to take risks. However, we view the issues there will be structural factors outside of our control, that will limit us.

Vulnerable Populations

Consideration of issues of structure and agency may lead one to suppose that vulnerability is not simply an individual experience but a collective one, that there are populations and communities that are vulnerable. This idea that whole groups can be vulnerable is not without its issue or problems and it can be that in calling groups vulnerable one could be stigmatising them (Frohlic and Potvin 2010). Groups like the unemployed or single mothers can be stigmatised whilst at the same time considered vulnerable and their very vulnerability can mark them out in negative ways. Griffiths, Calabria and Bailey refer elsewhere in this volume to the work of Brady and Brown (2013) who challenges presumptive and negative definitions concerning teenage pregnancy and young parenthood. It is good to be mindful of too easily defining groups in narrow ways and perhaps making it a defining characteristic of a group rather than something arising out of inequalities.

Sources and Types of Vulnerability

Here are some sources of vulnerability, consider each one in turn.

- Issues of poverty and/or inequalities along the lines of race or ethnicity can encourage vulnerability. So too can restricted educational attainment over the life course coupled with low income and when these ideas overlap there is a sense of them intersecting and working together to exclude (Mechanic and Tanner 2007).

- Vulnerability can also be multi-faceted (Scrambler 2019) with social factors or mechanisms combining with biological factors, with one form of vulnerability acting upon another. It could be suggested for example that people may be made vulnerable by disability. We may have to also acknowledge that the social environment plays a considerable part in giving meaning and significance to that vulnerability particularly when the social and physical environment is hostile or not accessible. Such ideas are supported by the social model of disability (Anastasiou and Kauffman 2013) which tends to downplay the biological aspects of disability. There can also be intersections or cross over between different inequalities, such as that between disability and gender. Women with disabilities can experience complex relationships between disability and gender with women facing problems in relation to different forms of interlinked discrimination. It may be, for example, that a woman may be presumed to undertake the caring for relatives in a family whilst she at the same time may have a disability that is 'unseen' restricting her ability to physically care for another. Her individuality as a woman and her own strengths and weaknesses as a person ignored and she faces gender and disability discrimination concurrently.
- We may also be able to locate vulnerability within the circumstantial and locate it geographically or in the transition from place to place. O'Higgins (2012) refers to the case of refugees who are taken into care by social services. The author questions if these people are vulnerable but their vulnerability can be explained by their movement from place to place, as they cross borders and their status by age. Some will be 'under ages' in that they will be under 18 years of age and will thus be under the guidance of a social worker. The social worker will decide on the kind of help they are able to receive with a greater chance of support if 'underage' (O'Higgins 2012) and given a discretionary right to remain until aged 17 and a half. O'Higgins argues that understanding their vulnerability means knowing of the circumstance, where they are geographically, which services they encounter and how they are defined.
- Vulnerability may be temporary or persistent (Mechanic and Tanner 2007), can occur in fluctuation, be fleeting or lifelong induced by acute illness, bereavement, family related or linked to wider community factors.

Making Decisions - Vaccines

Whilst there are different sources of vulnerability and different aspects to it and indeed different ways of imagining or making sense it there are also practical dilemmas and questions. Individuals or groups of people may be experiencing illness or concerned to get a vaccine, others will be manufacturing and distributing them. Who should get priority for them and what criteria would be used to decide?

You may have decided in the exercise above (Figure 13.2) and have your own value base that informed your decision making. Whatever your argument not all people agree with or want to take vaccines. Doherty et al. (2016) says that take up of vaccines is not always as high as one may anticipate and they point to the situation in the USA where those aged 65 years or more are taking vaccines at relatively small numbers, 67% took the vaccine in the winter of 2014–15. That may seem high but when you consider that influenza is a significant illness one may

Vaccine is a way of responding to illness by pre-empting or acting to prevent people getting illnesses but one question that can occur is how we prioritise those needing vaccines and where should vulnerability come into the equation.

We take an early look at issues facing groups and that is the issue of vaccination, and the question of who should be vaccinated against disease, we must think what the criteria should be for getting immunization or having it administered?

Should it be
a. Age –many age-related diseases or at least 'frailty' is an issue
b. Likelihood of contracting the disease or illness
c. vulnerability
d. Income-if you can afford to pay
e. Need in any event-regardless of cost or anything else
f. If the vaccine works or is likely to (effectiveness)
g. Behaviour-if you are prepared to 'help yourself' generally?

Are there other reasons for giving vaccination?

Figure 13.2 What would you do?

expect that number to be higher. This is despite the Global Vaccination plan 2011–2020 recommending wide vaccination to protect people against illness. Of course, these debates around vaccine and who should qualify have been most prominent since the global pandemic which started in 2020. Smith et al. (2020) highlight these issues to argue that those groups most at risk should be prioritised. They argue that those suffering hyper -tension or obesity or other clinical conditions should be given first access but also those in poverty (Smith et al. 2020), or practitioners with key worker status (Smith et al. 2020). There are arguments to support the prioritisation of vulnerable groups be they because of social inequities or through clinical risk. Some medics favour prioritising very specific groups such as those with learning difficulties for they argue they are at much greater risk from covid 19 (British Medical Journal 2021). Whilst it can be argued that children are at less risk from the disease, they also cite the dangers to children of contracting paediatric inflammatory multisystem syndrome (Wong et al. 2021) and from that view they should be high priority. There are many competing arguments and vulnerability, whether it from social or biological vantage points, or a combination of both, is often at the centre of the debates. These vulnerabilities are contextual, concerning the social contexts in which people live as well as the physiological aspects (Figures 13.3 and 13.4).

If you are an older person, how do you see yourself, vulnerable? But what if you're in a very early stage of the life course, how will you see yourself? Will you want to see yourself as vulnerable or not? Will it have advantages, or does it label you in ways you would not like? How as a professional may you see older people? Are their differences in how you see the genders?

Figure 13.3 Moment of reflection. Will you see yourself as vulnerable?

Clive is an 85-year-old man from the Caribbean originally but moved to England when he was 28 to take a job with Birmingham Transport before retiring aged 65.

He has always seen himself as 'strong' and resisted support from social services even though getting around his two-storey terraced house was getting more difficult. His social worker noticed he was having problems with the stairs and suggested a move to supported housing and a bungalow. He was resistant but his social worker noticed steep decline but equal resistance to her advice. He had a fall one afternoon and at that point he seemed to be 'reaching out to me' he said for help but then 'he changed just as quickly and said he was strong and was fine'

She fears that he may leave it 'too late', and he may have to relinquish his independence and move to more communal living, perhaps in a worse state for he had neglected his own needs and accumulated risk. Does she talk more with him or leave it to when he says he is 'ready'?

Figure 13.4 Case study: Clive: When to intervene?

Engaging Older People

There could be many ways of responding to or engaging vulnerable people but one of the problems in doing so is to reach understandings with people that they are or are not vulnerable.

The question of how one sees oneself is complex. Many older people do not accept the term 'vulnerable' when applied to themselves (Age UK 2015). Bennett says that there is an assumption within governments that people over the age of 65 are vulnerable. It can be assumed that they need targeted or special support. Bennett takes issue with that. She says that only a relatively small number need a lot of support or services, access to a doctor, financial, legal, or housing help. Bennett suggests that attitudes towards older people and their vulnerability and relation to services differ widely. She argues from her research that older widows are offered varying degrees of support but that men she said are offered more support than women and this raises the question of why this is so. Bennett offers three possible explanations. First, men simply do need more support. Second, she suggests that traditional gender roles shape such expectations and responses, and that volunteers and professionals hold different ideas about the genders and how they relate to help.

The point is not elaborated upon but perhaps women are regarded as more resourceful or maybe there are other reasons for this. The 3rd expectation is that women are offered support but do not take advantage of it. These are curious issues and perhaps suggest that people's perceptions of themselves and other perceptions of them are fraught with ideas about themselves and others that are somewhat confusing and bounded in stereotypes and mismatches of ideas. If you are trying to engage older people in services it may well be that you faced with challenges to try and unpack many different attitudes and expectations around ageing and vulnerability, images of self and other.

In the case study above the social worker may well have a dilemma and find it hard to push Clive or respect his wishes. Bennett (2015) says that in any intervention the timing must be appropriate. She said that in her study of widowers many saw themselves as resilient but there were what she called 'turning points' and help or advice needed to be given at such critical times rather than 'too early' or indeed 'too late'. She raises the issue of what happens when the older person has a perception of themselves as more resilient than they are, do we challenge them? Perceptions be-tween professionals, helpers, and older people themselves can vary.

There are also important issues of diversity exemplified by the work of Gordon 2015 who finds that Caribbean men's attitude towards their masculinity can be one of seeing themselves as strong, self-reliant and as 'breadwinner' (Roopnarine 2004). Roopnarine and chase (2015) goes on to argue that these factors plus a range of other issues such as discriminatory practice and migration issues can impact negatively upon their health. Interventions can be harder, meeting perhaps resistance from a proud service user can thus be more difficult. There can be resistance to health be-haviours which may serve them well but are not in tandem with their idea of their own self (Roopnarine and chase 2015). They may be committed to their 'bread-winner' role so much that the extra work may endanger their own health but may be reluctant to desist from this for reasons partly concerned with self-image. Of course, one cannot make these behaviours the preserve of one ethnic group or one gender, but research can unearth such trends and they can be important if one is to under-stand issues of health, health interventions and outcomes. Perceptions of self and the need to not show vulnerability but strength can be important issues when considering health and health behaviours and patterns.

The Safeguarding Agenda and Personalisation

The issue of vulnerability is very pertinent and critical if services are to find or know the 'best' way of supporting or engaging people who may be considered at risk and/or in need of safeguarding. How we 'see' people who are deemed vulnerable and how we go about responding to or engaging with these people is at the heart of safeguarding law and the personalisation agenda. The personalisation movement developed in the early 1980s in the USA and then the UK (Dickenson and Glasby 2010) and was promoted by people with a disability. Disabled people have since then been leaders or drivers of personalisation and they have championed a movement towards direct payments whereby they receive cash payments in lieu of directly provided services. It has been argued (Dickenson and Glasby 2010) that this policy has been developed, put into practice, and then developed by people with disability themselves.

The **personalisation agenda** asserts that issues of choice and control are at the centre (Carr 2013). She argues that the service user needs dignity and well-being, a sense of self determination and a need for self-directed care. This agenda sits alongside the safe-guarding one, which arguably is more about protection than autonomy, and you may reflect on the question of how far these agendas are compatible. Schwehr (2010) out-lines how the legal framework in relation to safeguarding has not changed in the UK in the sense in that whilst legislation may evolve the emphasis on supporting or protecting those people who lack capacity as assessed under the Mental Capacity Act 2005 is a constant principle underlying the law. The change of emphasis is that there has been a move towards the service user or citizen undertaking some self- assessment and self-directed support (Stevens et al. 2016). The 'best interests' of the service user should always take high priority in deciding what the service user is entitled to the local au-thority must decide as to if to provide the direct payments or the managed budgets. Schwehr (2010) states that the direct payments are not offered as a duty, but the au-thority must decide if that is the best route. Whilst the personalisation agenda is im-portant with the client to be at the centre, the regulations also state that the council should be mindful of the risks to the client if a third-party offering services to them appear dubious in some way. The council may be blamed if the person is abused, and they do have a 'duty of care' and will not want to be negligent.

Schwehr, emphasises that:

- An Independent Safeguarding Authority (ISA) must ensure that any client working for the service user obtains a Criminal Record Bureau check
- The Safeguarding Vulnerable Groups Act 2006 will provide the new framework for this new ISA scheme

It may be added here that a more in depth look at the personalisation is available in the person-centred intervention chapter of this volume. Given all this you may consider if the safeguarding and indeed personalisation agenda can work successfully with a variety of clients who may be regarded as vulnerable. What are the issues in this case, as below?

There are many issues involved in the story above (Figure 13.5) and it throws light upon the whole issue of vulnerability and the 'best way' of working with people who are vulnerable, aiming to support and empower them, whilst safeguarding.

Working with or engaging people who are vulnerable can be particularly difficult if the person lacks capacity or consent in any way. This is made particularly graphic when it comes to the very personal and sensitive area of sexual relations for people with disabilities, embodied in the article above (Figure 13.5). This will be a sensitive issue with or without payment, with or without legality. This may be a taboo area for some but for people with learning disabilities may need education on matters such as contraceptive use and this within the context of a Mental Capacity Act 2005 is brought to the fore. There are also human rights issues, and the Human Rights Act (Fenwick and Phillipson 2006) and a need to strike a balance between upholding the right of disabled people to have sexual relations and protecting or safeguarding them from abuse. Indeed, there is much evidence of people with physical disabilities being

---

You may want to consider the story below, what are the rights and wrongs, the arguments for and against in this story from 2010

It was reported in the 'Daily Telegraph', August 2010 that

'Councils pay prostitutes for the disabled'

'Taxpayer's money is being spent on prostitutes, lap dancing clubs and exotic holidays under Schemes designed to give more independence for the disabled'

https://www.telegraph.co.uk/news/health/7945785/Councils-pay-for-prostitutes-for-the-disabled.html

(Accessed on line 29: 10: 2020)

With the proviso that the 'Daily Telegraph' may be misreporting or misinterpreting one can debate the ethics here. You may want to consider who is vulnerable and how, the women themselves as sex workers, the council, the disabled people themselves and/or their careers, perhaps others?

Figure 13.5 Reflective moment: Sexual relations, vulnerability and Direct payments.

abused. Nosek et al. (2001) found in their research with 501 disabled women responding to questions of abuse in their relationships as many as 181 cited abuse, emotional, physical, and sexual.

Calus (2012) similarly found that those people with disabilities are more likely to have known sexual violence than people who are not disabled. The writer does however take issue with the idea that people with learning disabilities should be viewed as 'vulnerable', arguing that they become more exposed to risk when segregated or overly protected. She believes that people with learning disabilities should be taught to safeguard themselves and in doing so be more able to manage their own risk. DiGangi et al. asked people to 'frame' the issue of learning disability and their sexual relations in new and more challenging ways. Their rights, it is argued, are frequently ignored by those working with people who they say have been labelled as having 'learning disabilities'. Their argument is not pertaining narrowly to the issue of payment for sexual relations, as in the case study, but more widely into the area of what they call 'intimate citizenship', the right to make personal decisions about intimate relationships. Loving relationships they argue offer protection not only from unfair treatment but from loneliness and abuse. You may argue that there can still be issues with capacity and consent but Hollomotz (2011) argues with the premise that people with vulnerabilities are naturally or inherently vulnerable but rather it is situational. Environments can respond to people in negative and restrictive ways when people are given the label 'learning disabilities. Her approach is born of a so called 'ecological model' that asserts that vulnerability is fostered or played up and in doing so this disempowers people, makes them more passive and less inclined towards advocating for their own change.

Social Policies-Making a Difference?

If we want to consider vulnerability within the context of receipt of services for health and social care one may get no better example of a situation that can induce or exacerbate vulnerability it is the state of being homeless. Of course, one can argue that vulnerability was the very reason they became homeless in the first place and that homelessness is a symptom of being vulnerable, others may see it as a cause. One could point to wider social policies and economic austerity as key to understanding the vulnerability of young people to homelessness (Heerde and Patton 2020). In that sense homelessness is viewed as inciting vulnerability and that vulnerability is viewed as situational rather than residing within the person. This then gives rise to other vulnerabilities or vulnerable contexts in which education, employment and strong social networks are compromised. Working with this understanding Heerden and Patton argue that researchers, policy makers and practitioners of all kinds should come together more to build solutions. This emphasises less the vulnerability as a trait within people but within situations and thereby becomes seen as situational and contextual. The language of the legislation does however suggest that the 'person' is vulnerable and that such a person can have priority need, as such.

The legislation emphasises the issue of vulnerability for under the Housing Act 1996 local councils have a legal responsibility to support people who are homeless and in priority need (Housing Rights 2015), under section 189 (1)c:

'a person who is vulnerable because of old age, mental illness or handicap or physical disability or other special relation, or with whom such a person resides or might reasonably be expected to reside'.

But can social policies make a difference? Asian news monitor (2019) report that in the UK the numbers of people sleeping rough have reduced because of the rolling out of 'sleeping rough' initiatives with the claim that the numbers sleeping rough have reduced by a third or 32% because of the government putting in £400 million in funding. The plan was implemented in the spring of 2018 and the question may arise perhaps of to what extent is it the policy that has made the difference and to what extent have other factors such as changes in the demographics of those homeless or circumstances that policies don't directly affect. Alternatively, one can suggest that one cannot make easy associations between a reduction of a social issue or problem like homelessness because of a particular policy or the instatement of a particular service. Whilst Corinth (2017) found for example that in the United States there was a decrease in the numbers of homeless as supportive housing for the homeless increased the impact of this increase of supported housing was relatively small as the support was poorly targeted and many left this housing to enter the private sector housing.

Summary or Review

After reading this chapter you should now be able to:

- Understand how vulnerability can be seen in different ways depending on time, place, setting and circumstance. There are different sources and different types of vulnerability related to people and wider social structures
- Appreciate people may be defined (and who defines them) in terms of their vulnerability, can impact on if and how they receive or interact with services
- Consider different ways in which it is possible to engage or reach out to people who are vulnerable, whether it be prioritising the vulnerable for vaccines, housing them as priority, safeguarding them or enabling them to take risks through personalised approaches
- Understand how social policies can make a difference to the lives of people considered vulnerable with recognition that there may be other factors also shaping those lives beyond policies

References

Age UK, 2015. *Improving later life. Vulnerability and resilience in older people [online]*. London: Age UK. Available at: https://www.ageuk.org.uk/globalassets/age-uk/documents/reports-and-publications/reports-and-briefings/health–wellbeing/rb_april15_vulnerability_resilience_improving_later_life.pdf

Anastasiou, D., and Kauffman, J.M., 2013. The Social Model of Disability: Dichotomy between impairment and disability. *Journal of Medicine and Philosophy: a forum for biothics and Philosophy Medicine*, 38 (4), 441–459.

Berger, P., and Luckmann, T., 1991. *The social construction of reality*. London: Penguin Books.

Birkmann, J., and Welle, T., 2014. Theoretical and conceptual framework for the assessment of vulnerability in natural hazards and climate change in Europe. In: Birkmann, J., Kienberger, S., and Alexander, D.E., eds. *Assessment of Vulnerability to natural hazards, a European perspective*. London: Elsevier, 2014, pp. 1–19.

Brady, G., and Brown, G. 2013. Rewarding but let's talk about the challenges: Using arts based methods in research with young mothers. *Methodological Innovations Online*, 8 (1), 99–112.

Burr, V., 1995. *An introduction to social construction*. London: Routledge.

Calus, A.M., 2012. Learning disabilities and sexual vulnerability: a social approach. *Disability and Society*, 27 (2).

Carr, S., 2013. *SCIE Report 20: Personalisation: a rough guide* [online]. London: Social Care Institute for Excellence. Available at: https://shropshire-disability.net/wp-content/uploads/2012/03/Personalisation-Report-for-Practitioners.pdf [Accessed 29 October 2020].

Corinth, K., 2017. The impact of permanent supported housing on homeless populations. *Journal of Housing Economics* [online], 35 (March), 69–84. Available via: https://www.sciencedirect.com/science/article/abs/pii/S1051137715300474 [Accessed 29 October 2020].

Dickenson, H., and Glasby, J., 2010. *The personalisation agenda, implications for the third sector* [online]. Birmingham: Third Sector Research Centre. Available at: file:///C:/Users/SWK3FOSTEB/OneDrive%20-%20Nottingham%20Trent%20University/Key%20Themes%20Editing%20Project/NTU%20Citing%20References%20Guide%2010th%20ed%202016.pdf

Doherty, M., Schmidt-Ott, R., Santos, J.I., Stanberry, L.R., Hoffsteter, A.M., Rosenthal, S.L., and Cunningham, A.L., 2016. Vaccination of special populations: Protecting the vulnerable. *Vaccine*, 34 (52), 6681–6690.

Erola, J., Jalonen, S., and Lehti, H., 2016. Parental education, class and income over early life course and children's achievements. *Research in Social Stratification and Mobility*, 44, 33–43.

Fenwick, H.M., and Phillipson, G., 2006. Media freedom under the Human Rights Act. Oxford: Oxford University Press.

Frohlic, K.L., and Potvin, L., 2010. Commentary: structure or agency? The importance of both for addressing social inequalities in health. *International Journal of Epidemiology*, 39 (2), 378–379.

Hassan-Smith, Z., Hanif, W., and Khunti, K., 2020. Who should be prioritised for COVID-19 vaccines?. *Lancet*, 396 (10264), 1732–1733.

Heerde, J.A., and Patton, J.C., 2020. The vulnerability of young homeless people. *The Lancet*, 5 (6) (June), e302–e303. Available via: https://www.thelancet.com/journals/lanpub/article/PIIS2468-2667(20)30121-3/fulltext [Accessed 29 October 2020].

Hollomotz, A., 2011. *Learning disabilities and sexual vulnerability- a social approach*. London: Jessica Kingsley Publishers.

Housing Rights, 2015. *Homelessness - priority need and meaning of vulnerability reassessed* [online]. Belfast: Housing Rights. Available at: https://www.housingrights.org.uk/news/homelessness---priority-need-and-meaning-vulnerability-reassessed [Accessed 29 October 2020].

Larkin, M., 2009. *Vulnerable groups in health and social care*. London: Sage.

Mechanic, D., and Tanner, J., 2007. Vulnerable people, groups and populations: societal view. *Health Affairs (Project Hope)*, 26 (5), 1220–1230.

Merriam Webster Dictionary 2020. Available at: www.merriam-webster.com

Nosek, M., Clubb Foley, C., Hughes, R.B. and Howland, C.A., 2001. Vulnerabilities for abuse among women with disabilities. *Sexuality and Disability*, 19 (3) (January), 177–189. Available via: 10.1023/A:1013152530758 [Accessed 28 October 2020].

O'Higgins, 2012. Vulnerability and agency: Beyond an irreconcilable dichotomy for social service providers working with young refugees in the UK. *New Directions for Child and Adult Development*, 2012 (136), 79–91.

Roopnarine, J. L. 2004. African American and African Caribbean fathers: Level, quality, and meaning of involvement. In Lamb, M. E. (Ed.), *The role of the father in child development* (pp. 58–97). John Wiley & Sons Inc.

Segre, S., 2016. Social Constructionism as a Sociological Approach. *A Journal for Philosophy and the Social Sciences*, 39 (1), 93–99.

Seppala, E., 2012. Vulnerability, the secret to intimacy, psychology today. *The Science of Health, Happiness & Success* [online blog], September 5. Available at: https://emmaseppala.com/vulnerability-the-secret-to-intimacy-2/ [Accessed on line October 27 2020].

Schwehr, B., 2010. Safeguarding and personalisation. *The Journal of Adult Protection* [online], 12 (2) (May), 43–51. Available via: https://search.proquest.com/docview/527740925?pq-origsite=gscholar&fromopenview=true [Accessed 27 October 2020].

Scambler, G. 2019. Sociology, social class, health inequalities, and the avoidance of "Classism". *Frontiers in Sociology*, 4, 56. doi:10.3389/fsoc.2019.00056. PMID: 33869379; PMCID: PMC8022477.

Stevens, M., Woolham J., Manthorpe, J., Aspinall, F., Hussein, S., Baxter, K., Samsi, K., and Ismail, M., 2016. Implementing safeguarding and personalisation in social work, findings from practice. *Journal of Social Work*, 18 (1), 3–22.

Virokanaas, E., Liuski, S., and Kuronen, M., 2018. The contested concept of vulnerability- a literature review. *European Journal of Social Work*, 23 (2), 327–339.

Wong, B.L.H., Ramsay, L.E., and Ladhani, S.H., 2021. Should children be vaccinated against COVID-19 now?. *Archives of Disease in Childhood* [online], 2021 (106), 1147–1148. DOI: 10.1136/archdischild-2020-321225 [Accessed October 11 2021].

14 Children's and Young People's Mental Health

Jessica Arnold, Amy Allen, Dolores Ellidge, and Richard Machin

Chapter aims:

- Explore the impact of Adverse Childhood Experiences (ACE's) on later mental health
- Examine the relationship between parental and child mental health
- Evaluate the role of schools in relation to children's and young people's mental health
- Examine current provision from Child and Adolescent Mental Health Services (CAMHS) in England

Introduction

This chapter reflects a growing concern about the state of services for children and young people with mental health problems and the need to develop strategies for promoting and sustaining mental wellbeing. The chapter is divided into four distinct sections, addressing four current issues related to the mental wellbeing of children and young people in the UK. The link between Adverse Childhood Experiences (ACEs) and later mental illness is explored, with emphasis on the impact such experiences can have on child development. With alerting the reality of suicide attempts and unhealthy coping behaviours being triggered when ACEs have been evident in a child's life.

The impact of parental mental health on children is discussed, with a summary of recent evidence exploring this complex relationship. The third section explores the role of schools in the monitoring and management of the mental well-being of children and adolescents, examining current policy and provision.

The final section of this chapter explores how Child and Adolescent Mental Health Services (CAMHS) provide support and interventions for young people with mental illness within England and wider parts of the UK.

Children and Young People's Mental Health

It is estimated that 1 in 6 children aged 6–17 years old in the UK have a mental disorder (NHS Digital 2021). Whilst the causes of mental illness are varied and complex, it is clear that more needs to be done to prevent such a high proportion of

DOI: 10.4324/9781003079873-17

young people experiencing psychological distress. This chapter focuses on four key topics related to the mental wellbeing of children and adolescents in the UK, giving an introduction to some of the current debate surrounding this issue.

Experiencing traumatic events has been identified as a predisposing factor in the development of a wide range of psychiatric illnesses. This link was first explored following the First World War, with vast numbers of soldiers developing what was then labelled as 'shell-shock' (Shatkin 2015). In recent years, there has been a wealth of research demonstrating the impact of trauma, abuse and neglect in early childhood on life-long mental health. The Office for National Statistics (ONS 2019) has identified an alarming trend which shows that young people suffering adversity are more susceptible to mental illness than any other disorder. The first section of this chapter examines the mechanisms by which early trauma can lead to a range of mental illnesses.

The notion that early interactions between parents (or caregivers) and infants are critical in the development of the child is not a new one. The work of John Bowlby (1952) emphasised the importance of consistent, responsive and meaningful engagement in the formation of early attachments which then provide a model for future relationships. The '1001 Critical Days' (HM Government 2021) campaign further emphasises the impact of a baby's early life experiences and how it shapes the foundations for their childhood cognitive, physical and emotional growth and development. Unfortunately, mental illness can make it difficult for a parent to form these early bonds with their child. The second section of this chapter explores the reasons for this, the impact a parent's mental health can have on the mental wellbeing of the child and examines interventions aimed at tackling this difficult issue. Perinatal mental health is a focus here, exploring the effect that the mental health of a primary care giver in the early stages of life can have on a child's development.

It is known that by the age of 14 half of all mental health problems are established (Arnold and Baker, 2018 and NHS Long Term Plan 2019) rising to 75% by the age of 18 (NHS England 2014a). Early intervention is pivotal to ensuring appropriate treatment for children and young people who present with mental ill health. NHS England (2014a) recommends that support from professionals is sought as soon as possible, the aim is to provide early intervention and to prevent escalation to the point where specialist intervention is needed.

Education plays a pivotal role in the lives of children and adolescents, not just in relation to their academic attainment, but also their emotional and social development. Humphrey et al. (2016) presents a compelling argument that schools play a vital role in setting the scene for positive mental health. Schools are uniquely positioned to be able to identify signs of psychological distress, equip young people with the tools needed to maintain mental wellbeing and perhaps even provide early intervention for mental illness. However, current policy in relation to the responsibility of school's mental health lacks clarity, with provision varying from school to school.

Adverse Childhood Experiences and Mental Ill Health

There is growing evidence worldwide that Adverse Childhood Experiences (ACEs) contribute to mental ill health in children and young people often persisting into adulthood (Chang et al. 2019; Duin et al. 2018 and Hughes et al. 2016).

Many traumatic experiences in childhood are instigated by a child's caregiver (Feltz-Cornelis 2019) when they have been exposed to harm or stressful events by their parents or caregivers. Further to this, Cheong (2017) asserts threats to harm being a stressful life event for a child.

Public Health Scotland (PHS 2021) define ACEs as stressful events or environments relating to childhood, including, for example: - Domestic violence - Parental abandonment due to separation or divorce - Victim of abuse (physical, sexual and/or emotional) - Victim of neglect (physical or emotional) - Member of the household in prison - Household in which adults are experiencing alcohol and drug use problems (PHS 2021).

ACEs have been described as 'stressful events during childhood that can have a profound impact on an individual's present and future health' (NHS Health Scotland 2019). If a child experiences long-term exposure to four or more of the factors listed above, the cumulative stress can impact upon overall mental and physical health throughout a lifetime. Traumatic events in early childhood play a significant role in the development of later stress-related symptoms and mental ill health (Steck and Steck, 2016 and Nemeroff and Binder 2014). Kerker et al. (2015) state that exposure to 'toxic stress' at a young age stimulates the release of stress hormones in the brain and can impact upon brain development. Kendall-Tackett (2002) also observes that childhood abuse can have direct consequences for brain development. Research has concluded that traumatic experiences in early life compromise the normal development of a child's cerebral cortex and limbic system (Steck and Steck 2016). Thus, trauma alters the primitive parts of the brain and impacts upon a person's ability to control their own behaviour and impulses. Exposure to early stress and trauma can therefore lead to long-term negative consequences for brain development.

McLaughlin et al. (2010) state that exposure to ACEs increases a young person's vulnerabilities and decreases their ability to cope with and manage stressful life events which may occur in adulthood. There is evidence of greater risk taking and engagement in risky behaviours if childhood adversity has taken place, and adoption of unhealthy coping mechanisms and lifestyles are often observed (Kerker et al. 2015 and Kendall-Tackett 2002). Moreover, victims remain vulnerable to unusual levels low self-esteem, insecure attachment styles and poor coping skills such as self-harming and substance misuse (Anda et al. 2005).

An association between ACEs and suicide attempts remains significant and depression and depressive disorders alone account for many links between mental illness and childhood sexual and/or physical abuse (Fuller-Thomson et al. (2016) and Anda et al. 2005). Childhood trauma is also a risk factor for lifelong suicide attempts (Zatti et al. 2017 and Anda et al. 2005). Zatti et al. (2017) identify four prominent risk factors for suicide attempts later in life - physical abuse, sexual abuse, neglect and the witnessing of domestic violence during childhood (Zatti et al. 2017).

Trauma and stress related disorders are listed in the Diagnostic and Statistical Manual of Mental Disorders (DSM-5) (American Psychiatric Association 2013). The range of diagnoses includes reactive attachment disorder, post-traumatic stress disorder (PTSD), adjustment disorders and acute stress disorders (American Psychiatric Association 2013). In order to receive a formal mental health diagnosis for trauma, children and young adults are assessed within Tier 3 CAMHS. A definitive diagnosis is required from a psychiatrist. This level of CAMHS service has been discussed in further detail within this chapter.

Impact on Parents' Mental Ill Health on Children

The World Health Organisation (2019) report that 5% of adults globally experience depression whilst in the UK 25% of adults have at least one diagnosable mental health condition and 10% of children between the ages of five and sixteen have a diagnosable mental health condition (Kings Fund 2019). The cost of perinatal mental illness is significant not just in terms of outcomes for parents and their children but the financial cost to society and health and social care services. Bauer et al. (2014) calculated that perinatal mental illness costs £8.1 billion per year in the UK with 28% of these costs related to the mother and 72% related to the child.

Mental health across the lifespan deteriorated during the COVID-19 pandemic with Pierce et al.'s study (2020) identifying that people within the UK on a low income, unemployed and women with children at home (particularly pre-school children) had an increased risk of deterioration. The increase for mental health support has been evident through PANDAS Foundation (2021). This UK based charity providing peer support for parents experiencing mental health symptoms, report a 240% increase in calls to their helpline and 150% increase in email contacts during the period of March 2020 – March 2021. With the prevalence of mental health conditions so high it is unsurprising that many parents experience mental health needs during key stages of their children's life.

Poor maternal mental health in pregnancy and postnatal care has been recognised as disadvantageous to infant and family well-being for decades new evidence is starting to emerge about baby's brain development following birth. Long term impacts on children's well-being in response to their early childhood experience is now starting to become recognised of vital importance. Babies are born primed to learn but are dependent on parents, family, and other carers to gain experiences which will promote healthy brain growth and optimise their development. Developing an emotional attachment in childhood is associated with the ability to develop positive relationships throughout life (Marks, Murray, and Vida Estacio 2018) therefore babies whose parents respond readily to their needs and provide positive stimulation through communication and play are more likely to develop the skills required for independent and successful lives.

Parents with poor mental health may be less responsive to their babies or children. For example, anxiety and depression affects 13% of women antenatally and up to 20% of women in the year following birth (NICE 2016). In addition, it is now increasingly recognised that fathers' can also experience depression during and following the pregnancy. Around 10% of fathers experience postnatal depression and up to 18% experience anxiety in the perinatal period (Leach et al. 2016). However, prevalence of perinatal mental illness in fathers (PMI) increases significantly to 25–50% when mothers are also experiencing perinatal mental illness (PMI) (Goodman 2004). A significant risk factor for a father to develop depression following their babies' birth has been feeling excluded from the bond between mother and baby (Kim and Swain 2007). Further to this, McDonald et al. (2021) has suggested that men who do become fathers can be at greater risk of mental health problems if they themselves did not have a secure attachment with their own caregiver (mother) as a baby and child.

A trait of depression is that the individual tends to be more self-absorbed and self-focused. In parents this may result in a decreased focus on their child's feelings

(Hanley and Williams 2020) rather than being attentive or nurturing. In addition, parental depression can lead to a baby being exposed to toxic stress which may result in distorted stress responses in later life from the child (Leadsom et al. 2013). Therefore, babies who are exposed to stress, trauma, and who experience delayed or unmet needs are likely to have long term negative impact from their early years experiences resulting in poorer life outcomes (Leadsom et al. 2013). Although children of parents with PMI do not automatically experience poorer outcomes, children whose mothers experienced psychological distress have an increased risk of developing an emotional disorder. Parry-Langdon (2008) proposes that a mothers' poor mental health negatively affects the child's cognitive and emotional development which creates a five times higher risk of the child developing mental health problems in later life. Both parents experiencing mental illness increases the risk to the child's development and long -term psychological well-being. When adverse experiences in childhood are not recalled they still have the potential to impact on cognitive functioning in adulthood (Reuben et al. 2016).

Parents' poor mental health is a contributing factor to attachment disorder and adverse childhood experiences both of which have life-long impacts on health and well-being. Hanley and Williams (2020) identified some evidence that maternal anxiety at thirty-two weeks gestation increased the risk of the child experiencing poor behavioural outcomes and diagnosis of ADHD. Links between poor behavioural outcomes and parental mental health are also supported by Hoeve (2012) who considered how Bowlby's 1973 attachment theory identifies that if attachment between parent and children is disrupted children can experience relationship difficulties, delinquency and aggressive behaviour.

Links between parental mood disorders and children experiencing mental illness are also evidenced. A study by Vandeleur et al. (2012) identified that children whose parents had a major depressive disorder had an increased risk of developing a mood disorder and anxiety with separation anxiety disorder most commonly affecting children aged 6–11 years. They also found an increased risk in female children of developing alcohol dependency disorder with male children having an increased risk of cannabis abuse. Sandstrom et al. (2020) also reported that children of parents with a major depressive disorder displayed increased anxiety. Their findings suggested that language, thought processing, oppositional behaviour and attention difficulties were frequently observed and could be utilised as observation-based indicators of risk of the child developing externalising disorders and cognitive impairment. Similarly to Sandstrom et al. (2020), supporting the use of child observations, Verderhus et al. (2021) proposes screening for ACE's can make a difference to facilitating effective and early interventions for health conditions such as PTSD, depression and substance misuse.

No Health Without Mental Health promotes the importance of positive parenting in providing the best start to life. They identify that a "good start in life and positive parenting are fundamental to good mental health and wellbeing, and to lifelong resilience to adversity" (HM Government 2011 p. 10). Supporting parents to be able to care for their infants warmly, responsively and safely is essential to reduce the impact of parents' mental health and adverse life conditions. Leadsom et al.'s 1001 Critical Days (2013) emphasises the need for preventative services to reduce the risk of parents mental health to their children particularly important when it is evidenced that the 50% of lifelong mental health conditions start before the age of 14 years

(HM Government 2011). The four-tiered approach of the initiative promotes timely access to local universal and specialist for women at risk of or experiencing mental health problems along with access to antenatal classes for all parents however despite the evidence of father's mental health there is little focus on their needs. Hopefully evaluation of the initiative will result in fathers needs also being considered. This is particularly important as Nomaguchi et al. (2017) suggest that fathers can buffer the impact of maternal stress on young infants by contributing towards caretaking activities and providing practical support for the mother, both of which reduce pressure on the mother and therefore decrease the infant's exposure to stress.

Mental Health in School

Schools play a key role in the mental health and well-being of children and young people. The Children's Society (2020) state that schools provide a safe space for pupils, a support network where signs of abuse and neglect can be detected and young carers can be supported, and a well-being boost providing important opportunities for socialisation and play.

Schools have a statutory duty to promote the welfare of pupils; this includes preventing the impairment of a child's health or development and taking steps to ensure best outcomes for all (Department for Education 2021). However, the Department for Education advice in relation to mental health is non-statutory and schools have a significant amount of flexibility to decide how they provide mental health support (Department for Education 2018). It is estimated that 52% of English primary schools provide counselling services, and 70% of secondary schools (Parkin and Long 2021). Schools do not need to have a discreet mental health policy but are required to produce a range of policies which clearly promote mental health and well-being. It is important for schools to be aware that the Equality Act (2010) places a legal duty to support pupils with a mental health condition if it has a long-term impact on normal day-to-day activity, in these circumstances reasonable adjustments must be made. The guidance emphasises that mental health problems affect many pupils and that schools have a responsibility to develop a whole-school approach (Public Health England 2021). For example, discussions around mental health can be embedded in teaching sessions on relationships, citizenship, sex, and health. Schools should develop ways to appropriately use the pupil premium (additional funding for disadvantaged children in schools in England) and special educational needs (SEN) budgets to support pupils with mental health issues. The guidance recognises that there are often links between mental health and behavioural issues. For example, pupils may present as being withdrawn, anxious or disruptive, and schools are expected to identify and support in these situations. Professionals working in the education sector are not expected to be mental health experts. However, all staff within a school should be able to identify potential mental health problems and be aware of systems which allow for referral and escalation of issues. These responsibilities are placed not only on direct teaching staff but also school leaders, safeguarding leads and governors. Schools are encouraged to adopt the following Department for Education (2018) model:

- Prevent: creating a safe and positive environment through the teaching and ethos of the school
- Identification: recognising mental health issues in a timely and appropriate manner

- Early support: helping pupils to promptly access mental health support
- Referral to specialist support: ensuring referrals are made to external agencies such as CAMHS, GP, and voluntary agencies. Putting pupils, families, and carers in touch with local and/or national organisations that offer support and guidance

Of course, all pupils will experience some levels of stress during their school careers, often related to examination periods or key transition stages. The Department for Education (2018) identify mental health problems or disorders when children and young people experience emotional and/or behavioural problems which are beyond the scope to be expected at any given age. This can include, but is not limited to, depression, anxiety, attachment disorders, trauma disorders, eating disorders, habit disorders, and psychotic disorders. The 2020 Mental Health of Children and Young People (MHCYP) survey (Vizard et al. 2020), assessed different types of mental health issues and asked parents, children, and young people to judge whether it is unlikely, possible, or probable that a mental disorder is present. The findings of this survey showed that 14.4% of primary school children (5- to 10-year-olds) had a probable mental disorder, an increase of 5% since 2017. For children of secondary school age (11- to 16-year-olds), 17.6% were assessed as having a probable mental disorder, again a 5% increase since 2017. This survey highlighted the significance of school support, with 62.6% of children and young people aged between 5 and 16 with a probable mental disorder receiving support from school or college. Despite this, it should be recognised that providing mental health support in schools can be challenging. Gee et al. (2021) recognise that staff delivering mental health support in schools, and senior educational leaders, must receive high-quality training, and that young people themselves should be involved in the design of school-based support. The Care Quality Commission (CQC) (2017) report found that mental health provision in schools is inconsistent and that the mental health of pupils is adversely affected where access to high-quality counselling is unavailable. School leaders expressed within the report they do not have the 'expertise or time' to deliver this level of support themselves and counselling is the highly desired option to be embedded in all schools (CQC 2017, p. 24)

The Social Policy chapter in this book discusses the ways in which school closures during the COVID-19 lockdowns had a damaging impact on many children and young people, particularly disadvantaged pupils. These inequalities in experience were also evident for pupils with mental health problems. Children and young people aged 11–16 with a probable mental disorder were more likely to say that lockdown had made their life worse (54.1%) than those unlikely to have a mental disorder (39.2%). Public Health experts have questioned the value of closing schools during the COVID-19 pandemic. It is argued that there was an insufficient evidence base to link school closures with a reduction in COVID-19 rates, and that school closures exacerbate mental health problems and social isolation (Lewis et al. 2021). There are certainly long-term educational and mental health consequences of the 2020 COVID-19 lockdowns. It has been identified that students' mental health should be prioritised alongside academic targets (Widnall et al. 2020). Access to mental health support services is vital for children and young people but the pandemic impeded access to this support; it was reported that nearly 45% of 17–22 year olds with probable mental health problems did not seek help as a result of COVID-19 (Newlove-Delgado et al. 2021).

In May 2021, the government committed to providing an additional £17 million funding to improve mental health and wellbeing in education. This funding can be used to train a mental health lead, and to provide support and resources to staff working with children and young people whose mental health has been adversely affected by the pandemic (Department for Education 2021). This sits alongside government commitments to improve mental health in schools following the Green Paper 'Transforming children and young people's mental health provision' (Department of Health and Social Care and Department of Education 2017). However, there have been criticisms that these commitments are not backed up with adequate resources, that there remains a lack of joined-up work with other community mental health services, and that key groups such as young women and those from minority ethnic groups are not sufficiently prioritised (Khan 2017).

Mental Health Risk and Protective Factors

In an educational setting there are a number of risk factors which mean pupils are more likely to experience mental health problems, and protective factors which can promote resilience (Department for Education 2018). It is important to explore these risk and protective factors as they tell us a great deal not just about mental health and schools, but also about the mental health of children and young people in a broader sense. Discrimination and stigma are significant risk factors associated with mental health issues. Gronholm et al. (2017) powerfully describe the impact of mental health discrimination and the complex, multi-faceted ways that it can lead to social exclusion, including reduced educational opportunities. They emphasise that the impact of discrimination can be as significant as mental ill health itself and the stigma associated with this. One of the six objectives of the UK government's 'No Health Without Mental Health' policy is that fewer people will experience stigma and discrimination (HM Government 2011). Bullying, including online bullying, is a significant risk factor for young people's mental health. It has been found that an unsupportive school environment and negative body image can create a susceptibility to bullying, especially for girls (Landstedt and Persson 2014). This research called for improvements to the school environment and the promotion of anti-violence educational programmes. This mirrors the protective factors identified by the Department for Education (2018) to respond to discrimination, stigma and bullying which include promoting positive peer relationships, having robust safeguarding and child protection policies, and ensuring effective partnership work for specialist referrals.

There are clear links between socio-economic disadvantage and childhood mental health issues with significant impacts on children and young people in a school and home setting. A study by University College London (Deighton et al. 2019), of over 28,000 pupils in year 7 (aged 11–12) and year 9 (aged 13–14) in state secondary schools found that the prevalence of mental health in England is greater than previously thought. 40% of pupils scored above abnormal thresholds for emotional problems, conduct problem and hyperactivity. Socio-economic disadvantage (measured in this study by entitlement to Free School Meals) was identified as a significant mental health risk. Whitehead, Taylor-Robinson, and Barr (2021, p. 1) highlight the links between child poverty and mental health problems, stating that 'child poverty is already the biggest threat to child health and development in the UK'.

They emphasise that the COVID-19 pandemic has exacerbated existing inequalities with lockdown measures disproportionately affecting children from low-income families. There are particularly close links between homelessness and mental health problems. The national homeless charity Centrepoint (2021) report that over 50% of homeless young people reported mental health issues, with anxiety, depression and stress most commonly reported. This is compounded by the fact that many young, homeless people with mental health problems are reluctant to, or find it hard to access support services (Black et al. 2018). A number of protective factors in the school environment can help to mitigate social disadvantage. They include promoting effective support networks, effectively using the pupil premium, ensuring the take-up of free school meals, and providing leisure and sport activities. Ultimately, the socio-economic influence on childhood mental health problems is directly linked to policy decisions. It is acknowledged that anti-poverty programmes and direct cash transfers can improve mental health. Measures such as providing higher levels of means-tested benefits, increasing the pupil premium, and investing in preventive services (such as Sure Start children's centres) would reduce financial insecurity and improve childhood mental health (Whitehead, Taylor-Robinson, and Barr 2021).

It is recognised that challenging family circumstances can adversely affect childhood mental health and present a significant educational risk factor. A large-scale study of over 10,000 mothers with children born between 2000 and 2002 highlighted the enduring influence that parent's relationship has on childhood mental health (Benson and McKay 2017). Family breakdown has a critical, and gendered, impact on childhood mental health. This research found that for girls family breakdown has the greatest single impact on mental health, and for boys it is the equal top influence; girls are more likely to display emotional problems, while boys are more likely to exhibit behavioural problems. An earlier study emphasised the adverse impact of family breakdown on mental health but cautioned that the focus should not only be on family types but also on 'family functions' such as communication between parents, level of conflict, financial insecurity, existing mental health issues within the family, and parent-child relationships (Mooney, Oliver and Smith 2009). Similarly, the links between childhood mental health and domestic violence are well-established. Holt, Buckley, and Whelan (2008) highlight that young people living with domestic violence are at increased risk of experiencing emotional and behavioural problems, and that these issues can have an enduring impact and intersect with other challenges in a young person's life.

Childhood maltreatment, including sexual or physical abuse and neglect, not only has a very significant impact on the school life of children and young people but is also a serious public health and human rights issue (Lazenbatt 2010). Childhood maltreatment can be linked not only to educational failure but can 'have major long-term effects on all aspects of a child's health, growth and intellectual development and mental wellbeing' (Lazenbatt 2010, p. 2). Research has shown that childhood maltreatment is linked to a wide range of adverse outcomes for young people including serious mental health problems, educational deficit, addiction issues, and sexual health problems (Strathearn et al. 2020).

One of the most challenging family circumstances is bereavement. The Childhood Bereavement Network (2016) found that in 2015 approximately 41,000 children in the UK lost a parent before their eighteenth birthday; this equates to a child experiencing parental bereavement every 22 minutes. Weinstock et al. (2021) report that COVID-19 bereavements have created a 'grief pandemic' affecting over 1 million children and young people. They highlight that adolescents are at risk of complicated grief during the pandemic, especially those from disadvantaged backgrounds. McLaughlin, Lytje and Holliday (2019) stress that bereavement, while painful, is part of the human experience. However, there are bereavement related-risk markers of mental and behavioural problems. Young people experiencing multiple-death bereavement have a higher post-traumatic stress score than those bereaved by a single death. Where suicide is the cause of bereavement, young people themselves are more likely to experience suicidal thoughts/behaviours. Young people who are parentally bereaved are more likely to experience depression than those who experience the death of other adults (Kaplow et al. 2020).

There are a number of ways in which schools, and agencies in the Health Care social sector, can respond to challenging family circumstances. The Department for Education (2018) outline the following as protective factors: affection, clear and consistent discipline, stable long-term relationships, the presence of at least one supportive adult, celebrating success, and experience of secure attachment. Lazenbatt (2010) emphasises the key role that staff in schools have in recognising and responding to maltreated children and being aware of signs of abuse and neglect. It should be recognised that schools need to work in collaboration with other services to build a strong network of support around pupils (Mowat 2019). Good practice should centre on holistic, person-centred assessment and individualised responses to the challenges that young people face (Holt, Buckley, and Whelan 2008). McLaughlin, Lytje and Holliday (2019) emphasise the supportive role that schools can provide to bereaved children. Often the capacity of the immediate family to support children can be limited as they too are grieving. Staff at schools should be available to talk to pupils and this can promote resilience and reduce the potential for high-risk behaviour. The COVID-19 pandemic provides an opportunity for schools, and other health and social care agencies, to 'reinvigorate collective structures that can help vulnerable young people through their darkest moments' (Weinstock et al. 2021, p. 5).

Child Adolescent Mental Health Services (CAMHS)

CAMHS is a specialist mental health service for young people up to the age of 18. Different localities describe levels of service available using a four-tier model (Figure 14.1). Terminology and boundaries between tiers do vary slightly across the country (Scie 2012).

CAMHS Tiers

CAMHS is predominantly classified as a Tier 3 and 4 service. As shown in Figure 14.1, Tier 3 denotes a specialist service and Tier 4 a highly specialist inpatient unit. Historically, CAMHS provided a Tier 2 'Emotional Wellbeing Service' for young people presenting with mild to moderate difficulties, eg. low self-esteem or anger management issues. This tier still operates in some localities such as Hertfordshire and Calderdale, West Yorkshire, but it is now largely covered by early intervention services within the third sector - voluntary agencies or charities and

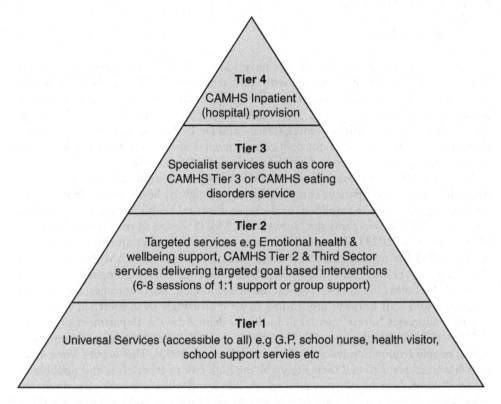

Figure 14.1 Child Adolescent Mental Health Services (CAMHS).

Source: *(Adapted from Healthy Young Minds, 2021).*

counselling services who offer 'goal based' short term interventions. Salmond and Jim (2007) state that Tier 2 services provide early assessment and thus tend to work with younger clients. Regardless of provider, however, early intervention is of paramount importance.

Within Tier 3 young people present with significant and complex problems. These often have a profound impact upon mental health causing difficulties in accomplishing daily tasks. NHS England (2014b) observes that Tier 3 patients typically present with one or more of the following symptoms:

- Emotional and behavioural disorders (moderate or severe)
- Conduct disorder and oppositional defiant disorder
- Psychosis (14 years plus)
- Obsessive-compulsive disorder (OCD)
- Self-harm
- Suicidal ideation
- Dual diagnosis including co-morbid drug and alcohol use
- Neuropsychiatric conditions
- Attachment disorders
- Post-traumatic stress disorders

- Development disorders
- Anxiety and mood disorders
- Eating disorders

Symptoms may differ, but all patients have unhealthy ways of coping with mental distress. Young people often present with self-harm which can be repetitive, ritualistic and compulsive. Examples include, self-cutting, scratching, burning or scalding, head- banging or hair-pulling, over/under-medicating, punching/hitting/bruising, swallowing objects, or self-poisoning (Derby and Derbyshire Safeguarding Children's Partnership 2020). Although not defined as a mental illness, self-harm is a symptom of poor coping mechanisms and emotional distress (Lancet 2016).

Tier 3 clients are supported by a CAMHS clinician within the community and normally attend an outpatient clinic weekly or fortnightly. Sessions and contact may increase if patient risk is amplified, or decrease if mental health becomes more stable. During the 2020 Covid pandemic, however, CAMHS moved to remote consultations (Bhardwaj et al. 2021). The pandemic was seen as a 'perfect storm' (Danese and Smith, 2020) for mental health services, placing a strain on CAMHS nationwide (Bentham, Driver and Stark 2020). This could have an alarming impact on referral rates. McNicholas (2018) observes that under-resourcing, staff shortages, recruitment challenges and staff burnout are leading to an increasingly over-stretched service.

Tier 4 addresses 'severe' mental ill health as defined by the Department of Health (DH) necessitating 'highly specialist' inpatient care (DH 2003). Only a small number of young people require admission to Tier 4 (McDougall 2008). This occurs when a patient has fixed plans to end their life involving high risk to themselves and possibly to others. Patients have usually moved through Tier 3 and will move back after discharge from Tier 4. Tier 4 can act as assessment only or assessment and treatment for those needing time on a secure psychiatric unit. 24/7 care is overseen by nurses whose observations prevent self-injury, ensure a safe environment and promote interpersonal interventions to encourage recovery (Foster and Smedley 2019). At all stages, a multidisciplinary approach is essential to planning care (Partridge et al. 2010).

Teams within CAMHS

Tier 3 CAMHS is community based and is usually divided into two teams; 'Core CAMHS' addresses generic mental illness (including conditions listed earlier in this chapter), and a second team works exclusively with 'Eating Disorders'. In addition to this, a CAMHS out of hours crisis team and a hospital liaison team may operate to respond to situations where a young person presents in immediate life-threatening danger – for example, overdose, strangulation, ligature attempts, hallucination, self-harm requiring medical attention or suicidal plans with the intent to end life (Wright et al. 2010 cited in Richardson). The existence of emergency teams depends on commissioning within a particular locality, but the NHS Long Term Plan (2019) intends to expand age appropriate crisis services across England.

Who is Employed within CAMHS?

CAMHS employs professionals with extensive knowledge of children and young people within the context of mental health and illness. Historically, community Tier 3

CAMHS employed Mental Health Nurses, however, this expanded to include professionals from other disciplines, for example, social workers, occupational therapists, adult trained nurses, systematic family therapists, cognitive behavioural therapists (CBT) and psychiatrists. In some situations, the law requires interventions to be made by specialised professionals. For example, Psychiatrists can prescribe medication and detain and legally section a patient under the Mental Health Act and cognitive behavioural therapy (CBT) can only be delivered by therapists registered by a professional body.

Access to CAMHS

An increasing number of CAMHS units in England are adopting a streamlined 'in house' referral route straight into CAMHS known as the 'Single Point of Access' (SPA). This allows CAMHS to be an 'active gatekeeper' (Rocks et al. 2020) by screening referrals. It also allows clinicians to proactively engage with professionals, carers or young people who may raise queries about a referral. Adopting this model can 'simplify' access to direct support and help to remove barriers to mental health services (Rocks et al. 2020).

It is however a contentious issue with accessibility into this level of mental health provision within a CAMH service. Hiller and Clair (2018) asserts that many young people experiencing early onset of mental health issues are not adequately supported by services and professionals in a timely manner. As a result of being left untreated, this can develop into chronic mental ill health conditions as suggested by Hiller et al. (2018) and for some young people this leads to sectioning under the Mental Health Act. Even when children and young people are accepted into CAMHS there are high thresholds for treatment which can mean that they are placed at the end of lengthy waiting lists (CQC 2017 and House of Commons 2016). Further to this, it has been evidenced for many years that mental health services are turning away vulnerable young people who are residing in care because they do not have what is considered to be a 'stable placement' (House of Commons 2016, p. 7). This has been seen to be a challenging issue with those children in care not being able to access the mental health treatment they require due to movement across different placements and new referrals being issued into different CAMH teams (House of Commons 2016; NSPCC Learning 2021). This is an ongoing challenge for children in care to be able to access support required. CAMHS teams are structured very differently across the UK depending on the Clinical Commissioning Groups (CCG) with only a few CAMHS still having a dedicated Looked After Children (LAC) Team situated within their service provision. As it seems, those teams which do still operate have been 'ring-fenced' to provide this service in some areas within the UK for children who are in local authority care, and require a mental health service with mental health practitioners who have expertise with children in the care system (House of Commons 2016).

What is CAMHS Commissioned to Deliver?

The DH 'Future in Mind' report (2015) prioritises the NHS's 'Five Year Forward View' (5YFV) strategy (2015) which sets targets for a system-wide transformation of CAMHS embedding the principles of Children and Young People Improving Access to Psychological Therapies (CYP-IAPT). Each CAMHS area has a transformation plan to ensure therapeutic interventions are evidence based. (Fonagy and Pugh, 2017). This seeks to align therapeutic talking provided by CAMHS with adult mental health services which deliver IAPT (Ludlow, Hurn and Lansdell 2020). Ludlow et al. (2020) state that this high intensity workforce would deliver CBT to young people with moderate to severe anxiety and help guard against vulnerabilities in later life. Improving care through evidence-based practice (EBP) and measuring outcomes reflects the foundational principles of CYP-IAT (Burn et al. 2020).

Conclusion

To conclude, this chapter has alerted, toxic stress during infancy and throughout childhood can be damaging to a child's overall mental health and wellbeing. As discussed in the chapter, children and young people who have been exposed to ACEs can develop increased vulnerabilities where there is a likelihood that they will engage in risky behaviour and even suicidal attempts across their lifespan.

A parent's bond is vital for babies to have the stimulation they require in the infancy years as highlighted in the Government (2021) campaign. This once again raises the attention to the importance of those early years in a baby's life which can then impact on their overall health and development. Recognising deterioration in the parent's mental health has been raised within this chapter as being crucial.

As this book chapter illustrates, mental ill health in childhood can be complex and vary greatly. Understanding which service can support a child's mental health presentation can be challenging. CAMHS Tier 3 is the one primarily accessed for treatment and diagnosis. Other emotional services are available and should be sourced to ensure the correct route of referrals is made to best meet the child's individual needs. The policy and provision discussed further supports the need for education providers to have trained and qualified staff who have appropriate skills, knowledge, and experience to make referrals to appropriate emotional wellbeing services.

Once again, the complexities and barriers with accessing CAMHS particularly for children who reside in the care system has been raised, this of course varies vastly across the UK and more consideration needs to be given to these vulnerable children to access the specialist mental health support they need.

References

American Psychiatric Association, 2013. *Diagnostic and statistical Manual of mental Disorders (DSM-5)* [eBook type]. 5th ed. Washing DC, America: American Psychiatric Publishing. Available via: https://ebookcentral.proquest.com/lib/ntuuk/detail.action?docID=1811753 [Accessed 10 September 2021].

Anda, R., Felitti, V., Bremner, D., Walker, J., Whitfield, C., Perry, B., Dube, S., and Giles, W., 2005. The enduring effects of abuse and related adverse experiences in childhood. A convergence of evidence from neurobiology and epidemiology. *European Archives of Psychiatry and Clinical Neuroscience* [online], 256, 174–186. DOI: 10.1007/s00406-005-0624-4. [Accessed 10 September 2021].

Arnold, J., and Baker, C., 2018. The role of mental health nurses in supporting young people's mental health: a review of the literature. *Mental Health Review Journal* [online], 23 (3), 197–220. DOI: 10.1108/MHRJ-09-2017-0039. [Accessed 07 August 2021].

Audit Scotland. 2019. NHS in Scotland.

Bauer, A., Parsonage, M., Knapp, M., Lemmi, V., and Adelaja, B., 2014. *Costs of perinatal mental health problems* [online]. London: Centre for Mental Health. Available at: https://www.centreformentalhealth.org.uk/sites/default/files/2018-09/costsofperinatal.pdf [Accessed 8 October 2021].

Benson, H., and McKay, S., 2017. *Family breakdown and teenage mental health* [online]. Romford, UK: Marriage Foundation. Available at: https://marriagefoundation.org.uk/wp-content/uploads/2017/11/MF-paper-Family-breakdown-and-teenage-mental-health-FINAL.pdf

Bentham, C., Driver, J., and Stark, D., 2020. Wellbeing of CAMHS staff and changes in working practices during the COVID-19 pandemic. *Journal of Child and Adolescent Psychiatric Nursing* [online], 34 (3), 225–235. DOI: 10.1111/jcap.12311. [Accessed 01 September 2021].

Bhardwaj, A., Moore, A., Cardinal, R.N., Bradley, C., Cross, L., and Ford, T.J., 2021. Survey of CAMHS clinicians about their experience of remote consultation: brief report. *BJPsych Open* [online], 7 (1), 1–4. DOI: 10.1192/bjo.2020.160. [Accessed 28 August 2021].

Black, E., Fedyszyn, I., Mildred, H., Perkin, R., Lough, R., Brann, P., and Ritter, C., 2018. Homeless youth: Barriers and facilitators for service referrals. *Evaluation and Program Planning* [online], 68, 7–12. DOI: 10.1016/j.evalprogplan.2018.02.009.

Burn, A.M., Vainre, M., Humphrey, A., and Howarth, E., 2020. Evaluating the CYP-IAPT transformation of child and adolescent mental health services in Cambridgeshire, UK: a qualitative implementation study. *Implementation Science Communications* [online], 1(89), 1–13. DOI: 10.1186/s43058-020-00078-6. [Accessed 10 August 2021].

Care Quality Commission (CQC), 2017. *Review of children and young people's mental health services* [online]. London: Care Quality Commission. Available at: https://www.cqc.org.uk/sites/default/files/20171103_cypmhphase1_report.pdf

Centrepoint, 2021. *The mental health needs of homeless young people* [online]. London: Centrepoint. Available at: https://centrepoint.org.uk/media/4650/prevalence-of-mental-health-need-report.pdf

Chang, X., Jiang, X., Mkandarwire, T., and Shen, M., 2019. Associations between adverse childhood experiences and health outcomes in adults aged 18–59 years. *PloS one* [online], 14 (2), e0211850. DOI: 10.1371/journal.pone.0211850. [Accessed 14 May 2022].

Cheong, E.V., Sinnott. C., Dahly. D., and Kearney, P.M., 2017. Adverse childhood experiences (ACEs) and later-life depression: perceived social support as a potential protective factor. *BMJ Open* [online], 7 (9), 1–11. DOI: 10.1136/bmjopen-2016-013228. [Accessed 18 May 2022].

Childhood Bereavement Network, 2016. *Key estimated statistics on childhood bereavement.* London: Childhood Bereavement Network. Available at: https://childhoodbereavementnetwork.org.uk/about-1/what-we-do/research-evidence/key-statistics

Danese, A., and Smith, P., 2020. Debate: Recognising and responding to the mental health needs of young people in the era of COVID-19. *Child and Adolescent Mental Health* [online], 25 (3), 169–170. DOI: 10.1111/camh.12414. [Accessed 01 September 2021].

Deighton, J., Lereya, S., Casey, P., Patalay, P., Humphrey, N., and Wolpert, M., 2019. Prevalence of mental health problems in schools: Poverty and other risk factors among 28 000 adolescents in England. *British Journal of Psychiatry* [online], 215 (3), 565–567. DOI:1 0.1192/bjp.2019.19

Department for Education, 2018. *Mental health and behaviour in schools.* London: Department for Education. Available at: https://assets.publishing.service.gov.uk/government/uploads/system/uploads/attachment_data/file/755135/Mental_health_and_behaviour_in_schools__.pdf

Department for Education, 2021. *Keeping children safe in education 2021 Statutory guidance for schools and colleges* [online]. London: Department for Education. Available at: https://assets.publishing.service.gov.uk/government/uploads/system/uploads/attachment_data/file/1021914/KCSIE_2021_September_guidance.pdf

Department for Education, 2021. *Schools and colleges to benefit from boost in expert mental health support* [online]. London: Department for Education. Available at: https://www.gov.uk/government/news/schools-and-colleges-to-benefit-from-boost-in-expert-mental-health-support

Department of Health [DH], 2003. *Specialised Services National Definition Set: 23 specialised services for children.* London: HMSO.

Department of Health [DH], 2015. *Future in mind; Promoting, protecting and improving our children and young people's mental health and wellbeing* [online]. London: Department of Health. Available at: https://assets.publishing.service.gov.uk/government/uploads/system/uploads/attachment_data/file/414024/Childrens_Mental_Health.pdf

Department of Health and Social Care and Department of Education, 2017. *Transforming children and young people's mental health provision: a green paper* [online]. London: Department of Health. Available at: https://www.gov.uk/government/consultations/transforming-children-and-young-peoples-mental-health-provision-a-green-paper

Derby and Derbyshire Safeguarding Children Partnership, 2020. *Self-harm and Suicidal Behaviour Guidance Working with children and young people in Derby City and Derbyshire* [online]. Derby: Derby and Derbyshire Safeguarding Children Partnership. Available at: https://www.proceduresonline.com/derbyshire/scbs/user_controlled_lcms_area/uploaded_files/Self%20Harm%20and%20Suicidal%20Behaviour%20Support%20Guidance%20September%202020.pdf [Accessed 01 September 2021].

Duin, V.L., Bevaart, F., Zijlmans, J., Luijks, M.J.A., Doreleijers, T.A.H., Oldehinkel, A., Marhe, R., and Popma, A., 2018. The role of adverse childhood experiences and mental health care use in psychological dysfunctioning of male multi-problem young adults. *European Journal of Child and Adolescent Psychiatry* [online], 28, 1065–1078. DOI: 10.1007/s00787-018-1263-4. [Accessed 16 May 2022].

Feltz-Cornelis, C., Potters, E., Dam, A., Koorndijk, R., Elfeddali, I., and Sluijs, J., 2019. Adverse Childhood Experiences (ACE) in outpatients with anxiety and depressive disorders and their association with psychiatric and somatic comorbidity and revictimization. Cross-sectional observational study. *Journal of Affective Disorders* [online], 246, 458–464. DOI: 10.1016/j.jad.2018.12.096. [Accessed 10 September 2021].

Fonagy, P., and Pugh, K., 2017. Editorial: CAMHS goes mainstream. *Child and adolescent mental health* [online], 22(1), 1–3. DOI: 10.1111/camh.12209. [Accessed 10 August 2021].

Foster, C., and Smedley, K., 2019. Understanding the nature of mental health nursing within CAMHS PICU: 1. Identifying nursing interventions that contribute to the recovery journey of young people. *Journal of psychiatric intensive care* [online], 15 (2), 87–102. DOI: https://doi-org.ntu.idm.oclc.org/10.20299/jpi.2019.012. [Accessed 27 August 2021].

Fuller-Thomson, E., Baird, S.L., Dhrodia, R., and Brennenstuhl, S., 2016. The association between adverse childhood experiences (ACEs) and suicide attempts in a population-based study. *Child: Care, Health and Development* [online] 42(5), 725–734. DOI: 10.1111/cch.12351. [Accessed 10 September 2021].

Gee, B., Wilson, J., Clarke, T., Farthing, S., Carroll, B., Jackson, C., King, K., Murdoch, J., Fonagy, P., and Notley, C., 2021, Review: Delivering mental health support within schools and colleges – a thematic synthesis of barriers and facilitators to implementation of indicated psychological interventions for adolescents. *Child and Adolescent Mental Health* [online], 26 (1), 34–46. 10.1111/camh.12381

Goodman, J., 2004. Paternal postpartum depression, its relationship to maternal postpartum depression, and implications for family health. *Journal of Advanced Nursing* [online], 45 (1), 26–35. DOI: https://doi-org.libezproxy.open.ac.uk/10.1046/j.1365-2648.2003.02857.x. [Accessed 8 October 2021].

Gronholm, P.C., Henderson, C., Deb, T., and Thornicroft, G., 2017. Interventions to reduce discrimination and stigma: the state of the art. *Social Psychiatry and Psychiatric Epidemiology* [online], 52 (3), 249–258. DOI: 10.1007/s00127-017-1341-9.

Hanley, J., and Williams, M., 2020. *Fathers and Perinatal Mental Health A Guide for Recognition, Treatment and Management.* Oxen: Routledge.

Hiller, R.M., and Clair, M.C., 2018. The emotional and behavioural symptom trajectories of children in long-term out-of-home care in an English local authority. *Child Abuse & Neglect* [online], 81, 106–117. DOI: 10.1016/j.chiabu.2018.04.017. [Accessed 03 April 2022].

HM Government, 2011. *No Health Without Mental Health. A cross-government mental health outcomes strategy for people of all ages* [online]. London: HM Government. Available at: https://assets.publishing.service.gov.uk/government/uploads/system/uploads/attachment_data/file/138253/dh_124058.pdf

HM Government, 2021. *The best start for life: a vision for 1,001 critical days.* London: HM Government. Available at: https://assets.publishing.service.gov.uk/government/uploads/system/uploads/attachment_data/file/973112/The_best_start_for_life_a_vision_for_the_1_001_critical_days.pdf. [Accessed 04 November 2021].

Hoeve, M., Stams, G.J., van der Put, C.E., Dubas, J.S., van der Laan, P.H., and Gerris, J.R., 2012. A meta-analysis of attachment to parents and delinquency. *Journal of abnormal child psychology* [online], 40(5), 771–785. DOI: 10.1007/s10802-011-9608-1. [Accessed 8 October 2021].

Holt, S., Buckley, H., and Whelan, S., 2008. The impact of exposure to domestic violence on children and young people: A review of the literature. *Child Abuse & Neglect* [online], 32 (8), 797–810. DOI: 10.1016/j.chiabu.2008.02.004.

House of Commons, 2016. *House of Commons Education Committee: mental health and well-being of looked-after children (Hc481)* [online]. London: House of Commons. Available at: https://publications.parliament.uk/pa/cm201516/cmselect/cmeduc/481/481.pdf. [Accessed 18 May 2022].

Hughes, K.E., Lowey, H., Quigg, Z., and Bellis, M.A., 2016. Relationships between adverse childhood experiences and adult mental well-being: results from an English national household survey. *BMC Public Health* [online], 16, 222. DOI: 10.1186/s12889-016-2906-3. [Accessed 16 May 2022].

Humphrey, N., Lendrum, A., Ashworth, E., Frearson, K., Buck, R., and Kerr, K. 2016. *Implementation and process evaluation (IPE) for interventions in educational settings: A synthesis of the literature.* London: EEF.

Kendall-Tackett, K., 2002. The health effects of childhood abuse: four pathways by which abuse can influence health. *Child Abuse Neglect* [online], 26 (6–7), 715–729. DOI: 10.1016/s0145-2134(02)00343-5. [Accessed 17 September 2021].

Kerker, B., Zhang, J., Nadeem, E., Stein, R., Hurlburt, M., Heneghan, A., Landsverk, J., and Horwitz, S., 2015. Adverse childhood experiences and mental health, chronic medical conditions, and development in young children, academic pediatrics. *Adverse Childhood Experiences* [online], 15(5), 510–517. DOI: 10.1016/j.acap.2015.05.005. [Accessed 10 September 2021].

Khan, L., 2017. *Transforming children's mental health? Reflections on the government's green paper.* London: Centre for Mental Health. Available at: https://www.centreformentalhealth.org.uk/blogs/transforming-childrens-mental-health-reflections-governments-green-paper

Kim, P., and Swain, J.E., 2007. Sad dads: paternal postpartum depression. *Psychiatry (Edgmont)* [online], 4 (2), 35–47. Available via: https://pubmed.ncbi.nlm.nih.gov/20805898/ [Accessed 15 May 2022].

Kings Fund, 2019. *Mental health: our position* [online]. London: The Kings Fund. Available at: https://www.kingsfund.org.uk/projects/positions/mental-health#:~:text=One%20in%20four%20adults%20have,a%20diagnosable%20mental%20health%20problem [accessed 8 October 2021].

Lancet, T., 2016. Making the most out of crisis: child and adolescent mental health in the emergency department. *The Lancet* [online], 388 (10048), 935–935. DOI: 10.1016/S0140-6736(16)31520-3. [Accessed 01 September 2021].

Landstedt, E., Persson, S., 2014. Bullying, cyberbullying, and mental health in young people. *Scandinavian Journal of Public Health* [online], 42(4), 393–399. DOI: 10.1177/1403494 814525004. [Accessed 05 August 2021].

Lazenbatt, A., 2010. *The impact of abuse and neglect on the health and mental health of children and young people* [online]. Belfast: NSPCC. Available via: https://www.researchgate.net/ publication/238772406_The_impact_of_abuse_and_neglect_on_the_health_and_mental_ health_of_children_and_young_people [Accessed 10 May 2021].

Leach, L.S., Poyser, C., Cooklin, A.R., and Giallo, R., 2016. Prevalence and course of anxiety disorders (and symptom levels) in men across the perinatal period: A systematic review. *Journal of Affective Disorders* [online], 190, 675–686. DOI: 10.1016/j.jad.2015.09.063. [Accessed 8 October 2021].

Leadsom, A., Field, F., Burstow, P., and Lucas, C., 2013. *The 1,001 critical days: the importance of the conception to age two period: a cross party manifesto* [online]. London: Department of Health. Available at: https://www.nwcscnsenate.nhs.uk/files/8614/7325/ 1138/1001cdmanifesto.pdf [Accessed 8 October 2021].

Lewis, S.J., Munro, A.P.S., Smith, G.D., and Pollock, A.M., 2021. Closing schools is not evidence based and harms children. *British Medical Journal* [online], 372, n521. DOI: 10.1136/bmj.n521

Ludlow, C., Hurn, R., and Lansdell, S., 2020. A current review of the children and young people's improving access to psychological therapies (CYP IAPT) program: perspectives on developing an accessible workforce. *Adolescent Health, Medicine And Therapeutics* [online], 11, 21–28. DOI: 10.2147/AHMT.S196492. [Accessed 10 August 2021].

Macdonald, J.A., Greenwood, C.J., Letcher, P., Spry, E.A., Mansour, K., McIntosh, J.E., Thomson, K.C., Deane, C., Biden, E.J., Edwards, B., Hutchinson, D., Cleary, J., Toumbourou, J.W., Sanson, A.V., and Olsson, C.A., 2021. Parent and peer attachments in adolescence and paternal postpartum mental health: findings from the ATP generation 3 study. *Frontiers In Psychology* [online], (12), 672174– 672174. DOI: 10.3389/fpsyg.2021. 672174. [Accessed 01 December 2021].

Marks, D.F., Murray, M., and Vida Estacio, E., 2018. *Health Psychology Theory, Research and Practice*. 5th ed. London: Sage.

McDougall, T., Worrall-Davies, A., Hewson, L., Richardson, G., and Cotgrove, A., 2008. Tier 4 child and adolescent mental health services (CAMHS) - inpatient care, day services and alternatives: an overview of tier 4 CAMHS provision in the UK. *Child and Adolescent Mental Health* [online], 13 (4), 173–180. DOI: 10.1111/j.1475-3588.2007.00481.x. [Accessed 01 September 2021].

McLaughlin, C., Lytje, M., and Holliday, C. 2019. Consequences of childhood bereavement in the context of the British school system. Report for the Faculty of Education, University of Cambridge.

McLaughlin, K., Conron, K., Koenen, K., and Gilman, S., 2010. Childhood adversity, adult stressful life events, and risk of past-year psychiatric disorder: a test of the stress sensitization hypothesis in a population-based sample of adults. *Psychological Medicine* [online], 40 (10), 1647–1658. DOI: 10.1017/S0033291709992121. [Accessed 10 September 2021].

McNicholas, F., 2018. Child & adolescent emergency mental health crisis: a neglected cohort. *Irish Medical Journal* [online], 111(10), 841. Available via: https://imj.ie/child-adolescent-emergency-mental-health-crisis-a-neglected-cohort/

Mooney, A., Oliver, C., and Smith, M., 2009. *Impact of family breakdown on children's wellbeing evidence review* [online]. London: Department for Children, Schools and Families. Available at: https://core.ac.uk/download/pdf/4160412.pdf

Mowat, J.G., 2019. Exploring the impact of social inequality and poverty on the mental health and wellbeing and attainment of children and young people in Scotland. *Improving Schools* [online], 22 (3), 204–223. DOI: 10.1177/1365480219835323

Nemeroff, C., and Binder, E., 2014. The preeminent role of childhood abuse and neglect in vulnerability to major psychiatric disorders: toward elucidating the underlying neurobiological mechanisms. *Journal of the American Academy of Child and Adolescent Psychiatry* [online], 53 (4), 395–397. DOI: 10.1016/j.jaac.2014.02.004. [Accessed 10 September 2021].

Newlove-Delgado, T., McManus, S., Sadler, K., Thandi,S., Vizard, T., Cartwright, C., and Ford, T., 2021. Mental Health of Children and Young People group. Child mental health in England before and during the COVID-19 lockdown. *Lancet Psychiatry* [online], 8 (5), 353–354. DOI: 10.1016/S2215-0366(20)30570-8

NHS Digital, 2021. *Mental health of children and young people in England, 2021 wave 2 follow up to the 2017 survey* [online]. London: NHS Digital. Available at: https://digital.nhs.uk/data-and-information/publications/statistical/mental-health-of-children-and-young-people-in-england/2021-follow-up-to-the-2017-survey [Accessed 04 November 2021].

NHS England, 2014a. *Five year forward view* [online]. London: NHS England. Available at: https://www.england.nhs.uk/wp-content/uploads/2014/10/5yfv-web.pdf [Accessed 01 September 2021].

NHS England, 2014b. *Model child and adolescent mental health specification for targeted and specialist services (tiers 2 and 3)* [online]. London: NHS England. Available at: https://www.england.nhs.uk/wp-content/uploads/2018/04/mod-camhs-tier-2-3-spec.pdf [Accessed 26 August 2021].

NHS, 2019. *The NHS long term plan* [online]. London: NHS England. Available at: https://www.longtermplan.nhs.uk/publication/nhs-long-term-plan/ [Accessed 01 September 2021].

NICE, 2016. *Antenatal and postnatal mental health quality standard* [online]. London: National Institute for Health and Care Excellence. Available at: https://www.nice.org.uk/guidance/qs115/resources/antenatal-and-postnatal-mental-health-pdf-75545299789765 [Accessed 08 October 2021].

Nomaguchi, K., Brown, S.L., and Leyman, T.M., 2017. Fathers' participation in parenting and maternal parenting stress: variation by relationship status. *Journal of Family Issues* [online], 38(8), 1132–1156. DOI: 10.1177/0192513X15623586. [Accessed 18 May 2022].

NSPCC Learning, 2021. *The independent review of children's social care* [online]. London: NSPCC Learning. Available at: https://learning.nspcc.org.uk/media/2617/independent-review-childrens-social-care.pdf

Office for National Statistics (ONS), 2019. *Child Health* [online]. London: UK Statistics Authority. Available at: https://www.ons.gov.uk/peoplepopulationandcommunity/healthandsocialcare/childhealth/articles/childrenwhosefamiliesstruggletogetonaremorelikelytohavementaldisorders/2019-03-26 [Accessed 27 August 2021].

PANDAS Foundation, 2021. *Service User Contacts March 2020- March 2021; Unpublished report*. Oswestry: PANDAS Foundation.

Parkin, E., and Long, R., 2021. *Support for children and young people's mental health* [online]. London: House of Commons Library. Available at: https://researchbriefings.files.parliament.uk/documents/CBP-7196/CBP-7196.pdf

Parry-Langdon, N., (ed.), 2008. *Three years on: Survey of the development and emotional well-being of children and young people* [online]. Newport: Office for National Statistics. Available at: https://lx.iriss.org.uk/sites/default/files/resources/child_development_mental_health.pdf [Accessed 8 October 2021].

Partridge, I., Richardson, G., Casswell, G., and Jones, N., 2010. Multidisciplinary Working. In: Richardson, G., Partridge, I., Barrett, J., eds. *Child and Adolescent services: An operational handbook Paediatric Liaison*. 2nd ed. London: Royal College of Psychiatrists, 2010, pp. 69–78.

Pierce, M., Hope, H., Ford, T., Hatch, S., Hotopf, M., John, A., Kontopantelis, E., Webb, R., Wessely, S., McManus, S., and Abel, K.M., 2020. Mental health before and during the COVID-19 pandemic: a longitudinal probability sample survey of the UK population. *The Lancet* [online], 7 (10), 883–892. Available via: https://doi-org.libezproxy.open.ac.uk/10.1016/S2215-0366(20)30308-4 [Accessed 8 October 2021].

Public Health England [PHE], 2021. *Promoting children and young people's mental health and wellbeing: A whole school or college approach* [online]. London: Public Health England. Available at: https://assets.publishing.service.gov.uk/government/uploads/system/uploads/attachment_data/file/1020249/Promoting_children_and_young_people_s_mental_health_and_wellbeing.pdf [Accessed 16 May 2022].

Public Health Scotland [PHS], 2021. *Adverse Childhood Experiences (ACEs). Overview of ACE's* [online]. Scotland: Public Health Scotland. Available at: http://www.healthscotland.scot/population-groups/children/adverse-childhood-experiences-aces/overview-of-aces [Accessed 1 September 2021].

Reuben, A., Moffitt, T.E., Caspi, A., Belsky, D.W., Harrington, H., Schroeder, F., Hogan, S., Ramrakha, S., Poulton, R., and Danese, A., 2016. Lest we forget: comparing retrospective and prospective assessments of adverse childhood experiences in the prediction of adult health. *Journal of Child Psychology and Psychiatry* [online], 57 (10), 11-3-112. DOI: 10.1111/jcpp.12621. [Accessed 8 October 2021].

Review of Maternal care and mental health, 1952. [Review of the book *Maternal care and mental health*, by J. Bowlby]. *Journal of Consulting Psychology*, 16 (3), 232. DOI: 10.1037/h0050582

Rocks, S., Glogowska, M., Stepney, M., Tsiachristas, A., and Mina, F., 2020. Introducing a single point of access (SPA) to child and adolescent mental health services in England: a mixed-methods observational study. *BMC health services research* [online], 20 (1), 623–623. DOI: 10.1186/s12913-020-05463-4. [Accessed 19 August 2021].

Salmond, C., and Jim, J., 2007. A Characterisation of Tier 2 Services in Child and Adolescent Mental Health. *Child and Adolescent Mental Health Volume* [online], 12 (2), 87–93. DOI: https://acamh.onlinelibrary.wiley.com/doi/10.1111/j.1475-3588.2007.00440.x [Accessed 01 September 2021].

Sandstrom, A., MacKenzie, L., Pizzo, A., Fine, A., Rempel, S., Howard, C., Stephens, M., Patterson, V., Drobinin, V., Van Gestel, H., Howes Vallis, E., Zwicker, A., Propper, L., Abidi, S., Bagnel, A., Lovas, D., Cumby, J., Alda, M., Uher, R., and Pavlova, B., 2020. Observed psychopathology in offspring of parents with major depressive disorder, bipolar disorder and schizophrenia. *Psychological Medicine* [online], 50 (6), 1050–1056. DOI:10.1017/S0033291719001089. [Accessed 22 October 2021].

Shatkin, A., 2015. *Child and Adolescent Mental Health*. New York: W. W. Norton and Company.

Social Care Institute for Excellence [Scie], 2012. *Introduction to children's social care* [online]. London: SCIE. Available at: https://www.scie.org.uk/publications/introductionto/childrenssocialcare/furtherinformation.asp [Accessed 01 September 2021].

Steck, A., and Steck, B., 2016. *Brain and Mind Subjective Experience and Scientific Objectivity*. Switzerland: Springer publishing.

Strathearn, L., Giannotti, M., Mills, R., Kisely, S., Najman, J., and Abajobir, A. 2020. Long-term cognitive, psychological, and health outcomes associated with child abuse and neglect. *Pediatrics* [online], 146 (4), e20200438. DOI: 10.1542/peds.2020-0438

The Children's Society, 2020. *Schools: more than a drop-off point* [online]. London: The Children's Society. Available at: https://www.childrenssociety.org.uk/what-we-do/blogs/importance-of-schools.

Vandeleur, C., Rothen, S., Gholam-Rezaee, M., Castelao, E., Vidal, S., Favre, S., Ferrero, F., Halfon, O., Fumeaux, P., Merikangas, K.R., Aubry, J., Burstein, M., and Preisig, M., 2012. Mental disorders in offspring of parents with bipolar and major depressive disorders. *Bipolar Disorder* [online], 14, 641–653. DOI: 10.1111/j.1399-5618.2012.01048.x. [Accessed 22 October 2021].

Vererhus, J.K., Timko, C., and Haugland, S.H., 2021. Adverse childhood experiences and impact on quality of life in adulthood: development and validation of a short difficult childhood questionnaire in a large population-based health survey. *Quality of Life Research* [online], 30, 1769–1779. DOI: 10.1007/s11136-021-02761-0. [Accessed 8 October 2021].

Vizard, T., Sadler, K., Ford, T., Newlove-Delgado, T., McManus, S., Marcheselli, F., Davis, J., Williams, T., Leach, C., Mandalia, D., and Cartwright, C., 2020. *Mental health of children and young people in England, 2020* [online]. London: NHS Digital. Available at: https://files.digital.nhs.uk/CB/C41981/mhcyp_2020_rep.pdf

Weinstock, L., Dunda, D., Harrington, H., and Nelson, H., 2021. It's complicated-adolescent grief in the time of Covid-19. *Front Psychiatry* [online], 23 (12), 38940. DOI: 10.3389/fpsyt.2021.638940

Whitehead, M., Taylor-Robinson, D., and Barr, B., 2021. Poverty, health, and Covid-19. *British Medical Journal* [online], 12, 372–376. DOI: 10.1136/bmj.n376

Widnall, E., Winstone, L., Mars, B., Haworth, C., and Kidger, J., 2020. *Young people's mental health during the COVID-19 pandemic* [online]. Leeds: National Institute for Health Research. Available at: https://sphr.nihr.ac.uk/wp-content/uploads/2020/08/Young-People%E2%80%99s-Mental-Health-during-the-COVID-19-Pandemic-Research-Briefing.pdf

World Health Organisation. 2019. Mental Disorders. https://www.who.int/news-room/fact-sheets/detail/mental-disorders#:~:text=In%202019%2C%201%20in%20every,of%20the%20COVID%2D19%20pandemic

Wright, B., Kraemer, S., Wurr, K., and Williams, C., 2010. Paediatric Liaison. In: Richardson, G., Partridge, I., Barrett, J., eds. *Child and Adolescent services: An operational handbook*. 2nd ed. London: Royal College of Psychiatrists, 2010, pp. 151–162.

Zatti, C., Rosa, V., Barros, A., Valdivia, L., Calegaro, V., Freitas, L., Ceresér, K., Rocha, N., Bastos, A., and Schuch, F., 2017. Childhood trauma and suicide attempt: A meta-analysis of longitudinal studies from the last decade. *Psychiatry Research* [online], 256, 353–358. DOI: 10.1016/j.psychres.2017.06.082. [Accessed 17 September 2021].

15 Ageing in the 21st Century

Chris Towers

After reading this chapter you should be able to:

- Understand issues in ageing and the difference between the empirical realities of ageing and the social construction of older people, including some biological realities of ageing and myths and realities of later life
- Understand issues of agency and structure, diversity, inequality and choice as people move into later life
- Consider different perspectives on ageing across issues from housing to income, health and care

Introduction

This chapter starts with an exploration of what ageing means in terms of some biological realities but contrasts these with some ideas on how older people are perceived or constructed. We will then explore further how later life is understood within the context of issues of structure and agency. This chapter reflects different ways of seeing older people with an understanding of how social policies and wider social factors will structure or shape a life. This chapter explores how free people are to make active and meaningful choices and in doing so will highlight issues of inequality, diversity, and power. There will also be some focus on specific issues in ageing such as housing choices and issues of income. These will be looked at with due consideration to matters of diversity and the different ways in which people age, socially. This chapter refers to case studies to reflect how the wider issues may reflect on individuals and this will enable you to understand how these translate to everyday life.

Ageing and the Life Course: Myths and Realities

There has been an increase in the ageing of the population in the 20th and now the 21st century with improvements in public health and better living standards (Phillipson 2013). There were just 20 million people over the age of 60 in 1950 but by the year 2000, it was 550 million and by the year 2025, it is projected to be over 2 billion United Nations (2009 cited in Phillipson 2013). This ageing of the populace is a reality of ageing with consequences for society and the organisation of resources. But empirical data like this sits alongside all sorts of myths or social

DOI: 10.4324/9781003079873-18

constructions. Understanding issues of ageing means knowing the realities of ageing and separating empirical realities from social constructions of older people. One needs however to understand what is meant by social construction. Berger and Luckman (1991) argue that reality is socially defined in the sense that human beings construct their own notions of people and society and imagine them in certain ways that may not correlate with empirical truths. People can be constructed in negative ways, imagined as deviant in some ways (Becker 1963). Older people could be constructed as passive or less able and ascribed qualities that they as individuals may not adhere to. These constructions are ones shaped by the powerful (Burr 1995) with the more powerful pushing their vision of forms of reality. Social policies can also construct people, limiting their choices with restrictive housing options and poor pensions, encouraging dependent lives (Townsend 1981). Taylor and Earl (2016) suggest that older people can be viewed in particularly restrictive ways and that they can be in effect pushed into a retirement against their wishes and in ways that do not correspond to their needs. It can be that the narrow and reductionist ways of knowing older people may lead to restrictive or prejudiced social policies that limit their horizons or prospects.

Ageism is still very much around, a process whereby people make assumptions of people based on their chronological age and everyone becomes vulnerable to ageism the longer they live (Palmore 2015). Ageism is about stereotypes, the idea that people become more senile or sick (Palmore, Whittingham and Kunkel 2009 cited in Palmore 2015) as they age. Whilst everyone may not indeed become sick or in the same way the irony is that if older people internalise these ideas, they can then become more vulnerable to that very ill assumed to be a feature of growing older (Palmore 2015). Of course, this is not to deny the realities of ageing. The Covid-19 pandemic has focused hearts and minds on some critical issues in ageing in the 21st century and placed the spotlight on the circumstances and vulnerabilities of people as they age. The infection rates in care homes, the need for safeguarding, the needs, and uncertainties of relatives. Then there are the so-called 'underlying conditions' associated with age that can make people more vulnerable to disease. There has been attention to issues of ageing like no other issue, possibly since the Second World War. We have learned or had it confirmed through the pandemic that we age in different ways (Kirkwood 2011 cited in Walker 2014) and that ageing can be understood as complex interactions between physical and cultural processes (Bazalgette et al. 2011 cited in Walker 2014). We need then to look closer at the biology of ageing and some global trends, to explore some of the demographic trends in an ageing population and in doing so challenge some of the myths about older people.

Biology of Ageing

In exploring some of the realities of ageing it is important to state what we mean by the ageing process. Ageing can be understood as complex interactions between physical and cultural processes (Bazalgette et al. cited in Walker 2014). Yamni et al. said that these interactions can be categorised into three areas. First, changes in cells, blood and temperature. Second, there are changes in organ mass and third, we can notice a change and decline in the body's reserve systems. All these aspects of ageing are important to know but there can be a depletion of resources when the body undergoes trauma or loss of some sort. This becomes more apparent when the person has undergone a fall or experienced a long period of best rest. There are several common trends in ageing across the globe as outlined by the World Health Organisation (2018) such as hearing loss, back and neck pain, cataracts over eyes, depression, diabetes and dementia. With ageing it is likely that people can experience more than one of these conditions at the same time. Bishop et al. (2010) found that more than half of people over the age of 85 years experienced some degree of cognitive decline.

Dependence, Independence and the Dependency Ratio

Understanding ageing means having some understanding of physiological issues but also of the related concepts of dependence and independence and the relationship between the two. What does one mean by independence? The relationship between these concepts is complex and problematic and the two terms are indelibly inter-related. Glendinning (2005) argues that dependency is an inevitable part of the human situation to the extent that we are dependent on each other in terms of economics but also in psychological ways. Dependency is often considered negative or even shameful but people he argues are interdependent upon each other. People are involved in reciprocal exchanges, needing something from someone or some situation. The care receiver and caregiver are locked into a form of potential exchange or payback, a form of 'nested dependency' (Kittay 1999 cited in Glendinning 2005). With this in view we can perhaps accept that when we talk of ratios of dependency, we must consider that the term is not a given but problematic.

This ageing population will have many strengths as well as weaknesses and indeed it is important to reflect that view. It is possible to move away from seeing ageing and older people as simply problematic. It is more productive and fairer to not construct people in such reductionist terms but to see them as individuals facing all sorts of challenges as they age and to also acknowledge their strengths. These strengths can often be accrued from experience. With that said it must still be acknowledged that we are talking of an ageing population and we need to understand the ability of the population to provide effective health and social care for people as they age. The elderly dependency ratio (EDR) is essentially the number of people of working age, and we mean paid work (aged 15 to 64) to those aged 65 and over (Office of National Statistics 2019). We may add however that there are changes in populations and issues with migration across nations that makes this issue more complex. The dependency ratio is the ratio between those in paid employment and those not and so only recognises only the contributions people make to society through paid activity. This raises some questions about the nature of dependency including the issues of whether paid employment is simply synonymous with independence. Maybe people can be dependent in some ways but in paid employment and likewise in non-paid work and with a sense of independence. The terms independence and dependence are more complex than straightforward. We can of course be dependent on paid work for our independence. Indeed, the Office of National Statistics (2019) found that those people who appear to be 'economically active' may at the same time be independent in an economic sense. They also point out that those in work could well be reliant or in fact dependent on welfare benefits to remain in that paid work.

Patterns of Caring

Caring for people can support independence but caring can also take us away from the labour market and we may struggle financially at the same time. Older people can make more contributions than a dependency rate may allow or recognise, with its fixation on paid work. They engage in a lot of caring work, much of it either low-paid or not paid, between families. This is very much 'emotional labour' (James 1989, Brotheridge et al. 2010) where people invest their emotions in the 'work' and this can be exhausting and demanding, and women play a disproportionate role here. Poverty is hard to gauge and reasons or explanations for not working are complex, but research has shown that more than one in four women who don't work would like to work (Grant and Buckner 2006 cited in Hirsch et al. 2011). Whilst women's lives and employment careers can be punctuated by care in ways not always known by men, or at least not in the same way, it would be unwise to make too many generalisations. McCann et al. (2012) does however question assumptions that men play little part in caring roles. They may not always be the providers of care, but they are involved in the complex interfaces. There is research that suggests that men are so often in need of care with Vlachantoni et al. (2013) finding that 32% of men and 22% of women were reliant on informal support as they age (Breeze and Stafford 2019 in Vlachantoni et al. 2013).

Case Study: Rose

Issues of caring also bring into focus issues of independence and dependence. These are complex issues relevant throughout the life course. Let's consider the case of Rose, as discussed next.

Question: Would you describe Rose as independent? What are her needs and is she able to meet them or would you say she is struggling?

The question of independence has increasing importance as people age, but it is not easy to define. We discussed this earlier in the chapter when we looked at issues of dependence and independence and indeed it has many kinds of meanings and associations and is perhaps relative rather than absolute. There are in other words or degrees of it rather than it being one definitive concept (Bowers 2001, Tamaru et al. 2007 and Fox 2010 cited in Darawsheh 2015). A person may be able to do something like shop for themselves, but they may need transport to get there or as was the case in the case study of 'Rose'. They may have problems with internet shopping, but they can still make their own choices about what to purchase. They are neither dependent or independent, they are in essence 'interdependent' (Fine and Glendinning 2005). Rose needs the help of her neighbour and her physical problems means she has needs that must be met by others. Rose's income is a concern even if she owns the house and her economic dependence on her husband, when he was alive, has meant that she has marginal control of her financial situation.

Structure and Agency

Discussions around issues of dependence and independence can often lead into wider discussions around the nature of human action and questions of choice and control, relevant through the life course and into later life. Many things can structure those lives from social class to education, all can affect life chances, including parental influences (Erola et al. 2016).

There is the view that human agency is a more powerful force than one may care to imagine and that the human drive towards self-determination is evident early in the life course as the child learns about the world (Brim 1981 cited in Levy et al. 2005) with the early experiences and their meaning potentially trans-formed by later ones. The idea being that people are not just products of the world but are the ones that help make it or even transform it. Elder (1985 cited in Levy et al. 2005) talks of the concept of agency in relation to the notion of the life course and says that the notion of the life course is predicated on the idea of human agency or choice. Heinz (1996 cited in Levy et al. 2005) argues that there are not simply 'fateful' moments, with reference to Anthony Giddens, those moments can be controlled, they are times when the individual is not necessarily at the behest of events and they can't have any control over. People's ability to demonstrate agency can be strained as demonstrated by Coles and Vassarotti (2005 cited in Kilvington-Dowd and Robinson 2020) when they found that men struggled to maintain their sense of self as embodied in masculinity, resigning themselves to the physical declines of later life whilst trying to support others, notably their partners. Here we have an interplay between ageing and gender and the loss of agency that ageing can bring.

This analysis benefits from an understanding of both structure and agency and the relationship between the two. It is important to understand this relationship if one is to know something of later as well as earlier forms of life. Gunhild and Dykstra suggested, albeit arguing in the North American rather than UK context, that wo-men's and men's lives are not converging even if social policies may encourage convergence. They may not share childcare or employment opportunities in the same way. People can and will still show agency and make their own choices in relation to childcare and family matters although understanding the choices helps us to under-stand the actions of families and indeed and how structure and agency are linked. Giddens argues that people are not entirely lacking control of their own lives, they can structure them and make their own choices (Lamsal 2012) and yet, paradoxically their lives are structured, structured on the micro level by the structure of human relations and interactions but also by macro, institutional structures. The under-standing structure is dependent on knowing of issues of agency and vice-versa. Structures help us understand the context in which people exercise their agency. Dyke and Kearns (2006 cited in Aitken and Valentine 2006) argue that Giddens said that structure and agency as existing not in a dichotomous relationship but interwoven, one affecting the other.

Theories of Ageing and Life Course Perspectives

Some theories see matters of independence and dependence in relation to natural processes of ageing. Some theories may also suggest more influence of structure in people's lives or conversely, agency. Perhaps dependency is inevitable. Such an approach or attitude is consistent with the idea of **'disengagement theory'** espoused by (Cumming and Henry 1961) for they stressed that older people are regarded as role less in later life and becoming more and more removed from the instructions and relationships that gave meaning to their earlier lives. Such a view sees ageing and decline or retreat as 'natural' in their association. Other ideas question this perspective and see sociological understandings of how people age. This sees ageing as existing in relation to societal change and within social context rather than seeing any disengaging or indeed engaging as 'natural'. There are other theories that take a more sociological perspective and the idea that in later life people's lives are **structured as dependent** (Townsend 1981). People's lives are said to be shaped by limited access to independent housing, inadequate pensions and the organisation of community care services based on assumptions of dependency. One can adopt one of many perspectives to examine the issues of later life. The life course approach embraces the concepts of structure and agency, in other words, people experience social structures that shape a life. Family background, social policies, housing, location and neighbourhood all structure a life (Katz 2013) but people can also depart from these structures to some extent and show 'agency'. They can be partly architects of their own lives. Social gerontologists are, argues Katz, interested in the social aspects of ageing and this includes those things that influence a life such as the economy and these will have some impact on a person's agency through life, in effect their choices. But we can make a distinction between life course perspectives and the life cycle and it's useful to reflect, as we now will on the strengths and weaknesses of such terms (Figures 15.1 and 15.2).

Rose is 79 years of age. She was born in 1941 and was married for 40 years before her husband died quite suddenly in August of 2010 of a heart attack. She has remained in the same house they bought together in 1972, shortly after they married. The mortgage was paid off in 2008 and she remains there on her own, describing herself as 'house rich and income poor' for she has a small state pension and some money from the inheritance, but savings are small. The marriage was 'traditional' in that her husband used to do all the paid work and she looked after house and home, meaning no independent income or indeed work-based pension. She would like to still to do some paid work but struggles to get the chance as employers openly tell her 'you are too old' and this dismays here. She does some charity work for the homeless shelter in the city. Rose is physically quite active even if she has a few health concerns such as arthritis in her hands and she feels she increasingly needs to walk with the aid of a stick. She struggles sometimes with the buses. Buses are a challenge for moving around on them with her restricted mobility is not always good. Her neighbour is a close friend, and they provide emotional comfort to each other as they both complain of loneliness. They also shop for each other when one is having a bad time physically with her arthritis making it hard to shop. The interactions are a source of great comfort. Whilst her neighbour does internet food shops for her some time, she prefers to choose what she wants and writes down lists for her of her food requests.

Figure 15.1 Case study: Rose. With permission from the author.

Think of your life so far. How far has it been structured by laws, policies, family, background, your age, gender, ethnicity or fate, chance, your own efforts, or the actions of others? How may the events of early or mid-life effect later life? We will turn to these issues later in the chapter. How important is your education, housing etc in terms of structuring your life chances?

Figure 15.2 Moment of reflection. With permission from the author.

Life Cycle and Life Course

When we talk about the 'life cycle' we refer to maturational and generational processes in natural populations (O'Rand and Krecker 1990). We may want to contrast this with a definition of life course approaches, and these can be referred to as 'age graded sequence of roles, opportunities, constraints and events that shape the biography from birth to death' (Shanahan and Macmillan 2008, p. 40 cited in Alwin 2012). Is a life cycle a good way to understand issues in a person's life? Here is a definition of the life cycle, what are the strengths and weaknesses? What is missing from this understanding?

You might argue that the life course has a wider application and accounts for a range of human experiences and people. You may say that the life course is much wider a definition and is more useful as a means of examining the human experience. It serves as a means of highlighting events and the twists and turns of a life rather than simply looking at 'generational processes' that occur in populations (as reflected in Figure 15.3, as above). It allows one to consider the sociological aspects of a life and how much 'structure', 'agency' or choice may be a dominant feature. In short, the influence of the social world on the human being.

Poverty and Wealth, Food Access

My poem (as in Figure 15.4) 'talks' to the experience of living alone, accompanied by feelings of loneliness and grief. Isolation and loneliness can be key. Looking at issues of the life course it can be said that people through a life can reflect on their own lives, the phases, and the times of change. They can have perceptions of how they were, looking back at their younger selves or indeed they can also 'look forward'. They can be optimistic or downbeat (Pinkerton and Rooney 2014). These are the complex interplays of emotion and memory, the detail of people's private lives that sociological texts can easily miss. It is easy for example to miss the issue of poverty or to fail to account for this in examining the shape of a life. There are issues of poverty and we can frame these understandings within some general facts relating to patterns of consumption, poverty, wealth and food access.

There can be wide disparities in wealth and income as people age. Centre for Longitudinal Studies illustrates how people born in the late 1950s can have very

---

"Social mammals have three basic stages of postnatal development: infant, juvenile, and adult. Some species also have a brief female post-reproductive stage. The human life cycle, however, is best described by five stages: infant, child, juvenile, adolescent, and adult. Women in both traditional and industrial societies may also have a long post-reproductive stage. Analyses of bones and teeth of early hominids who died as subadults suggest that the evolution of the new life stages of childhood and adolescence are not of ancient origin. The current human pattern evolved after the appearance of *Homo erectus*. It is possible that evidence for the existence of the post-reproductive stage for women will also be recoverable from the fossil record because the hormonal changes associated with menopause have profound effects on bone density and histology of tubular bones. It is hypothesized that the new life stages of the human life cycle represent feeding and reproductive specializations of the *genus Homo*." (Bogin and Smith, 1996, p 703).

Figure 15.3 The life cycle: What's missing? Attributed permission from the author.

Only lonely on Sundays

I still sense it, his toast,
smelling like charcoal,
laden with butter,
lathered into the corners of the bread

I still hear it, his voice, crackling over the radio,
almost touch his slightly bruised red skin
and see his light blue shirt
with creases almost woven into it.

You ask me, I'll tell you of how I hear
the cistern, the water,
tick tock, dripping, almost,
into my skull.

But I'm ok thanks,
The weeks are fine.

I'm only lonely
on Sundays

Chris Towers, November, 2021

Figure 15.4 What does this poem tell you about life experience, what issues does this inspire
you as you read it? With permission from the author.

divided prospects with financial situations such that a significant element of them
expect to carry on working into their 60s.

This mixed evidence suggests that we are dealing with a less-homogenous group,
with older people experiencing very different lives. These factors can contribute
towards issues of quality of life but also suggest issues with diet but also isolated
lives which can increase the possibility of problems accessing food. There is also
poverty in later life. This can be partly an issue of social geography and we
must never assume that poverty is placed solely in urban areas. There are also
issues facing older people in rural locations (Walsh, O'Shea and Scharf 2020).
There are several factors that can combine to make older people living in rural
areas may be particularly susceptible to disadvantages such as sparse populations
that lead to a lack of social connections and with-it opportunities (Walker 2014;
Burholt and Scarf 2014 and Hennessy et al. 2014 cited in Walsh, O'Shea and
Scharf 2020).

Housing, Home, and the Life Course

We may reflect on issues of the life course in relation to particular social issues,
including that of 'housing'. Home is an important issue as we age, relevant to the
need not only for shelter but for meaning. Some research by Kearns et al. (2010) in
West Scotland discovered that home was considered a haven, a place where people

can express a sense of autonomy or meaning. They found that these issues cut across issues of housing tenure. Home had meaning wherever they lived and had its own meaning as people aged. This does not mean that older people want the same things from housing as they age for their diversity, with some wanting age-specific housing and others wanting housing from a wider supply of housing. People in rural places will also have different needs to those in cities. Whilst older people will differ in terms of housing it is often said that many older people would like to 'age in place' (Sixsmith and Sixsmith, 2008) or in other words remain where they are as they grow older. There are however mixed ideas on this concept. Rooney et al. (2017) said that some older people may need to make changes to the homes they currently occupy whilst others may like the idea of relocation. Ageing in place is not however straightforward.

Policy needs to be responsive towards changing needs as people move into later (Mackenzie et al. in Rooney et al. 2017) as people age and capabilities change. People may need to find a 'fit' between their physical situation and the environment that they now occupy or continue to occupy (Horstmann, Haaak and Iwarsson 2014 in Rooney et al. 2017). The concept of career is often applied to employment but that can be a narrow and misleading focus for people can have housing 'careers' within a life that can constitute a career within itself (Mulder and Hooimeijer, 1995). It is important to stress that each housing move needs to be understood within that wider sense of a career of relocations. Each move shaped by constraints and opportunities with some relocations painful as they struggle used to accept new environments (Clough et al. 2005).

Health and Matters of Choice Through the Life Course

A life course perspective also entails understanding the critical issue of health and the part health and health services play in a life. It could be argued that such matters expose once again issues of agency and structure. Some lives will be shaped by deprivation and there is much evidence that where a person lives will have an impact on their health outcomes with higher rates of mortality in some areas more than others. Shah and Cook (2008) found that older people who have low income and don't have a car tend to use NHS direct services more than more wealthy individuals in later life. Patterns of health and housing will play their part in shaping the early mid-life and the relationship between employment and mental health in mid-life can have consequences, with depression having a negative impact on one's ability to maintain work in mid-life (Rice et al. 2011). Rice et al. (2011) also found that there can be many explanations for why or how people are able to take early retirement, and these can include, advancing age, being female, the partner's retirement, pension wealth, high-income consumption and fair or poor health.

Retirement

Leaving paid work is a huge issue for many people, for economic but also social reasons. It has been considered a very significant event, a transition with many implications (Hyde et al. 2018).

Issues in Retirement: Gender, Ethnicity and Social Class

A life course approach to understanding later life supports an understanding of retirement for the pattern of a life including patterns of employment and caring can have an impact on the quality of the pension and the quality of a later life. Women's lives have historically and maybe even now been ones punctuated more by discontinuities and uncertainties than men's (Hyde et al. 2018). Understanding this means understanding that caring responsibilities break the idea of a 'career' as a smooth journey to retirement and a good pension and in that sense understandings of these issues tend to adopt a male or male breadwinner model (Duberley 2013). We make assumptions concerning the world of work and caring and can look upon these issues in many different ways. There are many issues of gender, social class and employment that can assist one to understand what retirement means for people as they age and to understand how the patterns of a life can have implications for later life, the times of change or disruption. Here are some other evidence around these issues:

- Ethnic minorities can have particularly poor financial situations approaching retirement (Hyde et al. 2018).
- Those with jobs with a high occupational status and more flexible patterns of work tend to carry on working beyond retirement (Dingemans and Mohring, 2019) and that inequalities across a life course continue beyond retirement.
- Housing careers through a lifetime can reach conclusions in later life when some may find themselves 'doing well' in terms of their housing but not so much in terms of their income. Many women who have divorced and inherited the house may also find that they are struggling in terms of income (Rowlingston 2006) with such a situation known as 'house rich and income poor'.
- Bardasi et al. (2002 cited in Kanabar 2017) found that the onset of retirement tends to mean for many the onset of poverty but in talking of the poverty of later life they also concluded that the period prior to later life was equally important to know. There are gender differences with men particularly likely to drop their standard of living from a period when they were in work to a retirement without it. For women the labour market history was less important to know but other factors were key such as if they lived in social housing, had an occupational pension or retired before the state pension age.

Continuing with the issue of poverty, there are issues for some people in terms of priority, what does one prioritise she asks, food or fuel? What would you choose?

The dilemma expressed in Figure 15.5, above, is not uncommon Many older people struggle to put the heating and eat properly such is their poverty in later life (O'Neil et al. 2006). If you choose the food you may then struggle with heating, and

---

Retirement may or perhaps may not seem a long way off for you but to what extent do you feel your gender, social class or ethnicity will have a bearing on the quality of your retirement?

Figure 15.5 Moment of reflection. With permission from the author.

as Hughes and Natarajan (2019) point out, 26,560 UK deaths occur amongst those aged 65 simply through the consequences of cold weather. You may also feel that Rupinder's ethnicity can be an issue in terms of disadvantage. We must acknowledge that many other groups may also experience problems of course and not all issues are strictly issues of ethnicity, that said, according to Evandrou et al. (2015) highlight, health disadvantages in later life seem most critical and most marked in the BME group with those from south Asia and Pakistan experiencing particular poverties and poor health outcomes.

Delfani, De Deken and De Wilde (2015) consider the relationship between housing status and income and poverty in later life within the UK and identified that a flat rate pension does go some way to alleviate poverty but the lack of consistent employment within the life, if less than 25 years, still has a profound effect upon poverty. Homeownership, particularly outright ownership alleviates poverty in that living rent-free then yields income in some ways or in part. Since the late 1980s, the percentage of pensioners *as a group* falling below the relative poverty line, whether defined at 50%, 60% or 70% of the median income, has continued to fall. Such a trend is mirrored in the fall of poverty among other groups in the population, such as working-age parents and children. Between 1991 and 2008, the percentage of pensioners who experienced persistent low income fell from 21% to 8%. Such trends are explained by a combination of successive cohorts of individuals reaching later life with a higher- amount of resources, but also changes in the welfare system which has increased the absolute value of the old-age pension over time, and a commitment from successive governments to tackling poverty and social exclusion in later life (Figure 15.6).

Intersectionality

Rupinder's situation in the case study (Figure 15.5) reflects an experience of poverty that takes in the issue of ethnicity. It is important to understand any cross-overs in later life between ageing, diversity and poverty. The idea of intersectionality is that there are interlocking or overlapping dimensions of power within lives, cutting across different oppressions and relations of power and key to understanding the relations between say gender and ethnicity or social class and disability. It is argued however that whilst all these diversities can overlap and converge it is also sometimes the case that one aspect of difference can be looked at in its own terms and not always in relation to others. Crenshaw (1991 cited in Twigg and Martin 2013) says that

---

Rupinder was born in 1934 in India and she moved with her husband and young family to the UK in 1959. Her husband worked on the buses and his income and pension were small, although he died prematurely at 59 and Rupinder, now 86, has been on her own some 27 years. Her children have moved away, and she doesn't feel she can rely on them for help anymore. She was a housewife and mother and was no occupational pension she struggles on a state pension. She lives in a housing association property just outside Birmingham in the West Midlands. She is torn between the need to keep her flat warm and buy enough good nutritious food. She sometimes goes cold so that she can afford to eat well enough and vice-versa

---

Figure 15.6 Fuel or food: Rupinder's dilemma. With permission from the author.

intersectionality allows one to link the twin experiences of racism and sexism into black women's lives and this overlapping experience allows more clarity and understanding of such lives rather than seeing a life through one prism. Whilst the intersections of ethnicity and gender or social class may explain some of the circumstances of later life one does not have to reduce understanding of later life with reference to the cumulative injustices of various inequalities. Men in old age, of any background, can face discrimination with old men, so often assumed to be the breadwinner pushed to the margins of society, considered non-productive, reliant on pension schemes (Phillipson 2013 cited in Twigg and Martin 2013). There can be aspects of say racial discrimination that exist themselves rather than always seen in relation to other structures (Bilge 2013). Intersectionality is never the less an important feature of experiences for identities can be complex rather than one-dimensional, as we age into later life. Lane et al. (2010) refer to how Chinese women who migrated to Britain in the 1950s and 1960s have had quite different experiences from subsequent generations of such migration with now older Chinese women experiencing poverty from early to later life.

Issue of Abuse, Mental Health and Safeguarding

Abuse and mental health are also important issues to consider when looking at issues in later life. These are safeguarding issues and important to know as older people can of course be vulnerable to abuse and discrimination by services, Anderson et al. (2013) note that Mental health services in the UK have developed into specialist services for older people, usually defined as those over the age of 64 years, and separate specialist services for adults aged 18–64 years. There is unequivocal evidence of discrimination against older people in mental health services in the UK fuelled by the approach to national policy implementation, which has promoted the needs of working-age adults and excluded older people (Anderson et al. 2009 in Anderson et al. 2013). Independent reports demonstrate that when older and younger adults in England with equivalent needs are compared, then older people have less access to mental health and social care services, and to redress that inequality would cost £2–4 billion of public money per year (Beecham et al. 2008 and Forder 2008 cited in Anderson et al. 2013). It might be surmised then that older people's mental health services are being compromised thus putting older people in more danger and someone like the case study having potentially less control and choice as he may have less options if experiencing mental health issues. Horton (2016) emphasises how important abuse is when considering older people and says that there are however some misconceptions Professionals believed that older people's 'interconnectedness' with family, social embeddedness in the community and 'meanings of the home' influenced help-seeking.

Dementia

Life course understandings of ageing and later life need to understand the impact of illness upon development. The brain changes and as people age there are changes of a vascular and cognitive kind (Peters 2006). The brain reduces in size as we age, and incidents of stroke and memory impairment become more common.

Dementia UK (2020) says that Dementia is an umbrella term for a range of progressive conditions that affect the brain. There are over 200 subtypes of dementia, but the five most common are Alzheimer's disease, vascular dementia, dementia with Lewy bodies, frontotemporal dementia and mixed dementia. Signs of Alzheimer's tend to develop gradually over time and can affect concentration, memory and communication. Dementia can affect a person at any age, but it is more commonly diagnosed in people over the age of 65 years. A person developing dementia before age 65 is said to have young-onset dementia. There are over 850,000 people living with dementia in the UK and this is set to rise to over one million by 2021 (Dementia UK 2020).

Understanding the life course and its impact on a person's later life means understanding the patterns of a life, the impact of social structures that can give shape to a life but also 'agency', the part the individual has played in that life, the decisions they have made from the choices available to them. The case studies and the commentary to follow should have helped you to place lives within contexts and to see how later lives, affected by physiology are also shaped by decisions made by self and others in complex interplays. Much more could have been said about dementia and physiological change and housing issues such as the move to residential care. There was no room to cover all issues, but this chapter has focused on just some of the issues affecting a life course and it is that life course approach that is the key to understanding many of those circumstances of later life.

Summary of Main Points

You should be able to:

- Understand that there are different perspectives on the life course from ones that emphasise psychological change to those that give more credence to sociological change and the influence of social structures and potentially social policies
- Recognise issues of independence, dependence and interdependence and patterns of care and caring as people age
- See how issues in early and mid-life can have an impact on late-life choices and circumstances including retirement, pension provision, poverty and housing

References

Aitken, S., and Valentine, G., 2006. *Approaches to human geography*. London: Sage.
Alwin, D.F., 2012. Integrating varieties of life course concepts. *The Journals of Gerontology: Series B* [online], 67B (2) (March), 206–220. DOI: 10.1093/geronb/gbr146
Anderson, D., Connelly, P., Meier, R., and McCracken, C., 2013. Mental health service discrimination against older people. *The Psychiatrist*, 37 (3), 98–103.
Becker, H., 1963. *Outsiders; Studies in the sociology of deviance*. London: Free Press Glencoe.
Berger, P., and Luckman, T. 1991. *The social construction of reality*. London: Anchor Books.
Bishop, N., Lu, T., and Yankner, B., 2010. Neural mechanisms of ageing and cognitive decline. *Nature* [online], 464, 529–535. DOI: 10.1038/nature08983
Brotheridge, C.M., and Lee, R.T., 2010. Development and validation of the emotional labour scale. *Occupational and Organisational Psychology*, 76 (3), 703–716.
Burr, V., 1995. *An introduction to social constructionism*. London: Routledge.

Clough, R., Leamy, M., Miller, V., and Bright, L., 2005. Housing decisions in later life. In: Clough, R., Leamy, M., Miller, V., and Bright, L., eds. *Housing decisions in later life*. London: Palgrave Macmillan, pp. 45–67.

Darawsheh, W., 2015. Towards culturally competent professional practice: exploring the concepts of independence and dependence. *Research, policy and planning* [online], 31 (1) (January), 3–17. Available at: http://ssrg.org.uk/members/files/2015/07/Darawsheh-Chard.pdf

Delfani, N., De Deken, J., and Dewilde, C., 2015. Poor because of low pensions or expensive housing? The combined impact of pension and housing systems on poverty among the elderly. *International Journal of Housing Policy*, 15 (3), 2–15.

Dementia UK, 2020. *What is dementia?* [online]. London: Dementia UK. Available at: https://www.dementiauk.org/get-support/diagnosis-and-next-steps/what-is-dementia/?gclid=Cj0KCQjwtZH7BRDzARIsAGjbK2bjyIrtNumOC7jhnbsFHSdKLI7xIcQ7GzbECDj_bDORDbF-VGPILqQaAok0EALw_wcB [Accessed 18 September 2020].

Dingemans, E., and Mohring, K., 2019. A life course perspective on working after retirement. *Advances in Life Course Research*, 39, 23–23.

Duberley, J., Carmichael, F., and Szmigin, 2013. Exploring women's retirement: Continuity, context and career transition. *Gender, Work and Organization*, 21 (1), 71–90.

Erola, J., Jalonen, S., and Leht, H., 2016. Parental education, class and income over early life course and children's achievements. *Research in Social Stratification and Mobility*, 44, 33–43.

Evandrou, M., Falkingham, J., Feng, Z., and Valchantoni, A., 2015. Ethnic inequalities in limiting health and self-reported health in later life. *Journal of Epidemiology and Public Health*, 70 (7), 653–662.

Fine, M., and Glendinning, C., 2005. Dependence, independence or inter-dependence? *Ageing in Society*, 25 (4), 601–621.

Hirsch, D., Phung, V.H., and Manful, E., 2011. *Poverty, ethnicity and caring*. York: Joseph Rowntree Foundation.

Horton, D.P., 2016. Tackling elder abuse and neglect: adult safeguarding under the care act 2014. *Elder LJ* [online], 349. Available via: https://heinonline.org/HOL/LandingPage?handle=hein.journals/eldlj2016&div=74&id=&page= [Accessed 17 September 2020].

Hughes, C., and Natarajan, C., 2019. The older I get, the colder I get' Older people's perspectives on coping in cold homes. *Journal of Housing for the Elderly*, 33 (4), 337–357.

Hyde, M., Cheshire-Allen, M., Damman, M., Henkens, K., Platts, L., Pritchard, A., and Reed, C., 2018. *The experience of the transition to retirement: rapid evidence review*. London: Centre for Ageing Better.

James, N., 1989. Skill and work in the social regulation of feelings. *The Sociological Review*, 37 (1), 15–42.

Kanabar, R., 2017. In or out? Poverty dynamics among older individuals in the UK. *Cambridge University Press*, 16 (4), 509–553.

Katz, S., 2013. Active and successful ageing, lifestyle as a gerontological idea. *Random Structures and Algorithms*, 44, 33–49.

Kearns, A., Whiteley, E., Tannahil, C., and Ellaway, E. 2010. Loneliness, social relations and health-being in deprived communities. *Psychology, Health & Medicine*, 20 (3), 332–344.

Kilvington-Dowd, L., and Robertson, S., 2020. "Let's duck out of the wind": Operationalising intersectionality to understand elderly men's caregiving experiences. *International Journal of Men's Social and Community Health*, 3 (2), 19–31.

Lamsal, M., 2012. The structuration approach of Anthony Giddens. *Himalayan Journal of Sociology and Anthropology*, 5, 111–112.

Lane, P., Tribe, R., and Hui, R., 2010. Intersectionality and the mental health of elderly Chinese women living in the UK. *International Journal of Migration, Health and Social Care*, 6 (4), 34–42.

Levy, R., Ghisleta, P., Le Goff, J.M., Spini, D., and Widmer, R., eds., 2005. *Towards an inter-disciplinary perspective on the life course*. Oxford: Elsevier.

Mcann, M., Donnelly, M., and O'Reilly, 2012. Gender differences in care home admission risk: partner's age explains the higher risk for women. *Age and Ageing*, 41(3), 416–419.

Mulder, C.H., and Hooimeijer, P., 1995. Moving into Owner-Occupation: Compositional and contextual effects on the propensity to become a homeowner. *Netherlands Journal of Housing and the Built Environment*, 10, 5–25.

O'Neil, T., Jinks, C., and Squire, A., 2006. 'Heating is more important than food', Older women's perceptions of fuel poverty. *Journal of Housing for the Elderly* [online], 20 (3), 95–108. DOI: 10.1300/J081v20n03_07 [Accessed 29 June 2020].

O'Rand, A.M., and Krecker, M.L., 1990. Concepts of the life cycle: their history, meanings and uses in the social sciences. *Annual Review of Sociology*, 16, 241–262.

Office of National Statistics, 2019. *Living longer and old-age dependency – what does the future hold?* [online]. Newport: Office for National Statistics. Available at: https://www.ons.gov.uk/peoplepopulationandcommunity/birthsdeathsandmarriages/ageing/articles/livinglongerandoldagedependencywhatdoesthefuturehold/2019-06-24 [Accessed 2 April 2020].

Palmore, E., 2015. Ageism comes of age. *The Journals of Gerontology: Series B*, 70 (6), 873–875. DOI: 10.1093/geronb/gbv079 [Accessed 2 April 2020].

Peters, R., 2006. Ageing and the brain. *Postgraduate Medical Journal* [online], 82 (964) (February), 84–88. Available via: https://pmj.bmj.com/content/82/964/84 [Accessed 19 October 2020].

Phillipson, C., 2013. *Ageing*. London: Policy Press.

Pinkerton, J., and Rooney, C., 2014. Care leavers' experiences of transition and turning points: findings from a biographical narrative study. *Social Work and Society: International Online Journal* [online], 12 (1) (January). Available at: https://www.scie-socialcareonline.org.uk/care-leavers-experiences-of-transition-and-turning-points-findings-from-a-biographical-narrative-study/r/a1CG0000003YWWiMAO ["Web exclusive content"].

Rice, N.E., Laing, I.A., Henley, W., and Melzer, D., 2011. Common health problems of early retirement: findings from the English Longitudinal Study of Ageing. *Age and Ageing*, 40 (1), 54–61.

Rooney, C., Hadjri, K., Faith, V., Rooney, M., McAllister, K., and Craig, C., 2017. Living Independently: exploring the experiences of visually impaired people living in age-related and lifetime housing through qualitative analysis. *Health Environments Research and Design Journal*, 11 (2), 56–71.

Rowlingston, K., 2006. 'Living poor to die Rich' or 'spending the kids' inheritance? Attitudes to assets and inheritance in later life. *Journal of Social Policy*, 35 (2), 175–192.

Shah, S.M., and Cook, D.G., 2008. Social economic determinants of casualty and NHS Direct use. *Journal of Public Health*, 30 (1), 75–81.

Sixsmith, A., and Sixsmith, J., 2008. Ageing in place in the United Kingdom. *Ageing International*, 32, 219–235. DOI: 10.1007/s12126-008-9019-y [Accessed 10 May 2020].

Taylor, P., and Earl, C., 2016. The social construction of retirement and evolving discourse on working longer. *Journal of Social Policy* [online], 45 (2), 215–268. DOI: 10.1017/S0047279415000665 [Accessed 20 April 2020].

Townsend, P., 1981. The structured dependency of the elderly: a creation of social policy in the twentieth century. *Ageing and Society* [online], 1 (1), 5–28. DOI: 10.1017/S0144686X81000020 [Accessed 20 April 2020].

Twigg, A., and Martin, W., 2013. *Routledge handbook of cultural gerontology*. London: Routledge.

Vlachantoni, A., Shaw, R.J., Evandrou, M., and Falkingham, J., 2013. The determinants of receiving social care in later life in England. *Ageing and Society*, 35, 321–345.

Walker, A., 2014. *The new science of ageing*. Bristol: Policy Press.

Walsh, K., O'Shea, E., and Scharf, T., 2020. Rural old-age social exclusion: A conceptual framework on mediators of exclusion across the life course. *Ageing and Society*, 40 (11), 2311–2337.

World Health Organisation, 2018. *Ageing and Health* [online]. Switzerland: World Health Organisation. Available at: https://www.who.int/news-room/fact-sheets/detail/ageing-and-health [Accessed 20 April 2020].

16 Transcultural Issues

Aslihan Nisanci, Adam Barnard, and Walters Tanifum

Chapter Aims

This chapter aims to examine factors and issues in transcultural communication and practice. Readers are expected to critically analyse stereotyped or essentialist views of culture and enhance their transnational cultural competence. Whether these are national, religious or otherwise socio-historically constructed, the goal is moving towards an understanding of communication, thought and action in a constantly fluctuating context where cultural identities are emergent, fluid and changing. It is hoped and expected that reading this chapter and completing the activities will bring about cultural and identity shifts, as well as changes in perceptions of culture, languages and practices to understand, adopt and utilise transcultural competence.

Introduction

The world is becoming increasingly diverse. Movement of peoples, movement of goods and services, globalisation, increasing heterogeneity replacing homogeneity and the development of social media and technology have led to a plural, multiple and complex world. The lived experiences of culture, how these experiences are received and perceived, thought about, acted upon demand a thorough understanding.

Ideas on anti-oppressive, anti-discriminatory, multicultural sensitivity and cultural competence approaches to practice enable providers to understand the cultural and ethnic barriers, conflicts and differences in societies so practice can respect people's individual and social identities and challenge oppression by dominant social groups. There is a need for everyone working in health and social care to develop an awareness of cultural competence and overcome the possible challenges that working with diverse communities can bring (Jones-Smith 2019; Marsiglia, Kulis, and Lechuga-Peña 2021; Sakamoto 2007). Health and social care workers are often located between traditional and cultural values, statutory and professional commitments and political demands. The modernisation, change, migration and modern world lead to distinct and significant changes for populations and professionals. The removal of oppressive and discriminatory thoughts, beliefs, actions that operate on personal, cultural and structural levels is vital element of health and social care work (Nzira and Williams, 2009).

In the UK, the legal basis for equality and diversity is the Human Rights Act 1998 and the Equality Act 2010. While the Human Rights Act 1998 protects the basic human rights of all individuals and provides equality, The Equality Act 2010 guarantees the equality and diversity service provision including health and social care services. Discrimination, harassment, victimisation and not making reasonable

DOI: 10.4324/9781003079873-19

adjustments are considered unlawful under the Act. The Act provides equality across nine protected characteristics:

- Age
- Disability
- Gender reassignment
- Marriage and civil partnership
- Pregnancy and maternity
- Race
- Religion or belief
- Sex
- Sexual orientation

Cultural competence requires a baseline of values that are centred on social justice, respect, dignity and worth of the person. Hence, it is central for health and social care. However, working toward cultural competence does not only mean learning about others' race or religion, but is a more complex process that includes self-reflection, an awareness of barriers to services, and changes in organisational procedures. Even the simple challenges with intercultural communication difficulties can become a barrier for clients from diverse cultural backgrounds (Marsiglia, Kulis, and Lechuga-Peña 2021). How can practitioners, workers and students navigate the minefield of potential communication mishaps? This chapter aims to address these challenging issues.

Drawing understanding from anti-oppressive views challenges the interests of social groups who have power and all othering exclusionary processes (Dominelli 2002; Nzira and Williams 2009). Multicultural sensitivity relates to issues of cultural competence and cultural awareness to understand and value devalued characteristics. Language is a central concern and 'political correctness' may silence the voices and concerns of the minority groups with the hegemonic use of the language imposed by the majority groups. The discussion around the term 'BAME' is a good example of the way a term can be problematic for different groups of people (BBC 2020). Therefore, it may become a backlash against progressive moves towards of more progressive services, thoughts, beliefs and actions.

This chapter reviews theoretical ideas to explore the issues and propose more inclusive, diverse and equal services. The chapter ends with reviewing the increased sophistication of oppressive views through 'dog whistle politics' and example activities.

Key Concepts, Theories and Models

Theories on cultural encounters emerged from growing concerns during the 1980s, about ethnic conflict in Western societies (Payne 2005: 375), social movements and the new millennia has seen silenced and marginalised groups respond to institutional and cultural forms of discrimination and oppression. Theoretical developments have posited the importance of intersectionality, critical theory, and critical race theory as theoretical frameworks to examine and challenge the overlapping and interdependent forms of personal, cultural and societal oppressions and challenges that people experience (Davis 2011; Delgado and Stefancic 2012; Marsiglia, Kulis, and

Lechuga-Peña 2021; Rossiter 1997; Salas, Sen, and Segal 2010). The search for equality and diversity in health and social care field led to new, practice-oriented concepts and theoretical approaches such as cultural competency, anti-discriminatory approach or anti-oppressive approach.

Equality, Diversity and Inclusion

The principle of equality ensures that everyone is treated with equal dignity by service providers, and no one is discriminated against based on their gender, ethnicity, ability status, health status or age. Diversity in health and social care means that the agencies and individual providers are aware of the effects of clients' different backgrounds and experiences on their lives, and they acknowledge and honour these differences. Agencies adopt Equality, Diversity and Inclusion (EDI) statements to reveal their stance on these issues.

Diversity has different dimensions some of which are subject to change and some of which are less subject to change. The dimensions that are less subject to change are called primary dimensions of diversity and listed as ethnicity, race, gender, physical ability, age and sexual orientation (Nahavandi 2022). The dimensions that can be changed are secondary dimensions of diversity and listed as religion, education, nationality, income, socioeconomic background, marital status, language, accent, family background, other group membership, professional background and region (Nahavandi 2022).

Stereotypes, Prejudice and Discrimination

As human beings, we want to comprehend our surrounding environment and assimilate our observations into categories in our minds. The cultural environment is no exception to this, and we hold categorical assumptions that all members of a given group have a particular trait. These assumptions are called 'stereotypes'. Stereotypes are mental shortcuts or overgeneralisations with a host of assumptions and beliefs, often based on incomplete and faulty information, about individuals and groups. Holding cultural stereotypes produces simplified understanding of groups and individuals that can become 'natural', 'normal' and unchallenged. Stereotypes can be positive or negative (Shiraev and Levy 2017). When they are negative, stereotypes form the basis of prejudice against certain groups of people, and they need to be effectively addressed to surface concerns and challenges built in prejudices, attitudes and beliefs. Based on these beliefs, we can treat people in discriminatory ways. Acting and behaving according to our negative views lead to oppressive practices. Discrimination can be practiced in easily understandable (overt discrimination) or subtle ways (covert discrimination) (Okitikpi and Aymer 2010) see Figure 16.1.

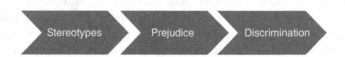

Figure 16.1 Stereotypes may lead to discrimination.

Source: Nahavandi (2022), p. 220. With permission from the author.

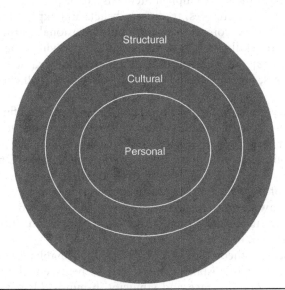

P: Personal, Psychological, Practice, Prejudice
C: Cultural, Communities, Conformity
S: Structural, Social division, Social forces, Socio-political

Figure 16.2 Thompson's (2012) Personal–Cultural–Structural (PCS) Model. With permission from the author.

Dalrymple and Burke (2009) and Thompson (2012) developed a practice model called **Personal–Cultural–Structural (PCS) Model** to understand discrimination within its social context. Originated in social work, the model informs transcultural practitioners on how to practice as an anti-discriminatory practitioner. The PCS model is useful to understand how thoughts, beliefs, opinions, behaviour and action exist on a personal/psychological level that blurs into cultural patterns or shares customs and habits and structural levels of organisations and institutions. Understanding how oppressive and discriminatory thinking, beliefs and action can be formed, maintained and sustained enable challenges to these ways of targeting particular groups and individuals (Figure 16.2).

Cultural Competence

Culture is the shared meanings, beliefs, opinions and understanding of groups or communities. It involves shared traditions, heritage and actions of a group. Cultural competence emerged in the 1980s—in America—as a framework for addressing the ethnocultural diversity produced by immigration and the need for social work to address the diversity (Danso 2016: 411). Since its emergence among social workers and counselling psychologists in the early 1980s (Greene-Moton and Minkler 2020, p. 142), the term cultural competence has continuously featured in the discourse of how health and social care providers can best demonstrate skills among different cultural service users they support. Cultural competence is 'the knowledge and in-terpersonal skills that allow providers to understand, appreciate, and work with individuals from cultures other than theirs' (Campbell-Stephens 2018, p. 1). It is to have a demonstrable awareness of other cultures, traditions, beliefs and experiences. In Jeffreys' (2010, p. 46) view, 'cultural competence is a multidimensional learning process that integrates transcultural skills in … three dimensions [involving] cognitive, practical, and affective [features]'. In other words, cultural competency refers to demonstrate the cultural awareness, knowledge and skills in working with all client systems (Jones-Smith 2019).

Self-awareness is one of the key dimensions of cultural competence and is defined as the practitioner's appreciation of their own and others' cultures. What you wear, how you greet others, what you eat, how you shower and what sport you like are all part of the cultural repertoire that you draw upon. Understanding these repertoires are part of cultural awareness. Being able to accommodate these needs into the delivery of care is part of becoming a transcultural practitioner. However, the practitioner should also be aware that there is no neutral position and it is not possible to suspend one's cultural background (Lum 2011; O'Hagan 2001; Yan and Wong, 2005) see Figure 16.3.

Culture is a contested construct, theoretically and politically (Bhabha 1994; Benhabib 1999, 2002). Sometimes, it is mistakenly perceived as being equal to a country's culture. Other times, it connotes race and ethnicity in minds. However, culture is a broader and complex term. Within the conceptualisation of cultural competency, culture includes multiple social positions including, but not limited to, gender, sexual orientation, age, ability status or religion.

Cultural competency has been criticised on several grounds. For example, it is criticised for being an apolitical term, which disregards the complex power dynamics in society (Sakamoto 2007). Furthermore, the term implicitly assumes that Whites are care providers as the norm and they are culture-free. However, we need to consider different dimensions of provider–client relationships when they deal with complex cultural encounters. For example, what do providers from minority ethnic background experience when they are working with White clients? What is it like for a provider to work with clients with disabilities? Examples can be diversified. Care providers should be aware that no one is exempt from culture(s) because culture has multiple

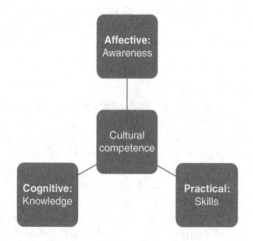

Figure 16.3 Three dimensions of cultural competence. With permission from the author.

dimensions. As a theoretical construct, intersectionality is suggested to comprehend these multiple dimensions including, but not limited to, class, gender, age, immigration status, mental health status, education status … etc. Intersectionality is a device or tool to help us analyse the complexities of the experiences (Davis 2011) and acknowledges that everyone has their unique experiences of discrimination and privilege (BASW 2022). Today, an intersectionality approach became part of professional guidelines on cultural competence (American Psychological Association 2017). In line with intersectionality, an anti-oppressive approach to cultural competency is suggested in order not to fall in the trap of disguising systems of oppression due to a neutral understanding of culture (Sakamoto 2007).

Another criticism is that cultural competence is an inadequate and potentially harmful model of professional development and health and social care provision as this is equated with simply having completed a past series of training sessions (Tervalon and Murray-Garcia 1998). Instead of cultural competence, cultural humility is suggested due to the risks of stigmatising and stereotyping posed by cultural competence (Lekas, Pahl, and Lewis 2020). Humility is often defined colloquially as 'freedom from arrogance and pride' but with a health and social care definition of 'a lifelong process of self-reflection and self-critique whereby the individual not only learns about another's culture, but one starts with an examination of her/his own beliefs and cultural identities'. Power imbalances should also be constantly checked in the provider–client relationship (Tervalon and Murray-Garcia, 1998, p. 119).

Cultural humility has also been criticised for not tackling structural issues and for including discussions on cultural congruence and anti-oppressive practice (Danso 2009, 2016). Despite these criticisms, we cannot deny the need for developing transcultural understanding and practice is a necessity for health and social care practitioners, trainees and workers.

Care providers need to know that cultures are in constant change, they are imagined territories and in ongoing dialogues with each other (Campbell-Stephens 2018). The process of constructing the other is one of the ways of recreating oppressive and discriminatory thought and action. The 'Other' confirms the recognition of their inherent dignity and intrinsic worth that are derived neither from my needs nor from my evaluation of their qualities. In other words, the relationship between myself and the 'Other' is infinitely beyond my comprehension, control and consumption (Kunz 1998). Therefore, developing cultural sensitivity, requires a rethinking of approaches that does not just consider cultural competence as more knowledge but a change in mindset, openness, humbleness to challenge oppressive and discriminatory thoughts and actions. To educate and train helping professionals, Ben-Ari and Strier (2010) advises that 'we should encourage the adoption of a position of complete openness in working with difference and diversity' (Ben-Ari and Strier, 2010, 10). They also suggest a humble attitude on the part of the professional along with an anti-oppressive perspective (Ben-Ari and Strier, 2010, 10).

Levinas' (1961) ethical ontology we have an embodied 'sensibility' for the other. He started with ethics rather than metaphysics (the philosophical theory that begins with first principles such as abstract concepts of being, knowing, identity, space and time) as a fundamental ontology or a description and interpretation of encountering another. A pre-conscious gives rise to spontaneous acts of responsibility to others via an embodied 'sensibility' (Hand 2001). The work necessary for an embodied sensibility is essential to transcultural competence, humility and sensitivity.

Intersectionality

Intersectionality invites services and providers to explore, understand and apprehend how service users, clients or patients experience oppression, discrimination and domination through diversity components such as race and ethnicity, immigration, refugee status, religion and spirituality, sexual orientation, gender identity and expression, social class, and mental or physical disabilities. Intersectionality challenges the perspectives that are solely gender or race-based (Marsiglia, Kulis, and Lechuga-Peña 2021). The diversity components are layered, multifaceted, and interrelated. Understanding these overlapping and interdependent social components, how they connect to make discrimination and disadvantage, and how to challenge and resolve these interactions are an essential part of equality, diversity and inclusion. For example, people may experience agism, racism and sexism collectively and individually at different times and in different environments. The goal is to see the whole person, and not seeing the person solely through their race, gender, socioeconomic status ... etc. Understanding the complex way the social components affect the individuals is vital to developing anti-discriminatory and anti-oppressive practice (BASW 2022).

Ideology

An ideology is a set of ideas associated with a particular set of social arrangements to 'legitimise the status quo', justify and protect vested interests and social arrangements, and lessen dissent and conflict. Thompson (2012) argues the power of ideas operates in the interests of power relations.

Hall (1986, 6) suggests 'ideology helps to sustain social order because it is part and parcel of the power relations in society – it influences how power works and how conflict is expressed and managed'. There are many ideologies at work in society that prioritise particular interests, and quieten others. As Marx says 'the ideas of the ruling class are, in every age, the ruling ideas'. Patriarchy, capitalism, imperialism are examples of dominant ideologies that have a structuring effect on people's and groups' experiences. The ability to define and sustain 'natural' and 'normal' have strong ideological overtones. For example, referring to 'the family' excludes the range and diversity of family forms and plays to Christian and right-wing positions.

Ideologically, critical theory fosters critical thinking (Jones-Devitt and Smith, 2007) that avoids assumptions (Brookfield 1990, 1991, 1994, 1995). Brookfield (1994, 204) suggests, on the one hand, critical thinking is 'able to penetrate hegemony, dominant cultural values and structural distortions with a single withering glance of pure clarity and, on the other hand, the learner as unquestioning dolt, duped into an uncritical acceptance of distorted meaning perspectives which have made structural oppression, economic inequity, racism, sexism and the silencing of divergent voices seem wholly natural'. Avoiding 'normalising' assumptions is the role for critical theory. Challenge and critique of these ideological constructions and taken-for-granted assumptions is a central element of critical theory. A significant part of ideological constructions are stereotypes and language and a need for critical thinking to explore, understand and challenge stereotypes and language.

Critical Theory

Critical theory is an umbrella term for the approaches that reveal power structures marginalising the individuals and communities. It uncovered the previously disguised oppressive relationships across categories of gender, race, ethnicity, physical ability and age. Rooted in the Frankfurt School in the 1930s, Critical Theory influenced the feminist theory and emancipation theory (Salas, Sen, and Segal 2010). It draws attention to the structural forces shaping individuals' lives. Critical theory argues that social problems are created and maintained by the structures of society and the cultural assumptions generated by dominant groups oppress and subordinate individuals and groups. Individual, psychological motivations are less important than the structure of society and focuses on structural rather than interpersonal and personal explanations of societal problems.

Critical theory transforms our perspectives regarding structural inequalities that systematically marginalise the individuals, groups, and communities. It underlines the macro level forces such as social, cultural, political, and environmental barriers in front of the individuals. Individuals interact with their environments.

In practice, critical theory is characterised by praxis, dialogue and 'conscientisation'.

- **Praxis** works with peoples' experience of oppression, injustice and inequality in the ideological understanding of how society works and agitates for social transformation.
- **Dialogue** works with equal relations with service users to exchange and discuss societal problems.
- **'Conscientisation'** is Paulo Freire's term for working with people to understand and analyse how social structures are implicated in people's oppression and discrimination. According to Freire, critical theory, people can transform society through self-awareness (Salas, Sen, and Segal 2010). Freire believed that regardless of their literacy levels, people can understand and change their realities through critical and reflective thinking (Christian and Jhala, 2015). Through empowerment, the oppressed can identify the oppressor they had been internalising, transform their realities, and experience liberation. This requires client participation in the service sectors.

Critical theory perspectives are concerned with empowering human beings to transcend the constraints placed on them by race, class and gender (Cresswell 2007; Fay 1987). We need to acknowledge our own power, engage in dialogues, and use theory to interpret or illuminate social action (Madison 2005). We would be interested in scientific study of social institutions and their transformations through interpreting the meanings of social life; the historical problems of domination, alienation, and social struggles; and a critique of society and the envisioning of new possibilities (Fay 1987; Morrow and Brown 1994). Service providers need to be aware and critical of perspectives that blame the individuals for all their problems and failures. The interventions that solely focus on the individuals are seen inefficient to tackle complex and deep-rooted social problems (Rossiter 1997). Service providers are called to address structural issues, social inequalities, and human rights violations (Garrett 2021). Pathologising the oppressed is criticised. Practice should be social justice oriented and carefully assess systemic level factors that marginalise the individuals. However, this does not mean that the only practice route is social change. Providers can both work with the individuals and be engaged in structural work. More importantly, the individual/social dichotomy is undermined, and more integrated ways of practice are suggested (Salas, Sen, and Segal 2010). Care providers are suggested to listen to the voices of the marginalised individuals and groups to understand the ways power operates and marginalises people.

From critical theory's standpoint, social care field is also a site of cultural construction and meaning-making (Rossiter 1997). In reflective practice, the care provider reflects upon the culture and meaning-making processes she is involved in during her interactions with the clients. In this sense, the provider is part of the power dynamics as well and should carefully consider her role in reproducing or challenging the oppressive practices.

Critical Race Theory

Critical Race Theory (CRT) started as a movement in the law in the United States in the 1970s and pointed to the subtler forms of racism despite the legal gains of the Civil Rights Movement (Delgado and Stefancic 2012). CRT emphasises the role of legal interventions to correct racial oppression and the need for additional support so people can realise their potential. The theory spread to disciplines and fields, whose contributions revealed the prevalence of racial disparities in education, housing, employment, health, mental health or justice (Sulé 2020). In the UK, the study by Bywaters (2020) is an example of the application of CRT to child welfare system as it reveals the inequalities based on race and ethnicity.

CRT incorporates both multicultural and oppression perspectives (Delgado and Stefancic, 2012), although does not sufficiently recognise structural oppression in neo-liberal economies (Cole 2009). The theory suggests that cultural competence and multiculturalism are only one step in the process of challenging oppressions. If we do not go further and do not realise subtle and persistent existence of racism in different domains of social life, multiculturalism only disguises racism and perpetuates the vicious cycle of structural inequalities (Constance-Huggins 2019). CRT informs health and social care practice in different ways:

- Providers become aware of the ways subtle forms of racism affect clients' lives, form barriers in front their access to services, and keep them trapped in the cycles of social inequalities
- Providers can advocate for their clients and take action towards social change to tackle subtle forms of racism
- Providers can empower their clients through informing them about the ways racism operates

Imagined Communities

Anderson's (1983) 'imagined communities' are sets of ideas that become recent and modern, universal and influential which all people are members of one or another community. Nations are socially constructed with members of imagined communities (such as Britishness), presented as political unities although carry the weight of colonisation and male privilege. Drawing these themes together, exploring, unpacking and deconstructing the construction of these forms of imagined communities enables challenges to be raised against ideology, oppression and discrimination in thoughts, beliefs and action.

Anti-oppressive Practice (AOP)

A broader definition of culture and going beyond diversity management by cultural competency require anti-oppressive approach (Sakamoto 2007). The radical social work movement of the 1970s and the subsequent structural, feminist and anti-racist social work movements set the ground for anti-oppressive social work (Dominelli 2009; Robbins 2011). Apparently, the approach has been influenced by conflict theory, critical theory, feminist theory, black feminist thought and the empowerment approach (Burke and Harrison, 1998; Robbins 2011; Sakamoto and Pitner 2005). Originating from British social work, the approach has become increasingly popular in Canada, Australia, New Zealand and other European countries from the 1990s onwards (Sakamoto and Pitner 2005).

Sharing the knowledge base of oppression theories (Robbins 2011), the main theoretical constructs of anti-oppressive social work are oppression, domination, privilege and multidimensionality of oppression (Dominelli 2009). The central emphasis is that private troubles are intricately linked to larger structural forces (Dominelli 2002) and oppressed people will not gain personal empowerment unless society makes transformations (Payne 2005). On this path, oppressive relationships and dynamics of oppressive power should be uncovered in all social domains (Dominelli 2002). The approach also includes global forces into analysis and strongly criticises today's global, neo-liberal market capitalism for reproducing poverty and social isolation (Dominelli 2002; Shera 2003). A postmodern interpretation of identity characterises this approach, formulising identity as a state of being in constant change (Dominelli 2002). Moreover, the postmodern emphasis that the oppressed groups should speak with their own voices is a basic principle. The multi-layered, multidimensional and complex nature of oppression also requires incorporating knowledge from various disciplines including psychology, sociology, political science, anthropology, economy and even history.

Anti-oppressive social work is also client-centred and empowerment-oriented. The client–provider relationship is supposed to be truly egalitarian, where the client, not the provider, is conceptualised as the expert over his or her reality. The provider only prepares the ground for the clients to develop their own stories with their own voices and tries to understand how hegemonic, oppressive discourses operate to suppress these stories (Dominelli 2002). At the same time, the practitioner avoids pathologising the client, does not try to normalise her and situates the client in the multi-layered context that surrounds her even when the intervention is at individual or family levels. More importantly, the intervention should be holistic: the client is viewed as the whole person, not only as an oppressed individual (Dominelli 2002). Providers should be aware both of the limits and capacities of their own and the client's agency and the constraints of the structure in a realistic fashion (Burke and Harrison 1998; Dominelli 2002).

The provider should also be aware of the political nature of the client–provider relationship and the dynamics of power. The provider pays attention to multiple subject positions of the client and herself (Sin and Yan 2003). Reflecting upon her own biases, assumptions, cultural views and various identities, provider use critical consciousness as an integral part of practice (Sakamoto and Pitner 2005). The overarching goal of the anti-oppressive practice as to highlight social injustice and find ways of eradicating it in both the social work practice field and in all social domains (Dominelli 2009). Dalrymple and Burke (2009), from an anti-oppressive perspective, suggest the aims are as follows:

- Overcoming barriers to [service users] achieving greater control of their lives
- Working in partnership with [service users] and including them in decision-making
- Minimal intervention, to reduce the impact of the oppressive and disempowering aspects of services
- Critical reflection and reflexivity of ourselves to understand how our values and biographies affect our practice relationships

Language

The way we express ourselves and the type of language are important to be open, humble and anti-oppressive. Language has the ability to name and identify specific objects, people and processes. However, it also has the power to affect and exclude individuals, groups and objects, or rename, repurpose and reproduce language. Language is not only descriptive, but also prescriptive (Shiraev and Levy 2017). Language is not open and transparent but carries with it a set of signifiers and virtue signalling.

Payne (2014, p. 379) provides a case example:

> Children in a group of private sector children's residential care homes were encouraged to celebrate the festivals of Diwali (Hindu/Jain), Christmas (Christmas), Pass-over (Jewish) and Ramadan (Islamic), which were relevant to some of the children in the home. However, there was no education about their importance in different cultural and historical contexts, and no attempt to ensure that children from different backgrounds realized the significance of a particular festival of their own cultural heritage. As a result, many of the children merely say the celebrations as a disconnected series of occasional celebrations, rather like birthday parties.

An inclusive, diverse and equal use of language promotes equality and recognises the value and worth of different uses of language. Providers need to be 'mindful' of the ways that language can be used to oppress and exclude particular individuals and groups. The normal rule of language (turn-taking, listening, valuing) needs to account for the different uses of language. We need to be open to others, humble and anti-oppressive in the type and use of language.

Decolonisation

Transcultural practice requires an opening of discussion around the culture, history and effects of colonisation and the way it is represented today. There is a need to go beyond micro-level cultural competency issues in professional–client relationship, reevaluate Western-centric ideologies and values (Mabvurira 2018), and address the structural inequalities affecting health and social care systems (Buyum et al. 2020).

The studies that show structural determinants of health and social care (Bywaters 2020; Sulé 2020) serve decolonising the systems. To decolonise practice; the materials, language and history of thoughts and practices need to be reconsidered. Decolonising the curriculum is also an important part of decolonisation efforts and has been frequently addressed (Al-Natour and Mears 2016; Begum and Saini 2019). It means creating spaces and resources for a dialogue among all members of the university on how to imagine and envision all cultures and knowledge systems in the curriculum and with respect to what is being taught and how it frames the world. Easy wins are through reordering the curriculum and make a diversity of peoples, places and thoughts available. More stringent demands are to make a 'fearless university' that attempts to open discussion and debate to a range of influences.

Awareness of cultural differences is the first step. Second, a range of different resources and open, free spaces are needed to provide an alternative view of how the world can be framed. This is an elegant way of challenging oppressive and discriminatory thoughts, beliefs and actions. Finally, celebration and valuing of transcultural values and experiences are necessary.

Without careful consideration, decolonisation is not without risks such as the risk of tokenism, superficiality and homogeneity. Decolonisation, as a movement, is criticised for not being critical enough and being used as a term to cover any socially progressive attempt (Dhillon 2021). If not carefully assessed, decolonisation has the risk of getting lost within liberal multiculturalism. For example, having a detailed knowledge and awareness of Judaism, Talmudic texts and orthodox practices does not automatically lead to culturally appropriate thoughts, behaviour and action. Taken for granted 'normality' can vary immensely from culture to culture, group to group and individual to individual. For example, what time do you get up sounds straightforward but is dependent on culture, employment, spirituality. Israel has a Sunday morning rush hour, which is difficult to comprehend in Western societies. BAME acronym, which is used for Black African and Minority Ethnic communities, is a catch all term. This acronym is homogenising the diverse experiences of a multitude of people and is being criticised widely.

Social Media

The various platforms of social media have offered unprecedented opportunities for open communication and practice but also the potential for discriminatory and oppressive language and action. The rise of 'hate-speech', 'hater' and the expression of discriminatory and oppression language and action has led to an exclusionary culture (Relia et al. 2019; Ekman 2018). Open, free speech is a good thing but making informed and critical judgments on what is being said, 'fact checking' and countering 'fake news' are new fault lines that have been drawn and that we need to respond to, so that complex social problems are not reduced to an individual level and 'blames the victim'.

Dog Whistle Politics

Just as cultures shift and change over time, the sophistication of discriminatory and oppression related to intersectionality has shifted and changed. In order to mobilise the support of their voters, politicians discovered ways of influencing their constituency while staying politically correct. This is called 'dog whistle' politics and is defined as 'speaking in code to a target audience' to talk about taboo subjects (Drakulich et al. 2020). The term refers to the ultrasonic sound only audible to dogs and relates to coded or suggestive language to marshal support for one group and denigrate another group. The message is not vocalised explicitly but remains unconscious and unspoken (López 2014). It works like subliminal advertising. For example, calling Obama as Barack Hussein Obama has a coded message of association for some sections of the United States. Used in this way, the hidden forms of assumptive thinking are built into cultural constructions.

The unspoken but alluded to messages of communication require an opening out or giving air the debate of challenging issues for open and clear communication, to 'bottom out' or thoroughly dissect the questions, constructions and issues that frame culture.

Conclusion

This chapter discussed cultural competency and the related dimensions. It presented critical perspectives on culture and called practitioners to challenge essentialist views. Cultural competency was viewed as a process which requires lifelong learning and critical self-reflection from the practitioner. The chapter also argued that transcultural practice is not limited to practitioner–client relationship and goes beyond practitioner's individual skills. Transcultural practice requires an anti-oppressive approach and an awareness of the structural determinants of health and social care. For this reason, perspectives such as critical race theory and intersectionality were presented along with the concepts like cultural competency and cultural humility. Personal–cultural–structural model, which combines individual and structural factors in transcultural practice, was also discussed. All approaches to multicultural sensitivity share common principles of a concern for rights, social justice and critical practice. Understanding of the ability to communicate across cultural and ethnic barriers protects the principles of inclusion, diversity and equality. Transcultural issues require assessing, planning, monitoring, evaluation and review to ensure that appropriate health and care services are being delivered to meet the needs of individuals, groups and communities. We are all in this together and all have a role to play in challenging oppression and discrimination for a more open, inclusive, diverse and equal way of being.

ACTIVITIES

Activity 1: Practice Example

There is a range of examples that show these processes at work. For example, scheduling meetings at times inconvenient for certain groups. Would you have a team meeting during Ramadan? Answering this you might suggest that as inconvenient as scheduling a meeting on Christmas Day. However, that would also prioritise Christian calendars and could be seen as an unspoken assertion of the privilege of Christianity. So marginalisation, discrimination and oppression are multi-levelled and in need of challenge. For a fully transnational cultural competence, a self-awareness and self-knowledge, understanding and respect for cultural differences and actions and behaviour that are inclusive need to be developed.

Activity 2: Case study/vignettes

Think of a moment where you were motivated to be with the other.

Think through what you are wearing. Where did it come from? What are the conditions under which it was produced? Is this an ethical piece of clothing? Where is your phone from?

In light of the previous discussion think through how you might provide guidance on services to be more inclusive.

What is the structure of feeling that emerges from these uncertain times? Raymond Williams has the 'structure of feeling' as part of the historical consciousness of contemporary times in material culture. The global pandemic has led to a range of changes in 'structures of feeling'.

Activity 3: Pause and Reflect

Think of a moment when you encountered oppressive or discriminatory thoughts, beliefs, opinions, behaviour or action. What was expressed? What assumptions did this have? Did you elegantly challenge the thought, behaviour, opinion, behaviour or action? Did you really explore in a critical and self-reflective way the challenges presented by the encounter?

Activity 4: The Stereotypes I Hold

The aim of this activity is to raise your self-awareness. You will fill out a form individually. Using Table 16.1, identify your stereotypes, their sources, and your experiences that confirmed the stereotype. You can add as many columns as you like.

In Table 16.2, reflect on the stereotypes you listed in the first table, and identify the disconfirming information:

Table 16.1 The stereotypes I hold (Part I)

Stereotypes	Source	Personal Experiences
1.		
2.		
3.		

Table 16.2 The stereotypes I hold (Part II)

Stereotype	Disconfirming Information
1.	
2.	
3.	

Indicative Reading

Baker, W., 2015. *Culture and identity through English as a Lingua Franca: rethinking concepts and goals in intercultural communication.* 8th ed. Berlin, DE: De Gruyter Mouton.

Jackson, J., 2014. *Introducing language and intercultural communication.* London: Routledge.

Jones-Devitt, S., and Smith, L., 2007. *Critical thinking for health and social care.* London: Sage.

Neuliep, J., 2012. *Intercultural communication: a contextual approach.* London: Sage.

Samovar, L., Porter, R., and Mc Daniel, E., 2006. *Intercultural communication: a reader.* Wandsworth: Cengage Learning.

Samovar, L., Porter, R., Roy, C., and Mc Daniel, E., 2017. *Communication between cultures.* 9th ed. Wandsworth: Cengage Learning.

References

Al-Natour, R., and Mears, J., 2016. Practice what you preach: creating partnerships and decolonising the social work curriculum. *Advances in Social Work and Welfare Education*, 18 (2), 52–65.

American Psychological Association, 2017. *Multicultural guidelines: An ecological approach to context, identity, and intersectionality* [online]. Washington, DC: American Psychological Association. Available at: http://www.apa.org/about/policy/multicultural-guidelines.pdf [Accessed 20 May 2022].

Anderson, B., 1983. *Imagined communities: reflections on the origin and spread of nationalism.* London: Verso.

BASW, 2022. *SWU Blog: Intersectionality is a valuable tool for social work practice* [online]. Birmingham: BASW. Available at: https://www.basw.co.uk/media/news/2022/feb/swu-blog-intersectionality-valuable-tool-social-work-practice [Accessed 29 May 2022].

BBC, 2020. *'Don't call me BAME': Why some people are rejecting the term* [online]. London: BBC News. Available at: https://www.bbc.com/news/uk-53194376 [Accessed 10 June 2022].

Begum, N., and Saini, R., 2019. Decolonising the curriculum. *Political Studies Review*, 17 (2), 196–201.

Ben-Ari, A., and Strier, R., 2010. Rethinking cultural competence: What can we learn from Levinas?. *British Journal of Social Work*, 40 (6), 1–13.

Benhabib, S., 2002. *The claims of culture: Equality and diversity in the global era.* New Jersey: Princeton University Press.

Bhabha, H., 1994. *The Location of Culture.* London: Routledge.

Brookfield, S., 1990. Using critical incidents to explore learners' assumptions. In: Mezirow, J., ed. *Fostering critical reflection in adulthood.* San Francisco: Jossey-Bass, 1990, pp. 177–193.

Brookfield, S., 1991. On ideology, pillage, language and risk: critical thinking and the tensions of critical practice. *Studies in Continuing Education*, 13 (1), 1–14.

Brookfield, S., 1994. Tales from the dark side: a phenomenography of adult critical reflection. *International Journal of Lifelong Education*, 13 (3), 203–216.

Brookfield, S., 1995. *Becoming a critically reflective teacher.* San Francisco: Jossey-Bass.

Burke, B., and Harrison, P., 1998. Anti-oppressive practice. In: Adams, R., Dominelli, L., and Payne, M., eds. *Social work, themes, issues, and critical debates.* Basingstoke, Hampshire: Palgrave Macmillan, 1998, pp. 229–239.

Buyum, A.M., Kenney, C., Koris, A., Mkumba, L., and Raveendran, Y., 2020. Decolonising global health: If not now, when?. *BMJ Glob Health*, 5 (8), 1–4.

Bywaters, P., 2020. *The child welfare inequalities project: Final report* [online]. Coventry: Child Welfare Inequalities Project. Available at: https://pure.hud.ac.uk/ws/files/21398145/CWIP_Final_Report.pdf [Accessed 13 August 2021].

Campbell-Stephens, R., 2018. *Cultural sensitivity in safeguarding* [online]. Nottinghamshire: RMC Consultants. Available at: https://www.slideshare.net/complianceandsafety/cultural-sensitivity-in-safeguarding-by-rmc [Accessed 12 November 2019].

Christian, A., and Jhala, N., 2015. Social work needs Paulo Frierie. *International Journal of Humanities and Social Science Invention*, 4 (6), 36–39.

Cole, M., 2009. *Critical race theory and education: A Marxist response.* Basingstoke: Macmillan.

Constance-Huggins, M., (2019). *Critical race theory and social work in Stephen Webb (2019). The Routledge handbook of social work.* London: Routledge, pp. 163–171.

Cresswell, J.W., 2007. *Qualitative inquiry and research design: Choosing among five traditions.* London: Sage.

Dalrymple, J., and Burke, B., 2009. *Anti-oppressive practice: Social care and the law.* Maidenhead: Open University Press.

Danso, R., 2009. Emancipating and empowering de-valued skilled immigrants: What hope does anti-oppressive social work practice offer? *British Journal of Social Work*, 39, 539–555.

Danso, R., 2016. Cultural competence and cultural humility: A critical reflection on key cultural diversity concepts. *Journal of Social Work*, 18 (4), 410–430.

Davis, K., 2011. Intersectionality as buzzword: A sociology of science perspective on what makes a feminist theory successful. In: Lutz, H., Vivar, M.T.H., and Supik, L. eds. *Framing intersectionality: debates on a multi-faceted concept in gender studies.* London: Routledge, 2011, pp. 67–85.

Delgado, R., and Stefancic, J., 2012. *Critical race theory: an introduction.* 2nd ed. New York: New York University Press.

Dhillon, S., 2021. An immanent critique of decolonisation projects. *The Journal of the Canadian Philosophy of Education Society*, 28 (3), 251–258.

Dominelli, L., 2002. *Anti-oppressive social work: theory and practice.* Basingstoke, Hampshire: Palgrave.

Dominelli, L., 2009. Anti-oppressive practice in context. In: Adams, R., Dominelli, L., and Payne, M., eds. *Social work, themes, issues, and critical debates.* New York: Palgrave Macmillan, 2009, pp. 3–19.

Drakulich, K., Wozniak, K.H., Hagan, J., and Johnson, D., 2020. Race and policing in the 2016 presidential election: Black Lives Matter, the police, and dog whistle politics. *Criminology*, 58 (2), 370–402.

Ekman, M., 2018. Anti-refugee mobilization in social media: The case of soldiers of Odin. *Social Media + Society*, 4 (1). DOI: 10.1177/2056305118764431

Fay, B., 1987. *Critical social science.* Ithaca, NY: Cornell University Press.

Garrett, P.M., 2021. *Dissenting social work.* London: Routledge.

Green-Moton, E., and Minkler, M., 2020. Cultural competence or cultural humility? Moving beyond the debate. *Health Promotion Practice* [online], 21 (1), 142–145. DOI: 10.1177/1524839919884912 [Accessed 4 April 2021].

Hall, S., 1986. Managing conflict, producing consent. Open University, Unit 21 of D102, Social Sciences; A Foundation Course.

Hand, S., ed., 2001. *The Levinas reader.* Oxford: Willey-Blackwell.

Jeffreys, M.R., 2010. *Teaching cultural competence in nursing and health care.* 2nd ed. New York: Springer Publishing Company.

Jones-Devitt, S., and Smith, L., 2007. *Critical thinking for health and social care.* London: Sage.

Jones-Smith, E., 2019. *Culturally diverse counseling: Theory and practice.* London: Sage Publications.

Kunz, G., 1998. *The paradox of power and weakness: Levinas and an alternative paradigm for psychology.* Albany, NY: State University of New York Press.

Lekas, H.M., Pahl, K., and Fuller Lewis, C., 2020. Rethinking cultural competence: Shifting to cultural humility. *Health Services Insights* [online], 13, e1178632920970580. DOI: 10.1177/1178632920970580

Levinas, E., 1961. *Totality and infinity.* London: Kluwer Academic Press.

López, I.H., 2014. *Dog whistle politics: how coded racial appeals have reinvented racism and wrecked the middle class.* Oxford: Oxford University Press.

Lum, D., 2011. *Culturally competent practice: a framework for understanding diverse groups and justice issues.* Pacific Grove, CA: Brooks/Cole.

Mabvurira, V., 2018. Making sense of African thought in social work practice in Zimbabwe: towards professional decolonisation. *International Social Work* [online], 63 (4), 419–430. DOI: 10.1177/0020872818797997

Madison, D.S., 2005. *Critical ethnography: methods, ethics, and performance.* Thousand Oaks, CA: Sage.

Marsiglia, F.F., Kulis, S.S., and Lechuga-Peña, S., 2021. *Diversity, oppression, and change: culturally grounded social work.* Oxford: Oxford University Press.

Morrow, R.A., and Brown, D.D., 1994. *Critical theory and methodology.* Thousand Oaks, CA: Sage.

Nahavandi, A., 2022. *The cultural mindset: managing people across cultures.* London: Sage Publications.

Nzira, V., and Williams, P., 2009. *Anti-oppressive practice in health and social care.* London: Sage Publications.

O'Hagan, K., 2001. *Cultural competence in the caring professions.* London: Jessica Kingsley.

Okitikpi, T., and Aymer, C., 2010. *Key concepts in anti-discriminatory social work.* London: SAGE Publications.

Payne, M., 2005. *Modern social work theory.* 3rd ed. Chicago: Lyceum.

Payne, M. 2014. *Modern social work theory.* 4th ed. Oxford: Oxford University Press.

Relia, K., Li, Z., Cook, S.H., and Chunara, R., 2019. Race, ethnicity and national origin-based discrimination in social media and hate crimes across 100 U.S Cities. *Proceedings of the International AAAI Conference on Web and Social Media* [online], 13 (01), 417–427. Available at: https://ojs.aaai.org/index.php/ICWSM/article/view/3354 [Accessed 19 June 2022].

Robbins, S.P., 2011. Oppression theory and social work treatment. In: Turner, F.J., ed. *Social work treatment.* 5th ed. New York: Oxford University Press, 2011, pp. 343–353.

Rossiter, A.B., 1997. A perspective on critical social work. *Journal of Progressive Human Services* [online], 7 (2), 23–41. DOI: 10.1300/J059v07n02_03

Sakamoto, I., 2007. An anti-oppressive approach to cultural competence. *Canadian Social Work Review,* 24 (1), 105–114.

Sakamoto, I., and Pitner, R.O., 2005. Use of critical consciousness in anti-oppressive social work practice: disentangling power dynamics at personal and structural levels. *The British Journal of Social Work,* 35, 435–452.

Salas, L.M., Sen, S., and Segal, E.A., 2010. Critical theory: pathway from dichotomous to integrated social work practice. *Families in Society: The Journal of Contemporary Social Services,* 91 (1), 91–96. DOI: 10.1606/1044-3894.3961

Shera, W., 2003. *Emerging perspectives on anti-oppressive practice.* Toronto: Canadian Scholars' Press.

Shiraev, E.B., and Levy, D.A., 2017. *Cross-cultural psychology: critical thinking and contemporary applications*. NJ: Pearson Inc.

Sin, R., and Yan, M.C., 2003. Margins as centres: a theory of social inclusion in anti-oppressive social work. In: Shera, W., ed. *Emerging perspectives on anti-oppressive practice*. Toronto: Canadian Scholars' Press, 2003, pp. 25–42.

Sulé, V.T., 2020. Critical race theory. *Encyclopedia of Social Work, e1329 [online]*. DOI: 10.1093/acrefore/9780199975839.013.1329

Tervalon, M., and Murray-Garcia, J., 1998. Cultural humility versus cultural competence: a critical distinction in defining physician training outcomes in multicultural education. *Journal of Health Care for the Poor and Underserved* [online], 9 (2), 117–125. DOI: 10.1353/hpu.2010.0233 [Accessed 5 April 2021].

Thompson, N., 2012. *Anti-discriminatory practice: equality, diversity and social justice*. 5th ed. Basingstoke: Macmillan.

Yan, M.C., and Wong, Y.R., 2005. Rethinking self-awareness in cultural competence: toward a dialogic self in cross-cultural social work. *Families in Society*, 86 (2), 181–188.

17 Leadership in Health and Social Care

Jennifer Sanders

This chapter aims to:

- Develop a critical understanding of traditional and emerging leadership paradigms
- Discuss key issues in leading integrated health and social care services
- Aid reflection and preparation for roles in health and social care

Objectives

After reading this chapter you should be able to:

- Understand the concept of leadership and teamwork
- Discuss the key themes linked to leading integrated health and social care services
- Reflect on your employability and graduate attributes

After reading this chapter you will know the meaning of the following terms: leadership, teamwork, motivation, partnership working, emotional intelligence. There is a Moment of Reflection at the end of the chapter.

Introduction

Management is usually based on authority, referring to a formally designated role which an individual is assigned within an organisation's structure. Management is about actions and processes, using systems and procedures to attain organisational goals and objectives (Mullins 2016). Good practice in the management of people and the challenges facing health and social care managers has been explored in Chapter 11, *Managing Health and Social Care*. Whilst there is no clear definition of leadership, it is associated with relationships through which one person influences the behaviour or actions of others. Across time there have been numerous theories, focusing on a leader's traits, behaviours, functions, and interactions with their followers (Mullins 2016). As such, leadership is inextricably linked to teamwork and understanding the motivations, personalities and behaviours of team members. These theories and concepts with be discussed in a way to demonstrate both the linear progression of understanding as well as the interconnected nature. The structure of our integrated health and social care sector will be briefly introduced, with a central focus on organisational culture, values and partnership working. Finally, the chapter

DOI: 10.4324/9781003079873-20

will conclude by reflecting on the importance of self-awareness and exploring the professional attributes and academic knowledge a health and social care graduate has to become a leader in their field.

Leadership Theory

A typical starting point to conceptualise and theorise 'leadership' is to ask, are leaders born or made? The great man theory (Spector 2016) holds that individuals are either born a great leader or not. To this end, any external factors such as upbringing, education and employment experiences are opportunities for you to model your leadership abilities, they are not responsible for making you a leader. As with the debate of whether criminals are born or made, there is no empirical research to support the notion leaders are born. Trait theory (Spector 2016) pertains that individuals are born with innate characteristics which predispose them to become leaders. As a result, these individuals seek our opportunities which fit these characteristics and therefore enable them to emerge as the leader they are destined to become. There is yet to be a definitive list of these leadership characteristics/qualities to support this theory. A key problem is these theories focus on the individual's biology or psychology and ignore factors such as behaviour and environment.

Behavioural theories explain leadership through what leaders do. Within this category is the early work by Lewin, Lippit and White (1939) on leadership styles. The major leadership styles were identified:

- Autocratic – rule through command and control, enables quick decision-making and decisive action, but limits creativity and can become dictatorial
- Laissez-faire – hands-off leadership, where group members – often experts – make decisions, which can lead to lack of personal responsibility and motivation
- Democratic – arguable the most successful style, participation from group members is valued, leading to high-quality contributions and commitment but can slow down decision-making through consideration of all ideas

Lewin, Lippit and White (1939), along with later researchers, argue leadership is not about the position or status of an individual, but the way activities are carried out and how the leader behaves towards the group. Blake and Mouton's (1964) managerial grid also identifies styles a leader can adopt, based on a continuum of whether the leader has more concern for the staff or the task at hand:

- Country club management – leader has little interest in task completion but a high concern for the social needs of staff.
- Task compliance management – leader has little concern for staff's needs. Their overwhelming concern is with achievement of task/targets.
- Impoverished management – leader has very little interest in either staff or task. They do the bare minimum to get by.
- Middle-of-the-road management – leader is content to compromise. They seek to satisfy rather than maximise both the well-being of staff and production.
- Team management – leader emphasises both the need for high levels of achievement and excellent staff relations, the suggested approach all leaders should use.

Blake and Mouton's (1964) leadership grid explains the style that a leader may adopt but does not give instruction on how this behaviour would be enacted. By ignoring a range of internal and external variables, the theory fails to explain why some leaders are successful in certain situations but not in others. For example, when a leader has a 'win' with one team but 'fails' with another. Here, team dynamics and development have impacted leadership style and effectiveness.

Contingency theory then considers the environment in which a leader exists. In Hersey and Blanchard's (1969) situational leadership theory, leadership effectiveness is dependent on the relationship between the task, interpersonal skills, and favourableness of the work environment. The style of leadership adopted is influenced by the competence and commitment of the team member, referred to as 'follower readiness' with four levels. The four approaches that can be employed are as follows:

- Coaching – leader provides high levels of direction and support
- Directing – leader provides high levels of direction but low levels of support
- Supporting – leader provides high levels of support but low levels of direction
- Delegating – leader provides low levels of support and direction

This theory guides leaders in how to behave through matching their style to the characteristics of the follower, a practical approach to motivating individuals. Whilst the theory enables flexibility, it ignores variables such as demographics of the follower and can be burdensome varying style by individual rather than group. For example, in a setting where there is a high staff turnover.

Another theory focusing on the relationship between leader and follower is the leader–member exchange theory (Bauer and Erdogan 2016). A high-quality relationship is trust-based, where the leader and member like each other and support the other's ability to succeed. In a low-quality relationship, whilst there is no active disliking, leaders and followers do not go above the job description to support each other. The theory highlights the importance relationship type has on a leader influencing others and can have positive outcomes. There is the possibility high-quality relationships are mistaken from friendships and lacks an explanation of how time and culture changes may impact the leader–member exchanges.

There are a number contemporary theories which have particular relevance to health and social care. Servant leadership (Greenleaf 1977), often demonstrated in charities, religious and humanitarian groups, puts the followers first. Focus is on serving the followers for their own good through co-production. A consideration of the context and culture, leader attributes, and follower's needs and desires manifest as ethical and empowering leadership behaviours which produce outcomes of personal growth for the follower and societal impact. Although there are positive impacts of the leadership style putting the follower first, it can be restrictive and not suitable for all situations/environments.

Transformational leadership (Bass 1985) has been demonstrated through generation and development of the NHS, as well as increasing use of the private sector, for example, Richard Branson and Virgin Care Ltd. This theory looks at the process between leaders and followers. The emphasis is on leading by example, encouraging growth and learning, being inspirational and empowering. Charisma (see Weber 1964) is often associated, questioning whether being 'transformational' in a trait rather than a behaviour one can adopt. As such, transformational leadership is difficult to define and measure.

Increasingly, value-based recruitment is utilised in health and social care, reflecting the continued emphasis of the importance of values. As such, congruent leadership (Stanley 2019) is emerging as the style health and social care leaders should adopt. Congruent leaders are driven to act in ways which are consistent with their values and beliefs, resulting in dedicated followership. To date, there is limited empirical research analysing this approach, but concern around the lack of focus on change has been voiced (Stanley 2019).

Management and Leadership in Health and Social Care, management and leadership are traditionally seen as two different concepts. Cunliffe (2021) however takes a critical stance: management is more than functions and competencies; it is about who you are, how we experience organisational life and relate to others – a notion central to the leadership theories discussed above. Cunliffe and Eriksen (2011) argue that the relational nature of leadership goes beyond that with followers, but to the wider world in which leaders exist. Leadership is fluid, dynamic, socially constructed with leaders/managers embed in communities of difference. Understanding the importance of relationships through this lens can lead to responsive and morally-responsible leadership. It requires managers to be reflexive, in recognising how we interact and how this shapes the 'realities' in which practice occurs. High-profile scandals such as Mid-Staffordshire (see Francis 2013) and life-changing events such as the COVID-19 pandemic, focus on the need for ethical leadership by health and social care leaders/managers because their decisions have consequences beyond organisational boundaries (Cunliffe 2021).

Suggested Further Reading

Schedlitzki, D., and Edwards, G., 2018. *Studying leadership: traditional and critical approaches*. 2nd ed. London: Sage.

Managing Change

Managing change is a crucial role for leaders in health and social care. Change needs to be managed to ensure organisational objectives are met, whilst securing staff commitment, both during and after implementation. Often, at the same time, business as usual needs to be maintained. These needs can present considerable challenges for leaders. One challenge is resistance to change, which may come from subordinates, colleagues, senior management, or stakeholders. There are many reasons for this resistance, which leaders need to understand, anticipate, and overcome. Models of change provide tools and techniques to manage change in challenging situations.

Lewin's (1997) model of change has three stages, which creates the perception that change is needed, moves towards the desired behaviour which then becomes the norm. These stages are:

1 Unfreeze – Diagnosing and classifying what the problem is. Communicating effectively what requires change, why it is necessary and the positive impact this change would have.

2   Change – Transitioning to the new behaviour/ways of working starts, with individuals reassured of the positive impact the change will have.
3   Refreeze – Reinforcing the new state following the change, where this is now accepted as the new norm.

Within Lewin's model is the tool 'Force Field Analysis', which analyses the situation and provides a framework for identifying how to overcome resistance to change. 'Driving' forces – those pushing for change – and 'restraining' forces – those resisting change – are identified and analysed to either strengthen (for driving forces) or weaken (for restraining forces) each influence. There are several strategies leaders can employ to overcome these resisting factors (Barr and Dowding 2019):

- Education and communication – for use when people are not well informed of the need for change
- Participation and involvement–when leaders actively involve those affected by change in decision-making process
- Facilitation and support – using training and supervision to support those struggling to adjust to change
- Negotiation and agreement – leaders listen to concerns and all involved come to an agreement
- Manipulation and co-option – for use when the change process is not working, giving hesitant individuals some ownership within the process
- Implicit or explicit coercion – a last resort, leaders could use their power to create rewards for adherence and punishment for resistance

Lewin's model is simple, easily applied and therefore an efficient method for leaders to manage change. However, it can be criticised for not providing detail on practical application. Additionally, the 'refreezing' stage is problematic as change is continual, particularly in health and social care.

Teamwork

As demonstrated above, leadership approach is influenced by the relationship a leader has with their followers. A leader is part of the team, rather than a manager who would be above in the hierarchy. Within an integrated health and social care system, working with individuals who have complex needs, teamwork is key. A team is a group of people working together to achieve common objectives and are willing to commit the energy necessary to ensure they are achieved (Gopee and Galloway 2017). Tuckman (1965) theorised that teams go through four stages of development:

1   Forming – this is where team members become familiar, identify individual strengths, clarify roles and assign tasks, as well as establish ways of working
2   Storming – a natural stage of team development where there may be disagreements, needing effective communication and conflict resolution strategies to result in negotiations and collaboration
3   Norming – the team has formed and shares belief they can achieve their objectives
4   Performing – good teamwork is demonstrated, objectives are achieved, reflections on the group process can be observed

Tuckman later added a fifth stage – adjourning – to acknowledge the disbanding of teams, and the evaluations which occur. This simple view of how teams develop aligns with Hersey and Blanchard's (1969) situational leadership theory: the leader moves through coaching, from directing to supporting and finally, delegating as the group navigates the four stages. Whilst Tuckman's (1965) model provides a simple, linear approach to team formation its application to large-scale, multidisciplinary, and virtual teams may be limited. DuFrene and Lehman (2016) provide an overview of the diversity challenges experienced in virtual teams. They also outline how selection of a capable leader, linking to Blake and Mouton's (1964) managerial grid, is key to virtual team success. Another key aspect is team membership: selecting the right people for virtual work.

In the 1970s, Belbin (2010) was involved in experiments in which team role theory emerged and remains significant in understanding effective team working. Belbin's (2010) theory states that successful teams are made of up a diverse mix of behaviours, captured in nine team roles across three classifications:

- Thinking roles: monitor evaluator, plant and speciality
- People roles: co-ordinator, resource investigator and team worker
- Action roles: implementer, shaper and completer finisher

Although the nine roles are required, it does not mean a team needs nine individuals. This is because most people will have two or three roles which they are most aligned. Each team role has its strengths and allowable weaknesses and is of equal importance. The team roles will emerge when required, based on the team objectives and tasks being completed. As with behavioural leadership, Belbin's theory focuses on adapting behaviours to the situation.

As with leadership, there have been attempts to identify which personalities are best suited to teamwork. Tests to measure an individual's personality are often used during the recruitment process. Understanding your personality can help you appreciate your own preferences and behaviour. This self-awareness can be crucial in teamwork. There are two schools of thought around personality: trait theory and type theory. The Myers-Briggs Type Indicator (MBTI), developed in the 1940s and based on Jung's theory of psychological types, measures four dichotomies (Myers and Briggs Foundation 2021):

- Favourite world: Do you prefer to focus on the outer world or on your own inner world? This is called *Extraversion or Introversion.*
- Information: Do you prefer to focus on the basic information you take in or do you prefer to interpret and add meaning? This is called *Sensing or Intuition.*
- Decisions: When making decisions, do you prefer to first look at logic and consistency or first look at the people and special circumstances? This is called *Thinking or Feeling.*
- Structure: In dealing with the outside world, do you prefer to get things decided or do you prefer to stay open to new information and options? This is called *Judging or Perceiving.*

These dichotomies produce 16 personality types, expressed as a code with four letters. As with Belbin's team roles, all personalities are equal and have their strengths and weaknesses. Although the MBTI has been extensively researched and remains popular in the world of consultancy, criticism has been levied at the typology: the assumption individuals fit into one category and that everyone in that category is the same. Within personality theory, there has been a move towards trait theory. Trait theory holds that human personality occurs along continuous dimensions rather than discrete categories (Martin, Carlson and Buskist 2013). The most popular trait theory is McCrea and Costa's Five-Factor Model, which measures an individual's level of Openness, Conscientiousness, Extraversion, Agreeableness and Neuroticism (McCrae and Costa 1987). This prevailing theory conceptualises traits on a spectrum, emphasises a biological basis for personality and acknowledges the influence the environment can have on behaviours.

Understanding an individual's personality can have huge benefits for leaders, including knowing how they are motivated. Motivation is multifaceted, with behaviours and actions of an individual influenced by internal or external factors. Extrinsic motivation is related to tangible rewards such as salary, promotion, conditions of work which are external to the individual. Intrinsic motivation is psychological rewards that her internal to the individual, such as a sense of challenge or achievement, receiving appreciation or positive recognition (Mullins 2016). Theories of motivation can be categorised as content – an emphasis on what motivates individuals – and process – emphasis on the actual process of motivation.

Maslow's (1943) hierarchy of needs is a traditional and enduring theory of individual development and motivation. Usually depicted as a pyramid, the theory holds that everyone has the same needs or desired that must be satisfied. At the peak of the pyramid is self-actualisation, which individuals can achieve once low-level needs have been satisfied. Once a lower need has been satisfied, it is no longer a motivator. Therefore, leaders should direct their attention to the next higher level to keep individuals motivated. Although Maslow indicates the order in which needs are required to be met, there may be instances when the hierarchy will be reversed. When applying to a work situation, some difficulties arise. Leaders should be aware that needs are not only satisfied through employment, but also people's personal and social lives. The value placed on each need may vary across individuals, and aspects of work may fulfil multiple needs.

Understanding the needs and motivations of their followers allows leaders to devise strategies to ensure effective team working, achievement of objectives and development of the individual. To this end, supervision and coaching are important. Within health and social care, supervision is there to ensure the practitioner is continuously developing themselves and their practice, resulting in high-quality care and client needs being met. As such, supervision should be regular, planned, accountable and reflective process (Field and Brown 2019). Coaching is a strategy which can be utilised during supervision. Coaching is non-directive, focusing on improving performance and developing individuals' skills. Downey (2003) developed the TGROW model, providing a framework for a coaching session:

Topic – setting the general themes

Goal – identify the objective(s) to be achieved, as well as the goal for the session

Reality – understanding what the current situation is for the individual in relation to the objective

Options – explore all possible solutions for moving forward and achieving to objective

Will – identifying and agreeing what will be done, when and with what support

Adopting a coaching technique creates an environment where individuals can think creatively, take responsibility for their own learning and area of work, as well as instilling a culture of self and alignment to team norms and values. Overall benefits include higher motivation at an individual and team level, as well as improved organisational performance.

Suggested Further Reading

MacKian, S., and Simons, J., 2014. *Leading, managing, caring: understanding leadership and management in health and social care*. Abingdon: Taylor and Francis Group.

Integrated Health and Social Care

Values are enduring beliefs or principled actions, which are learned and acquired through experiences with individuals and organisations (Mullins 2016). Organisations have values, which support the vision of that organisation and help shape its culture. As mentioned above, value-based recruitment is increasingly employed within health and social care, along with the rise of congruent leadership. The vision of an organisation describes what it will become in the future, usually broad and inspirational. Organisational culture is the 'way things are done' which influences the behaviours and attitudes of individuals. Several scholars have attempted to classify organisational culture, to aid understanding of a complex concept. Schein (1992) states that organisational culture is the most difficult attribute to change, often outlasting products, services, leaders and founders. Handy (1993) describes four types of culture, aligned to organisational structure:

- Power – power is held by a few individuals whose influence spreads throughout the organisation. Usually a strong culture, which enables quick decision-making but can turn toxic.
- Role – power is determined by an individual's position in a bureaucratic organisation.
- Task – power derives from expertise, within a team that has formed to address a specific problem. The right mix of skills, personalities and leadership is required.
- Person – rather than working as a team, individuals see themselves superior to the organisation and work individually.

Organisational culture, conceptualised through values, beliefs and attitudes, has a significant impact on organisational processes, staff motivation, team working and partnership working. Peck and Dickinson (2009) discuss organisational culture and partnership working, concluding that culture plays a significant part in the success or failure of partnerships.

Partnership working is an integral part of health and social care. A partnership has shared aims, objectives and vision between organisations who share rights, resources, and responsibilities. Working in partnership may mean new structures and processes are developed. Partnerships are often required to achieve continuity of care, deliver coordinated packages of services and tackle 'wicked issues' (Glasby and Dickinson 2008). As such there are a range of benefits:

For partners

- Meeting objectives
- Shared learning
- Economic use of resources
- Potential for innovation
- Access to a broader range of skills

And for users

- Higher standard of provision
- Improved outcomes
- Access to a range of skills, services and knowledge

Partnership working is not without its problems, with Cameron et al. (2012) identifying factors which hinder joint working in health and social care across three broad themes.

Organisational issues:

- Problems establishing a shared purpose, aims and objectives
- Lack of clarity about roles and responsibilities
- Competing organisational visions
- Lack of pooled/shared budget
- Differences in organisational policy
- Not communicating or sharing information effectively
- Co-location undermining practice
- Lack of strong management
- Lack of involving professionals in planning

Cultural and professional issues:

- Negative assessments and professional stereotypes
- Different professional philosophies
- Lack of trust and respect between professionals
- Absence or limited joint training and team-building
- Role boundaries

And contextual issues:

- Complex relationships between agencies
- Constant reorganisation and lack of geographical boundaries
- Financial uncertainty
- Difficulty in recruiting staff

Bailey, Mutale and Holland (2018) evaluated the integration of social care interventions into primary care teams working with older adults with complex care needs. A key finding identified conditions – which link to the barriers identified above – required for effective integrated care delivery: leadership, training, shared sense of belonging, sharing social care identity, and confidence in social care worker role. Within the study the integrated teams produced better outcomes (quality and economic) than the district teams. Such research has led to the development of a toolkit to aid integration and produce effective integrated teams (see Bailey, Mutale and Holland 2018).

There has long been calls and reason for a fully integrated health and social care system. The *Health and Social Care Act 2012* introduced a number of changes to promote better integration of services. However, some may argue the reforms further fragmented the sector and policy barriers to integration remained (The King's Fund n.d). The COVID-19 pandemic of 2020/21 further highlighted the need for integration and demonstrated how this can be achieved. Amidst the greatest challenge our health and social care system has ever faced collaboration across services increased, new partnerships were created, new technology was adopted, and new working cultures developed with new approaches to problem-solving. The government has restated its commitment to an integrated health and social care system through the White Paper *Integration and innovation: working together to improve health and social care for all* (Department of Health and Social Care 2021). The proposed legislation has two forms of integration: integration within the NHS to reduce bureaucratic barriers preventing collaboration and make joint working an organising principle; and to have greater collaboration between the NHS, local government and wider delivery partners. The introduction of statutory integrated care systems (ICSs) will see support for place-based joint working, place-level commissioning aligned geographically to local authority boundaries and measures to improve data sharing. Alongside broader reforms to social care and public health, there is hope for a truly integrated health and social care system.

Suggested Further Reading

Heenan, D., and Birell, D., 2018. *The integration of health and social care in the UK: policy and practice*. London: Palgrave.

Preparing for Employment

As mentioned earlier in the chapter, value-based recruitment is increasingly used within health and social care. The purpose is to identify individuals whose values align with that of the organisation. It is therefore important that you understand your own values, and that you have explored the values and vision of the organisation you are applying for. Organisations may utilise any of the following to ascertain your values and understanding of the organisation:

- Ask you to list/describe the organisation's values
- Ask a question which explores your knowledge of the organisation's values, and how your personal values align
- Present a scenario and ask you to describe how you would respond

As a result of this value-based approach, recruitment has moved away from sending in CVs and having interviews, to submitting detailed application forms and attending assessment centres or interviews with a practical element. As well as your values, organisations are assessing your competency to carry activities which will be key to your job role. It is therefore useful to have techniques to aid this. The STAR technique provides a structured way of describing your skills, and is particularly useful for competency-based questions, such as "describe a problem you've recently had to solve" or "tell us about a time you've worked well in a team" (Figure 17.1).

STAR is a tool to aid self-awareness and self-assessment. Although this technique may be used at the end of your studies when applying for jobs, there is a related skill which you should start to develop as early as you can: emotional intelligence. Emotional intelligence is the capacity to monitor and regulate our own and other's emotions (Salovey and Mayer 1990). Goleman (2009) built on this definition, and identified five basic elements:

Self-awareness: Understanding our emotions, using them to guide decision-making but not letting our feelings rule us. Having a realistic assessment of our strengths and weaknesses.

Self-regulation: Thinking before acting. Handling our emotions to facilitate rather than interfere with tasks.

Motivation: Using our preferences to guide us towards our goals and overcome obstacles.

Empathy: Ability to identify with and understand the wants, needs and viewpoints of those around us.

Social skills: Masters at building and maintaining relationships, using skills to persuade and lead, negotiate and settle disputes, being a team player.

Throughout your studies think about how you deal with challenges, how you react to people and how you come across to others. This will increase your emotional intelligence and ability to answer competency-based questions. Emotional intelligence is key to responsible, relational and reflexive leadership.

Your studies and experience at university are designed to provide you with the graduate attributes which employers are looking for. Hill, Walkington and France (2016) outline that these can be viewed as your skills, knowledge, attitudes and values, developing your academic, citizenship and career competencies. Common graduate attributes include critical thinking skills; effective communication; leadership and teamwork skills; research and inquiry skills; information and digital literacy; ethical, moral and social responsibility; and cross-cultural awareness. All of which contribute to effective leadership in health and social care.

Conclusion

This chapter has outlined the developing understanding and practice of leadership within health and social care. A selection of key theories has been described and critiqued, showing how leadership can be considered from a biological, functional, behavioural and relational stance. The link between leadership and followership has

STAR stands for situation, task, action, result[1]:

Situation: When/where?

Around 10% of your answer should be used to set the scene. Use examples from employment, work experience, university, voluntary work, gap year or anything that allows you to provide enough detail about the skill

- *"When at university ..."*
- *"A good example of team work is when I worked at a ..."*
- *"Whilst on my Gap year in ..."*

Task: What?

Around 10% should explain the task either set by yourself or another. In order to provide a detailed answer this should be specific, measurable and time-bound

- *"I was in overall charge of organising the ..."*
- *"I worked in the customer service team at ..., a customer had a problem with ... so I had to..."*
- *"When a mini bus booked to take the university rugby team to the game did not turn up at the allotted time, I had to ......"*

Action: How?

50% of your answer should describe what you did and the skills you used to do it. This is the most important section. Concentrate on *how* you completed the task, staying focused on the skill they have asked you about!

To provide the detail you will need to reflect back on what you did by breaking it down step by step.

- *"When forming our project group, one of the first actions I took was to..."*
- *"A major role was to manage and co-ordinate the staff which I did by ..."*
- *"When the mini bus I booked to transport the rugby team to a match 30 miles away did not turn up. I solved this problem by...."*

Result: So what?

Use the last 30% to give details of the outcome. This could be a tangible outcome (e.g. a grade at university) or something you have learnt about yourself – but try and be specific.

- *"The result was that every aspect of the event ran as planned, and I received numerous emails telling me what a great event I'd organised..."*

[1] Guidance provided by Nottingham Trent University's Employability Team

Figure 17.1 STAR stands for situation, task, action, result.

been identified, with theory of team development and group roles discussed. The importance of understanding personalities, motivations and values has been highlighted. Exploration of partnership working shows the benefits and barriers, whilst the latest commitment from the government to developing a truly integrated health and social care system ties together the concepts covered within this chapter and Chapter 10. The last part of the chapter focuses on preparing you for employment, and the importance of developing emotional intelligence as your progress through your studies. The STAR technique for demonstrating your competencies can be used in conjunction with the broader notion of reflection captured in Chapter 10.

Summary of Main Points

You should be able to:

- Outline what leadership in health and social care entails
- Describe key aspects of leading integrated health and social care services
- Reflect on your own emotional intelligence and leadership skills

Moment of Reflection

An example of a criterion from a person's specification could be

> Good interpersonal skills and an ability to communicate complex ideas effectively to a range of stakeholders.

Use the STAR technique outlined in this chapter to plan an answer for how you could demonstrate you meet this criterion in a job application or interview.

References

Bailey, D., Mutale, G.J., and Holland, D., 2018. *Toolkit to support the social care role in integrated health and social care teams* [online]. Nottingham: Nottingham Trent University. Available at: https://ncasc.info/wp-content/uploads/2018/11/WW1_Toolkit_nott_tu_notts_video_removed.pdf

Barr, J., and Dowding, L., 2019. *Leadership in health care.* 4th ed. London: Sage.

Bass, B.M., 1985. *Leadership and performance beyond expectations.* London: Collier Macmillan.

Bauer, T.N., and Erdogan, B., 2016. *The Oxford handbook of leader-member exchange.* Oxford: Oxford University Press.

Belbin, M.R., 2010. *Management teams: Why they succeed or fail.* 3rd ed. Oxford: Butterworth-Heinemann.

Blake, R., and Mouton, J., 1964. *The Managerial Grid: The key to leadership excellence.* Houston: Gulf Publishing Co.

Cameron, A., Lart, R., Bostock, L., and Coomber, C., 2012. Factors that promote and hinder joint and integrated working between health and social care services: a review of research literature. *Health & Social Care in the Community* [online], 22 (3), 225–223. Available at: https://www.crisiscareconcordat.org.uk/wp-content/uploads/2014/04/briefing41.pdf [Accessed 28 February 2021].

Cunliffe, A.L., and Eriksen, M., 2011. Relational leadership. *Human Relations* [online], 64 (11), 1425–1449. DOI: 10.1177/0018726711418388

Cunliffe, A.L., 2021. *A very short, fairly interesting and reasonably cheap book about management*. London: Sage.

Department of Health and Social Care, 2021. *Integration and innovation: Working together to improve health and social care for all* [online]. London: Department of Health & Social Care. Available at: https://www.gov.uk/government/publications/working-together-to-improve-health-and-social-care-for-all/integration-and-innovation-working-together-to-improve-health-and-social-care-for-all-html-version [Accessed 1 March 2021].

Downey, M., 2003. *Effective coaching: Lessons from the coach's coach*. 3rd ed. Knutsford: Texere Publishing.

DuFrene, D.D., and Lehman, C.M., 2016. *Managing virtual teams* [online]. 2nd ed. New York: Business Expert Press. Available at: https://catalog.libraries.psu.edu/catalog/8273493

Field, R., and Brown, K., 2019. *Effective leadership, management and supervision in health and social care*. 3rd ed. London: Learning Matters.

Francis, R., 2013. *Report of the mid Staffordshire NHS Foundation Trust public enquiry: Executive summary* [online]. London: GOV.UK. Available at: https://assets.publishing.service.gov.uk/government/uploads/system/uploads/attachment_data/file/279124/0947.pdf [Accessed 4 August 2021].

Glasby, J., and Dickinson, H., 2008. *Partnership working in health and social care (Better partnership working)*. Bristol: Policy Press.

Goleman, D., 2009. *Working with emotional intelligence*. London: Bloomsbury.

Gopee, N., and Galloway, J., 2017. *Leadership and management in healthcare*. 3rd ed. London: Sage.

Greenleaf, R.K., 1977. *Servant leadership: a journey into the nature of legitimate power and greatness*. New Jersey: Paulist Press.

Handy, C.B., 1993. *Understanding organizations*. 4th ed. London: Penguin.

Hersey, P., and Blanchard, K.H., 1969. Life-cycle theory of leadership. *Training and Development Journal*, 23 (5), 26–34.

Hill, J., Walkington, H., and France, D., 2016. Graduate attributes: implications for higher education practice and policy. *Journal of Geography in Higher Education* [online], 40 (2), 155–163. DOI: 10.1080/03098265.2016.1154932

Lewin, K., 1997. *Resolving social conflicts and field theory in social sciences*. Washington: American Psychological Society.

Lewin, K., Lippit, R., and White, R.K., 1939. Patterns of aggressive behavior in experimentally created "social climates". *Journal of Social Psychology* [online], 10 (2), 269–299. DOI: 10.1080/00224545.1939.9713366

Martin, G.N., Carlson, N.R., and Buskist, W., 2013. *Psychology*. 5th ed. London: Pearson.

Maslow, A.H., 1943. A theory of human motivation. *Psychological Review* [online], 50 (4), 370–396. DOI: 10.1037/h0054346

McCrae, R.R., and Costa, P.T., 1987. Validation of the five-factor model of personality across instruments and observers. *Journal of Personality and Social Psychology* [online], 52 (1), 81–90. DOI: 10.1037/0022-3514.52.1.81

Mullins, L.J., 2016. *Management and organisational behaviour*. 11th ed. London: Pearson.

Myers and Briggs Foundation, 2021. *MBTI Basics* [online]. Gainesville: The Myers and Briggs Foundation. Available at: https://www.myersbriggs.org/my-mbti-personality-type/mbti-basics/ [Accessed 28 February 2021].

Peck, E., and Dickinson, H., 2009. Partnership working and organisational culture. In: Glasby, J., and Dickinson, H., eds. *International perspectives on health and social care: partnership working in action*. Oxford: Wiley-Blackwell, 2011, pp. 10–26.

Salovey, P., and Mayer, J.D., 1990. Emotional intelligence. *Imagination, Cognition, and Personality* [online], 9 (3), 185–211. DOI: 10.2190/DUGG-P24E-52WK-6CDG

Schein, E.H., 1992. *Organisational culture and leadership*. 2nd ed. San Francisco: Jossey-Bass.

Spector, B.A., 2016. *Discourse on leaders: a critical appraisal.* Cambridge: Cambridge University Press.

Stanley, D., 2019. *Values-based leadership in healthcare: congruent leadership explored.* London: Sage.

The King's Fund [n.d]. *How far has the government gone towards integrating care?* [online]. London: The King's Fund. Available at: https://www.kingsfund.org.uk/projects/verdict/how-far-has-government-gone-towards-integrating-care [Accessed 1 March 2021].

Tuckman, B.W., 1965. Developmental sequence in small groups. *Psychological Bulletin* [online], 63 (6), 384–399. DOI: 10.1037/h0022100

Weber, M., 1964. *The theory of social and economic organization.* London: Collier Macmillan.

18 Conducting a Student Empirical Research Study in Health and Social Care

Louise Griffiths, Penny Siebert, and Alice Lee

An understanding of research paradigms has become increasingly important in Health and Social Care. This chapter explores how to conduct a small-scale Empirical Research Study (ERS), providing all the essential steps for completing a social research project. This chapter draws on research approaches to support students undertaking research for their first research projects such as dissertations, by briefly discussing quantitative and qualitative research approaches. The final part of the chapter presents the findings of an ERS dissertation into the impact of social networking sites on mental health.

Learning Outcomes for the Chapter

By end of this chapter, you will be able to:

- Consider the reasons for carrying out a piece of research
- Consider the practical issues involved when developing a research proposal into an empirical research study (ERS)
- Understand how to write an ERS including all the elements which are central to primary research including academic writing, referencing and citations
- Be supported with your ERS through advice (hints and tips) from a fellow student (Alice)

Embarking on your first ERS can be daunting for students and many find they struggle knowing exactly where to start. It is important to know that many students experience this during the first month or so of their ERS dissertation both at the undergraduate and postgraduate levels.

An Overview of the Purpose and Goal of Doing an Empirical Piece of Research

The main reason for doing a piece of research is to answer a **question**. This question needs to be based on an interest of that was triggered by your reading or from the information you gained from your studies. Research is about exploring and expanding on a question that you have started to ask yourself:

- Why are certain things happening?

DOI: 10.4324/9781003079873-21

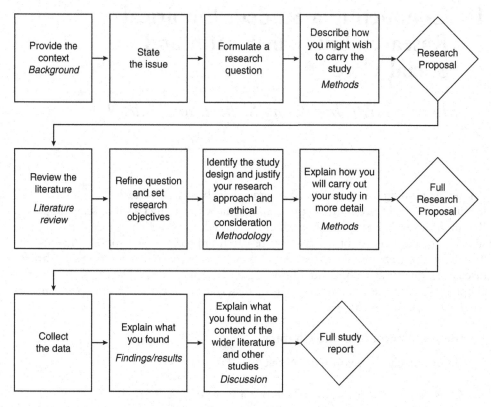

Figure 18.1 The research process. With permission from the author.
Source: (Siebert 2019).

- What is the nature of the connections between one aspect of social care and social conditions?
- What role do social physical and economic environment have on health outcomes?

Your research question helps to identify what research approach you should take. The research methods chapter provides an overview of the key research approaches and the kind of research questions that they can be used to address (Figure 18.1).

The Issues

Getting Started on Your ERS – The Research Proposal

The starting point for all research projects whether undergraduate or postgraduate is the research proposal. A proposal is the outline of your research idea that is written to present what you wish to research and how you think it can be explored. Indeed, the research proposal is the 'plan' for the final research project and should include a detailed plan from the start to the end of the project, whilst including key information such as the data collection tools used (such as interviews, questions, etc.), what type of analysis you will use and how you will write up the research into your final dissertation (Thomas 2017).

An important part of this stage of the process is exploring what has been written on the problem issue you have identified. Information gathered at this stage through an initial exploration of the literature, policy and other related data sources is used to describe the context in which an identified issue or problem you are interested is taking place. This provides your background to your research and helps you to start thinking about your research question. It also gives your reader an understanding of what are the core issues.

The proposal should include a descriptive title, literature review which includes the problem to be addressed, research aim and main research question, the proposed research design, methods, and ethical considerations (see Chapter 10, Valuing Health and Social Care for further details).

Case study example – Alice (Undergraduate student)

> Before I began conducting my study, I created a Gantt Chart to plan my research and findings, this gave me a timeline to work alongside, defining each aspect of my empirical research project from conducting the study to writing up my results. After this, I began by outlining the research through selecting the aims of each topic area. This outlines prior research that has already been conducted and identified gaps within the knowledge and outlines how my study could fill these.

Developing Your Research Proposal Into a Full Study Proposal

The next stage in the process of building on your research proposal is to develop the study into a feasible research study, this will take place after you have had the initial proposal reviewed and any feedback has been explored and addressed with your dissertation supervisor. A key focus at the stage of the process is refining and reframing your research question. This is helpful through searching and critically reviewing the exciting literature on your chosen topic. This will help you to identify the gap in the research and help you to focus you research question and refine your study design. Importantly the review of the literature helps you to decide in what ways your research will contribute to the evidence base. Based on what you have identified in the literature you have reviewed; you may decide that your research study can make a new contribution to the current evidence base because there is limited research on the issue you have chosen. Alternatively, you can decide that your study and potential findings can be used to build or contribute to the existing evidence base. These are important considerations to take as they will help when you come to write your discussion section of your dissertation, which will form a detailed discussion within this chapter. In Table 18.1 some of the other considerations to take into account are presented. An example is provided in Table 18.2.

Table 18.1 Research considerations

Key considerations	Yes	No	Notes
Are you keeping the same research topic as the proposal?			
Does the research topic need refining? E.g., proposal states 'mental health' does this need refining to a particular condition such as anxiety			
Return to the academic literature has there been any new research conducted?			
Assess the context of the research, has there been any changes which impact on the ethics and methods of the project, e.g., the impact of COVID-19 and the move to online research			
Do the methods of the project need adapting?			
How will you analyse the ERS?			
Review the project schedule/research plan and set weekly actions with your dissertation supervisor.			

EXAMPLE: Table 18.2

Table 18.2 Example

Research Term	Aims
Narcissism	This research project builds upon Andreassen's (2017) study surrounding the ideas of narcissistic behaviour online and how frequent users of SNSs utilise their SNS to promote their own achievements and express their aspirations, building upon narcissism being one of the 'big five' personality traits used online (Marshall et al. 2015). This research will utilise both quantitative and qualitative data to gain a personal insight into how the participants present themselves on SNSs.
Self-worth	The research explores the idea of self-worth and how participants value themselves through responsiveness upon SNSs. The research stems from Blease's theory of 'Facebook Depression' and aims to find trends amongst the amount of likes and the worthiness the participants feel (Blease 2015).
Self-image	This research aims to explore the impact of celebrity content on the insecurity surrounding the body image and the lifestyle of participants. Both genders are included in this study as current literature largely focuses upon the effects on females. This research aimed to find trends for both males and females regarding their insecurity towards lifestyle and body image after the presentation of content from celebrities.

Case study example – Alice (Undergraduate student) – Developing her research idea

Upon starting my research, I knew my area of interest was mental health due to my proposed career plan, so I decided on this as my topic for my dissertation. However, as a research topic, mental health is very broad, so from here, I began to take notes of current mental health issues being discussed within the media and topics, which I had studied throughout Health and Social Care to see if these would be viable for a research project. I found that social media was a current issue that was consistently mentioned alongside mental health which prompted me to conduct a literature search within this area.

I found a wealth of knowledge surrounding the impacts social media holds upon female body image, to bridge this gap within the knowledge I wanted to look at how men are impacted. Originally, my research topic was how far social media has influenced negative body image and disordered eating within males. After meeting with my dissertation supervisor, we discussed this question being too narrow, as at the time there was not enough literature on the topic, and it would be difficult to recruit participants. To improve my study, I recognised three trending patterns within the research where participants were most effected, these being narcissism, insecurity, and self-worth. This allowed me to tailor my question to encompass these three areas while comparing the different social networking sites and gender.

Following the initial review of the proposal some decision will need to be considered:

The next stage of any research process involves of developing, planning, and contextualising (Punch 2016). This is when you start to carefully think about the approaches you wish to take to answer your research question, which will consider why a particular study design or approach would best suit your research study, this forms your methodology and method sections (see Chapter 10 for further details).

Tip – The type of data you collect, and the way it is analysed is determined by the study design. The key thing to remember that the data you gather, analyse, and interpret will help you to answer your research question.

Second Stage: Writing Up Your ERS for Your Dissertation – Your First Full Draft

What Should Your Final Dissertation Look Like?

Title

This will start initially as a tentative title for your intended research in the early stages of the ERS. You will be able to revise your title during the course of your research and produce a final title in the final months of your ERS dissertation. The research title should clearly identify the focus of the research and include all the key elements of the ERS (Punch 2016).

Abstract

Abstract writing is the skill of providing a research summary within a paragraph or two, it is recognised that this can be a challenging task (Bell and Waters, 2018). The abstract should outline the importance of the research topic whilst highlighting how your ERS will contribute to the existing literature. The summary should include brief details of the methodology used (quantitative, qualitative, or mixed methods) alongside the details of the methods employed. Finally, a brief discussion of the key findings of your ERS should be provided here. The ERS abstract mirrors the abstracts you have been reading in journal articles as part of your university studies.

Case study example – Alice (Undergraduate student) – Abstract

Social Networking Sites (SNSs) have become an increasingly popular pastime for many young adults, gaining mainstream popularity within the last decade. While usage of SNSs does not appear problematic to many on a surface level, literature has begun to explain the impacts SNSs holds upon the mental health of its users. This empirical research study employs a Likert Scale questionnaire to examine the impact daily use of Facebook, Instagram, Twitter and Snapchat, and the effect these SNSs have upon their self-worth, self-esteem, and narcissistic tendencies amongst 120 participants aged 18–30. The results of this study concluded that the social capital held by celebrities on SNSs highly influenced the insecurity of participants surrounding their lifestyle and body image. This behaviour is also demonstrated within the participants through the creation of an online persona and the demonstration of narcissistic tendencies, although it is still unknown if this copied behaviour is due to celebrity influence. These results were consistent amongst literature and previous studies surrounding narcissism, self-worth, and low self-esteem on SNSs.

Research Background and Context/Introduction

In this section, you will describe the broad Health and Social Care background against which you will conduct your research. This should include a brief overview the size and nature of the problem within your chosen area of study.

RESEARCH AIM AND RESEARCH QUESTIONS

The introduction should also include the main research aim, your refined research question and your research objectives. This section should explain the purpose of the research and the importance within a few sentences (Bell and Waters, 2018).

This introduction should also provide the details of the theoretical perspective/theory that you are applying to your ERS dissertation. A theoretical perspective or theoretical framework is a theory that you are applying to your research, a lens which you are looking at the data through. This can be a challenging idea when first contemplating which theory relates to your research topic, indeed it is common for even the most experienced academics to consider several theoretical perspectives for their own research. An example, when researching women in prison a student/researcher may choose a feminist perspective as the research explores women in prison.

Case study example – Alice (Undergraduate student) – Theoretical Perspective

One of the most popular posts to SNSs is the selfie, a term deriving from the hypernym "self-portrait" to define an image of an individual taken by the individual on their smart phone or camera (Oxford Dictionaries 2013). Goffman's (1959) theory of self-presentation can be applied to the selfie, as many appear to package their behaviours and put on an "act" (p.31), which they present to the outside world through socialisation. This amplifies these behaviours which causes many to create an online persona for themselves, this can be seen through the Renfrew Centre Foundation (2014) study of selfie taking, this study found that 50% of their participants edit their selfies to appear more desirable. Unfortunately, gaps within the literature leave little reasoning as to why individuals create a persona for themselves, Kaplan and Haenlein (2010) speculate there are intentions of impressing those around them, however there is no de facto study that provides reasoning behind this.

This section should also signpost to the following chapters by providing a summary of what will be included in each chapter, e.g., chapter one explores the academic literature on the research topic of mental health. This illustrates good practice and enables the reader/marker to understand the ERS as a whole from the beginning.

Review of the Literature (Chapter 1)

This chapter involves taking a systematic approach to reviewing the literature, summarising the current state of knowledge and recent debates on the topic, as well as identifying gaps in knowledge. This will allow you to demonstrate a familiarity with the current evidence, theories, and opinions. This review will also demonstrate your ability to communicate clearly and concisely.

Firstly, you will need to conduct a literature search so that you have a knowledge of what literature exists and the ways in which your project will extend/contribute to such knowledge. When you are searching, the literature be critical, Henn et al. (2009) suggest asking the following questions when conducting a literature search:

- What research has already been conducted which is relevant to my research project?
- What are the main conclusions to be drawn from previous research?
- What were the main methods used by previous research?
- In which ways are the previous studies similar in terms of the conclusions and methods?
- In which ways are the conclusions and methods of previous studies different?
- Where are the gaps in the knowledge?

A suggested chapter structure is provided in Table 18.3.

Table 18.3 Suggested Chapter Structure

1 **Outline the purpose of your research** – What are you exploring/investigating?

2 **Why is research into this area important?** – Use official statistics here to illustrate the importance of your research from the offset if, for example, you were conducting your research project on obesity, you should add the rates of obesity at the level you think this information helps to describe the burden of disease or impact on services – 28% of adults in the UK are obese (Balogun et al. 2021).

3 **Provide definitions for the key concepts** – For example, if your research is on Homelessness and mental health, define these concepts.
  - What definitions are provided by the literature.
  - Discuss any disagreements regarding the definitions within the literature.
  - State which definition your research will use and provide a justification.

(Continued)

Table 18.3 (Continued)

4 Identify any policy responses from the government on your research topic – Is there an influential government report or has a policy been implemented?

For example, if your research was on homelessness and mental health the 'No Second Night Out policy' has been introduced. However, homelessness and mental health is still an area of concern so in this example you would briefly assess the impact of the policy, e.g., that it doesn't cover mental health to the extent that is required to support this condition in homeless people.

5 Discuss the (most influential/key) previous research on your topic and the production of key theories on your research topic.

6 State how your research will extend/contribute to the literature – Provide the justification for your research focus. In what ways, will your research contribute to the knowledge of the research area?

For example, there might be extensive national research into mental health and homelessness, however, your project explores participants locally within Nottingham, etc.

7 Rationale

Drawing on your literature review you should provide the justification for conducting your research, explaining why it is important and use this to help you to refine your research question.

You should explain the originality of your intended research. You should explain how your research builds on and adds to the current state of knowledge in the field or by setting out reasons why it is timely to research your proposed topic.

Case study example – Alice – Developing her Literature review

Upon conducting my literature review, I employed a Funnel Method which began with brainstorming ideas surrounding my topic of mental health. These were largely taken from what I had previously studied and current issues within the media. To gain a broader scope of the topic, I then began looking further afield at trusted mental health sources, for example Mind and Rethink to further narrow down my search. The idea of social media's impacts was continuously mentioned, so I began to use specialist research to formulate my literature review, through the use of books and journal articles and separated these into three categories. I used these to create the categories for my empirical research: Narcissistic Behaviour on Social Networking Sites, Self-worth and Depression through Online Likes, and Self-Image and its Comparison to Celebrities on Social Networking Sites.

Within my first draft of my literature review, I had the least information on Narcissistic Behaviour on Social Networking Sites due to a lack of connecting research in this area, with few studies being recent sources. I believed this would negatively impact my study and expressed my concerns about removing it altogether. However, being able to critique the studies allowed me to make connections between research on social networking and research on narcissism. I was able to use my study to try bridge this gap within the research.

Example of Alice's literature review:

> *Narcissism is defined in the DSM-5 by American Psychiatric Association (2013) as an individual who believes they are of greater value to those around them, are highly arrogant and lacks empathy towards others. Research has used the Goldberg (1990) 'Big Five' personality traits for structuring personality to find that there is a positive correlation between higher levels of narcissistic personality traits with higher usage of SNSs (Ryan and Xenos, 2011; Wang et al. 2012). These are highly accredited authors who have contributed repeatedly to the Journal of Computers in Human Behaviour and research surrounding SNSs and mental health, comparing both studies limits culture bias and progresses towards cultural relativism through the use of Rodgers (1957) Unconditional Positive Regard. Therefore, allowing both cultures within the studies to be viewed as equal.*

> *However, both literature sources acknowledged a lack of psychological theory surrounding narcistic behaviour on SNSs, showing there to be clear gaps within the literature. Andreassen et al. (2017) has tried to bridge this gap, using a funnel approach to apply the previous theoretical framework and add that many exhibit narcissistic personality traits online as SNSs allow for an expression of their aspirations and shows off their success, which the individual receives praise for in the number of likes, comments, or views that they receive. This research shows the speed in which SNSs, and the research surrounding it, have developed over the past few years.*

Research Methodology/Approach (Chapter 2)

Critically appraise the philosophical underpinning of your research design and methods to justify why your chosen research approach is appropriate to answer you research question. An important aspect for this section is the alignment of your study design, data collection approaches, analysis and interpretation. The chapter should initially discuss how you decided on your research approach of quantitative, qualitative, or mixed methods. This section should briefly outline the benefits/limitations of your chosen research approach in relation to your research topic.

   Case study example – Alice – Defining her Research Design

> *The research consisted of online Questionnaires, where participants were given a set of questions through an online software called 'SmartSurvey'. Utilising an online format allowed for participants to respond when it was appropriate for them to do, taking minimal time and boosting engagement (Wright 2005). However, Manfreda et al. (2006) theorised the two main issues with online data collection stemmed from a lack awareness with using the internet and potential for a lack of choice with using an online Likert Scale. Benfield and Szlemko (2006) further investigated this and concluded that a lack of familiarity is one of the most predominant issues surrounding online research, however, within this sample it is imperative that all participants must use SNSs, therefore implying they have a prior knowledge of using SNSs, which limits the issues presented.*

To combat any issues surrounding the format of the questionnaire or using an internet-based website to complete the questions, the questionnaire was given to five individuals within the target population as a pilot test before it was given to participants. This ensured it was completed on a small scale, using around 4% of the number of final participants. These pilot test participants did not take part within the final study and completed the questionnaire to check that even a participant with very little knowledge surrounding the topic could fully comprehend the questionnaire (Hassan, Schattner and Mazza 2006). This allowed for internal validity within the questionnaire, which is further highlighted through the fact that all participants within the study were able to fully complete the questionnaire.

Methods

This is the section where you should provide the detailed description of how the research will be carried out. Within this section, you should describe the research setting, participant recruitment and selection, data collection methods, data analysis and ethical considerations relevant for your research context. You should point out some of the potential challenges that the investigator may face in successfully completing the project and offer possible solutions to these challenges.

The research methods should demonstrate that the design of your project has been considered carefully and that the most appropriate approach has been selected.

A suggested chapter structure is provided in Table 18.4.

Table 18.4 Suggested Chapter Structure (2)

---

1 Briefly identify the focus of the research and the methods employed, e.g., Questionnaires, etc.
2 Provide details of the sampling strategy employed
3 Identify whether the methods you have used are qualitative or quantitative
4 Outline why the chosen methods have been selected? Why were these methods deemed most appropriate? E.g., considering the sensitivity of the research topic in-depth semi-structured interviews were deemed most appropriate as they enable disclosure to take place within a one-on-one interaction.
5 Provide justification for your methods by referencing the literature.
6 Acknowledge any associated limitations of the methods you have selected. Identify how the potential limitations will be overcome. E.g., a suggested limitation of using focus groups to collect data is that more confident participants dominate the discussions. Considering this limitation during the focus group all participants were encouraged to become involved in the discussions, etc.
7 Outline how you analysed your data? E.g., thematic analysis was employed to analyse the interview transcripts etc.
8 Provide details of what this form of analyse involved, e.g., selecting the themes from the data, etc.

   • Support the explanation with the literature

9 Provide justification for your selected method of analysis from the literature
10 Identify the ethical considerations of your research/support with the literature
11 Provide a brief critical reflections section – provide details of what you would improve within your research. E.g., if participants held misunderstandings of the research, you might critically reflect on this and state that on reflection if you had spent an increased amount of time during the research briefing explaining the focus of the research this could have been minimised, etc.

Case study example – Alice – Deciding on methods with consideration of ethical implications

> For my research, I employed an opportunity sample for my participants who were UK residents aged 18-30 who possessed at least one form of social networking. As my study required participants who are active users of social networking sites, I used these sites to recruit my participants. I used a questionnaire of both quantitative and qualitative questions, mainly focusing upon a Likert Scale where participants could rate their experiences based upon this scale. However, it was important to consider potential limitations with my research, as the questionnaire relied mostly upon quantitative data from Likert Scales, a potential limitation would be incomplete questionnaires due to the repetitive nature of the study.

Sample from Alice's ERS dissertation:

> To begin this study, the participant must have access to SNSs to view the advertisement. Next participants must meet an age requirement process, to align with the demographic. It is vital that the participant has some interest within mental health or the influences SNSs, meaning they have a desire to complete the study. Newington and Metcalfe (2014) found this to be one of the key contributing factors which make an individual more likely to want to participate within research. After this point, the questionnaire might be abandoned half-completed due to lack of time or sensitivity to the subject matter, leaving an incomplete set of results or the participant can complete the study. However, no questionnaires were left half-completed, and the target participant sample was exceeded by 59%. This was due to gaining a total of 120 participants, when the study only aimed to gain 50, giving the research a higher external validity as the sample size is larger and no questionnaires were abandoned.

Ethics

> For the ethical considerations of my dissertation, I complied to the ethical guidelines for research, as outlined by the Social Research Association (2003). This best suited my research, as it states participants must be protected through safety guidelines which will allow for high quality research within the social work and health sector.

> In addition to this, it was important that the data collected in my study complied to the GDPR, as it has been identified as a predominant issue surrounding social networking studies. Throughout the study, I maintained transparency with my participants through detailing what would be expected of them and of me as the researcher regarding anonymity and confidentiality.

Sample from Alice's ERS dissertation:

> To create anonymity within the research, participants will be asked to give an identification name, which consists of their first and last initials and the day they

were born. To do so, participants were instructed to combine their first initials of their first name and surname with the day of the month which they were born, therefore creating an identification name that a participant could easily be able to recall or be reminded of when prompted, if they wished exercise their right to withdraw up until a specified point within the research (Edwards 2005). Through the use of anonymous questionnaires, participants are more likely to give honest answers without fear of judgement as the answers will not be traced back to them (Ong and Weiss, 2000). Therefore, this can be applied within this study and allow for the validity to be increased, as answers contain more honesty which will hold a higher accuracy representation of real life.

Research Findings/Results (Chapter 3)

This section (chapter) provides the key findings from your ERS which will be differ depending on the research methodology/approach employed. If the ERS has used a qualitative approach this section may include the participant quotes which are used to support the selection of themes by you as the researcher. Alongside the use of participant quotes, this section if using a qualitative methodology will also include the analysis of the quotes which support the themes of the ERS. On the contrary if your ERS has used a quantitative methodology this chapter will present the detailed relationships between variables via graphs, charts and tables (Punch 2014).

Case study example – Alice identifying findings within my data

> *As I employed a Likert Scale method to examine qualitative date within my study, I was able to compare the dependent variable of the social networking platform upon how it impacted the wellbeing of the user. I was able to divide my results into three conclusions which were derived from my original aims, these were the separation of real life and the online identity, the need for validation to prove self-worth, and narcissistic behaviour through the creation of an online persona. I analysed the results using Microsoft Excel and concluded that 69% of participants changed or only showed certain aspects of their life online. This concluded the indication of narcissistic traits online and built upon original research into the motivations of using SNSs.*

Sample from Alice's ERS dissertation:

> *The four SNSs platforms chosen within this study are amongst the most popular amongst young generations, according to Smith and Anderson (2018). These four SNSs were deliberately chosen as sharing content on these sites allows for a greater potential for more 'followers' to engage, due to the increased users of these SNSs. This enables users to reinforce their ego, through the support they receive in the form of positive comments or 'likes' on their content which fits their online persona where they appear more favourably on SNSs. Therefore, this shows that platforms create a social arena where the users are able to fulfil a narcissistic need for affiliation that aligns with the positive version of themselves which they have created.*

Narcissistic behaviour online has been proven to manifest itself through the conversations surrounding personal achievements or emotions of the individual, due to the familiarity of anecdotes. Tamir and Mitchell (2012) used a categoric system and neuroimaging to place these categories of online content, which presented itself within this study through the creation of an online persona. Participants within this study gave qualitative evidence to determine their online persona, all information that was given was split into categories through thematic analysis, these categories all surrounded the individual and would include content surrounding the pragmatic context of the self. The behaviours shown within this study can be explained through the notion of posting more frequently on SNSs being linked to the nucleus accumbens, relating to the mesolimbic dopamine system showing that a pleasurable gain in mentioning the self-online (Schultz 2002). Consequently, demonstrating that this pleasurable gain serves as a motivator for the individual and drives them to post more content to receive further rewards.

Discussion (Chapter 4)

The findings of your research project need to be related to the academic literature which has been discussed in your literature review chapter. Once you have your findings you need to conduct a subsequent review of the literature. When returning to the literature you need to note whether the literature supports or contrasts with your research findings, in terms of the methods employed, the key findings and the conclusions. This section (chapter) should Identify within the literature any gaps in the knowledge that have been identified by your research.

Case study example – Alice relating my key findings to the academic literature

This research found that 69% of participants changed or only showed certain aspects of their lives to create an online persona on SNSs. Through doing this, participants showed a positive indication of narcissistic traits on SNSs where many enjoy posting content about their achievements or highlighting themselves within a positive light. This indicates that the role of narcissism is positively related to SNS usage, holding a clear presence amongst its users. Therefore, building upon work by Ryan and Xenos (2011) and Wang et al. 2012 where a correlation between higher SNSs usage and narcissistic personality traits were initially originated and Andreassen et al. (2017) which provided these results with reasoning as to personal motivations of why this content is shared.

Conclusion (Chapter 5)

This section is where you draw your research together and provide a final summary of your key findings. This section should also clearly state how you have answered your research objectives/hypothesis which you outlined at the beginning of your ERS. This section should also identify if something needs to change as a result of your research, e.g., policy or practice and make a call for action. Finally, the conclusion is the section to suggest how your research can be expanded on by suggesting areas of future research for a masters or PhD project.

Dissemination of Results

It is important to provide the reader with clear information of your plans for dissemination, in terms of what form of publication will you use to communicate your findings and who will be your audience. This is a key part of your research as now you have your findings you want to ensure key stakeholders hear about your research to support your proposed change and implementations.

References

It is also paramount to provide a reference list following the Harvard conventions or house style suggested by your University, ensure you check this with your dissertation supervisor to prevent being awarded a lower grade because of referencing errors.

Conclusion

This chapter builds on the 'Valuing Research in Health and Social Care chapter' to provide practical advice to develop your research proposal into an ERS with particular attention given to the write-up of the final research study. The use of an undergraduate case study provides useful 'hints and tips' for your own ERS but also provides insights into the decision process and supervisor relationship.

This chapter illustrates the importance of conducting research to positively impact Health and Social Care services and service users, whilst providing practical support from a student perspective to ensure the study you are considering as part of your degree (undergraduate or postgraduate) fills a gap in the existing knowledge.

References

American Psychiatric Association, 2013. *Diagnostic and statistical manual of mental disorders (DSM-5)*. 5th ed. Virginia: American Psychiatric Publishing. DOI: 10.1176/appi.books. 9780890425596 [Accessed 21 March 2022].

Andreassen, C.S., Pallesen, S., and Griffiths, M.D., 2017. The relationship between addictive use of social media, narcissism, and self-esteem: findings from a large national survey. *Journal of Addictive Behaviours*, 64, 287–293.

Balogun, B., Baker, C., Conway, L., Long, R., and Powell, T., 2021. *Obesity* [online]. London: House of Commons Library. Available at: https://researchbriefings.files.parliament.uk/documents/CBP-9049/CBP-9049.pdf. [Accessed 21 March 2022].

Bell, J., and Waters, S., 2018. *Doing your research project: a guide for first-time researchers*. 7th ed. London: Open University Press.

Benfield, J.A., and Szlemko, W.A., 2006. Research design: internet-based data collection: promises and realities. *Journal of Research*, 2 (2), 1–15.

Blease, C.R., 2015. Too many 'friends' and too few 'likes? Evolutionary psychology and 'facebook depression. *Review of General Psychology*, 19 (1), 1–13.

Edwards, S.J., 2005. Research participation and the right to withdraw. *Bioethics*, 19 (2), 112–130.

Goffman, E., 1959. *The presentation of self in everyday life*. New York: Anchor Books.

Goldberg, L.R., 1990. An alternative 'description of personality: The big-five factor structure. *Journal of Personality and Social Psychology*, 59, 1216–1229.

Hassan, Z.A., Schattner, P., and Mazza, D., 2006. Doing a pilot study: why is it essential. *Malaysian Family Physician*, 1 (2–3), 70–73.

Henn, M., Weinstein, M., and Foard, N., 2009. *A critical introduction to social research.* London: Sage Publications.

Kaplan, A.M., and Haenlein, M., 2010. Users of the world, unite! The challenges and opportunities of social media. *Business Horizons*, 53, 59–68.

Manfreda, K.L., Batageli, Z., and Vehovar, V., 2006. Design of web survey questionnaires: three basic experiments. *Journal of Computer Mediated Communication* [online], 7 (2). Available at: https://onlinelibrary.wiley.com/doi/full/10.1111/j.1083-6101.2002.tb00149.x

Marshall, T.C., Lefringhausen, K., and Ferenczi, N., 2015. The Big Five, self-esteem, and narcissism as predictors of the topics people write about in Facebook status updates. Personality and Individual Differences, 85, pp. 35–40.

Newington, L., and Metcalfe, A., 2014. Factors influencing recruitment to research: qualitative study of the experiences and perceptions of research teams. *BMC Medical Research Methodology*, 14 (10).

Ong, A.D., and Weiss, D.J., 2000. The impact of anonymity on responses to sensitive questions. *Journal of Applied Social Psychology*, 30 (8), 1691–1708.

Oxford Dictionaries, 2013. *Selfie* [online]. Oxford: Oxford University Press. Available at: http://oxforddictionaries.com/definition/english/selfie [Accessed 13 February 2019].

Punch, K., 2014. *Introduction to research methods in education.* 2nd ed. London: SAGE Publications.

Punch, K., 2016. *Developing effective research proposals.* 3rd ed. London: SAGE Publications.

Renfrew Centre Foundation, 2014. *Afraid to be your selfie?* [online]. Philadelphia: Renfrew Centre. Available at: http://renfrewcenter.com/news/afraid-be-your-selfie-survey-reveals-most-people-photoshop-their-images [Accessed 6 February 2019].

Ryan, T., and Xenos, S., 2011. Who uses Facebook? An investigation into the relationship between big five, shyness, narcissism, loneliness, and facebook usage. *Computers in Human Behaviour*, 27 (5), 1658–1664.

Schultz, W., 2002. Getting formal with dopamine and reward. *Neuron*, 36 (2), 241–263.

Smith, A., and Anderson, M., 2018. *Social Media Use in 2018* [online]. Washington: PEW Research Centre. Available at: https://www.pewresearch.org/internet/2018/03/01/social-media-use-in-2018/

Tamir, D.I., and Mitchel, J.P., 2012. Disclosing information about the self is intrinsically rewarding. *National Academy of Sciences of the United States of America*, 109 (21), 8038–8043.

Thomas, G., 2017. *Doing research.* 2nd ed. London: Macmillan Education UK.

Wang, J.L., Jackson, D.J., and Zharg, Z.Q., 2012. The relationships among big five personality factors, self-esteem, narcissism, and sensation-seeking to chinese university students, use of social networking. *Computers in Human Behaviour*, 28 (6), 2313–2319.

Wright, K.B., 2005. Researching internet-based populations: advantages and disadvantages of online survey research, online questionnaire authoring software packages and web survey services. *Journal of Computer-Mediated Communication*, 10 (3), 1–16.

19 Conclusion

Adam Barnard and Verusca Calabria

This chapter will:

- Discuss different types of knowledge
- Evaluate the importance of self-knowledge
- Draw the themes of this textbook together
- Reflect on the challenges ahead

Introduction

The journey through the key themes of health and social care has covered much terrain, distance, concepts, contours and themes. This chapter reviews the contribution that the individual chapters make and summarises the key themes that have been developed in each chapter. Having summarised the chapters, this chapter contains speculative ideas for future development in health and social care. The alternative models of health and social care, the values that underpin these models, the challenge of pandemics and the influence on mental health are considered.

This chapter should be read alongside Chapter 1 which sets out where themes are encountered in which chapter. This provides a route map for those who want to navigate a 'thematic reading' and explore in-depth specific issues in health and social care. Health and social care is complex and often mysterious. We hope this book has helped you navigate the terrain of the lived experience of health and social care and create and refine your picture of the highs and lows of health and social care.

This chapter summarises the contributions of each chapter and provides some indicative comments on the future of health and social care and the types of knowledge in health and social care. It also examines 'health and social care in pandemics', 'decolonising the curriculum', mental health, the current socio-economic system, political leadership, ethics and care, and what this means for practitioners and the future. Before, embarking on the speculation of what the future holds, a review of the book's chapters follows.

The knowledge, understanding and learning in this book moves between objective knowledge and subjective knowledge. Objective knowledge is the application of systematic and rigorous methods and methodology to produce knowledge that holds good and is the best yet knowledge we have. This type of knowledge one would hope, informs policy and practice across health and social care in the western world. Subjective knowledge is personal, shared, particular types of knowledge such as knowing what your baby wants, having intuitive understanding of a problem or tacit

DOI: 10.4324/9781003079873-22

form of what we need to do. Regardless of which position we identify we occupy. This book has opened the door to accessing 'objective' and 'subjective' knowledge for the research-minded practitioner.

The importance of self-knowledge is to value yourself in all your complexities and to be a fully functioning individual. To be able to support people in health and social care you need to be able to look after yourself and help yourself. Having a knowledge of self-awareness allows us to understand situations and occurrences from multiple perspectives and vantage points. It frees us from our pre-established assumptions and both conscious and unconscious biases. It helps us build better relationships with fellow professionals, service users and their significant others. It gives us a greater ability to regulate our emotions. Self-knowledge is a broad term which implies the awareness of one's feelings, attributes, motivations and abilities. It is important to note that self-knowledge is not a static type of information to acquire, but rather is as dynamic and constantly changing as you are.

The *first part* of the book laid the foundations for essential knowledge, understanding, skills and values in health and social care in the UK.

The *Foundations in Health & Social Care* brought to light how people's access to health and social care services is influenced by their lifestyle, needs, knowledge and experiences. Community resources support the development of an understanding of factors which influence individual health and well-being.

Human Growth and Development examined development through the life course. A theoretical understanding was developed to examine individual experiences of active, critical, discontinuity, and change in the life cycle.

Current Issues in Health and Social Care explored essential study skills around assisted dying, mandatory childhood vaccinations, and loneliness and isolation.

Working with People explored the complexity of working with service users and staff, for effective communication, examining equality and interpersonal communication in a reflexive way.

Social Policy examined two perspectives on exploring policy implications for health and social care and filmic representation and the role of emotions in learning.

The *second part* of the book extended breadth and depth of discussion for health and social care.

Health, Social Care and Crime proposed definitions, roles and the purpose of police, prosecution, courts, probation and prison service to provide an introduction to the criminal justice system of England and Wales. The chapter concluded by examining the explanation for, and impact of, criminal behaviour and challenging approaches of responding to criminal behaviour.

Person-Centred Interventions discussed the origins, principles and theory underpinning person-centred care and its link to humanistic and existential philosophy. A case study was presented which asked the reader to reflect on the ways in which they can develop their person-centred skills and apply them in a wide range of health and social care roles. These included coaching and guidance roles, professional supervision, negotiation and advocacy and care planning.

Valuing Research in Health and Social Care introduced key research concepts in the field are introduced whilst distinguishing between the producers and consumers within Health and Social Care research.

Managing Health and Social Care focused on the wider context in which health and social care services operate. The first section of this chapter explored how 'good practice' in the management of services can ensure high quality of care even in times of uncertainty. The second section examined specific challenges faced by managers within health and social care in recent years.

The *third part* of the book engaged with the specifics of health and social care.

Young People and Social Care examined service and intervention models were offered to support young people. Overarching frameworks and examples of best practice were offered.

Engaging with Vulnerable Groups explored social construction and structural aspects of vulnerable populations, and how decisions are influenced and made. Safeguarding and personalisation were explored.

Children's and Young People's Mental Health explored mental health conditions which commonly appear in childhood or adolescence and the role of biological, psychological, developmental and social factors in the formation of mental illness. Current policy and practice in the management of mental well-being and a range of therapeutic interventions of young people in the UK were explored.

Ageing in the 21st Century took a questioning stance to explore the experience of getting older and the choices and constraints that older people encounter.

Transcultural Issues examined how understanding factors and issues in transcultural thought, belief, communication, action and practice enables a transnational cultural competence to be developed. The chapter explored the paramount importance of both understanding anti-oppressive views and challenging the interests of social groups who have power. The chapter further explored how certain characteristics of individuals and groups in different positions are used to devalue them.

Leadership in Health and Social Care recommended that in an environment of increasing and more complex need, and decreasing staff levels and funding, the call for inspirational leadership has never been stronger. The chapter developed a critical understanding of traditional and emerging leadership paradigms, explored the challenges of leading integrated health and social care services.

Conducting a Student Empirical Research Study in Health and Social Care explored how to conduct a small-scale empirical research study in a stepped process. The chapter discussed quantitative and qualitative research the building blocks for a research study on social networking sites and mental health.

The next section of this chapter examines contemporary challenges and enablers in health and social care central to professional practice.

Health and Social Care in Pandemics

The unprecedented situation of the outbreak of COVID-19 presented a whole host of new challenges for health and social care, workers, friends and family. The most significant 'event' in writing this book has been the global pandemic and all the associated issues this has presented for individuals, groups, communities and society. There have been significant positives from this event. The way people pulled together through acts of reciprocity during the pandemic, the value of nature, the hope and optimism of people, the positive nature of most people. There have also been negative experiences with a huge number of people who died and limited attendance at funerals to mark and remember those that have died. The pandemic has revealed the stark inequalities endured by minoritised communities in the UK (health.org.uk). Existing inequalities have been shown in sharp relief and continue to endure.

The pandemic business boom has provided opportunities for some such as providers of lateral flow tests but distinct limitations and challenges for others such as losing relatives and loved ones. Political leadership appeared to be in turmoil at the time it was needed most.

For health and social care staff, working together has been a rewarding and joyful experience. Drawing on the strengths and expertise of others, addressing issues collectively and working through material to arrive at successful resolutions has been very satisfying. Using caution and confidence has been the watchword of negotiating through this pandemic. The pandemic has also been incredibly demanding and stressful for health and social care.

The Government leadership was questionable at best, with missed opportunities, poor planning of protective measures, the lack of personal protective equipment (PPE) and a slow response when compared to other countries. Herd mentality and herd immunisation became watchwords that seem reminiscent of farming analogies that dismiss the power of the masses and crowds. Social media and its attendant problems grew in significance feeding partial and misleading information. Partial and vested interests appeared to have benefited from the pandemic. Online retailers, delivery drivers and digital services have all done well.

The shift in values, ethics, people's moral compass and the ability to judge what is right and wrong and act accordingly was interesting to see. Things that had previously been valued (such as the value of work) were downgraded in their significance, and smaller, human things had grown in significance. Protest groups and activism like Black Lives Matter and climate change protests gathered momentum and importance. The prioritisation of well-being, reducing waste, considering resources like water and energy, and greater recycling have all represented a shift in values. The value of nature, music and self-care became priorities. Few people want to return to the ways of working and living pre-pandemic and the promise of a more modest future beckons. The existing inequalities have been given stark relief and thrown into focus. The everyday challenges people face, 'furloughing', the ability to house the homeless, the support and resilience networks that people are able to draw upon have all been prioritised. Those activities that some people used to see as important have shrunk into the background, those activities that are important have come into focus in the foreground. The pandemic has renewed the importance of approaching post-pandemic life encounters with empathy, humility and kindness. The shift in values and attitudes should be a move to openness and transparency, trust and support.

Well-being and people's mental health have received increased scrutiny that moved from a difficult situation pre-pandemic to a crisis situation in the pandemic. The rollout of vaccines has improved the situation and offer the possibility of a return to normal but what might that normal look like. The collateral damage of people and processes that was caused will have a lasting impact across health and social care.

The new normal has brought a range of contemporary anxieties, just as the global pandemic brought an extreme period of uncertainty, we are now experiencing new uncertainties as we transition into a post-pandemic world. Traditional boundaries and power relations will have changed, and it is hoped that increasing participation, democratisation and power-sharing will characterise post-pandemic worlds.

Celebrating diversity and being transparent should lead to greater cooperation and support for all of those involved. Becoming aware of personal, cultural and systemic forms of racism and disadvantage, are being called out and challenged to bring about social justice. Changes bring uncertainty, anxiety and concern. There is a need to address issues early in a meaningful and sustained action plan.

Decolonising the Curriculum

Teaching in health and social care needs to be inclusive, diverse and international. This can challenge the orthodoxy of current teaching and practices based on western knowledge and provide alternative models of understanding and delivery by exploring concepts of history, culture, nationalism, migration, gender and race in the context of post-colonial theories and literature. Examining how communities are imagined and created through a sense of belonging in time and place, interrogating culture and its relationship with individual memories and familial relationships, and how these emerge in powerful narratives of race and history we can develop a critical understanding of colonial and post-colonial constructs such as Orientalism, the global and transnational, the cosmopolitan and the international. This can inform current thinking and practice in health and social care.

Franz Fanon (1963, 1965) in *Black Skin, White Masks* (1967) explored how the colonial ideology of racism was imposed on children at a young age and the traumatic fracture of a dual consciousness for people of colour. Ross (1996) examines the ideology of hygiene applied to a decolonial war situation in Algeria. Mignolo (2003) argues decolonising involves a radical questioning of all epistemological structures which serve to privilege European ways of knowing imposed by the coloniser over the non-European ways of knowing of the colonised. Flexible epistemologies of practice-based applied research have gone some distance in mitigating against the colonial influence of knowledge production.

Academic language in learning and teaching requires us all to be mindful and take action to start to decolonise the curriculum. Three examples, 'get down to the nitty gritty', 'overseer' and 'barbarism' and to resist the symbolic violence in language. Nitty gritty is a derogatory term from slave ships. Getting down to the nitty gritty was when acts of sexual violence and abuse were perpetrated against slave women and so is a racist, violent and derogatory term. The idea of an overseer is to provide oversight and scrutiny on academic work, but the role of an overseer has a heritage as a general manager on slave plantations, so again is racist and derogatory term. Barbarism was a term applied to referencing systems that the 'work demonstrates only occasional barbarism'. External Examiners noted this use of the word. The motivation for using the word came from the *Socialisme ou Barbarism* the group of Postwar French intellectual's journal but was seen as racist in its use.

Health and Social Care struggles with these types of questions. How we teach students and practitioners (Bell 2018, Cesaire 2000) can address some of the vicarious learning where we experience something indirectly through another person. The challenge is that with a value-base that articulates, celebrates and promotes inclusivity, equality and diversity but works within policies, procedures and practices that replicate existing inequalities of power.

Mental Health

The challenges of psycho-social work environments across health and social care give rise to a range of problems such as sickness presenteeism as an expression of a strenuous life situation in total for some individuals, and/or one behavioural strategy among a wider set of stress-related behaviours (Bergström et al. 2009). New forms of solidarity amongst groups, and across different national states have emerged such as Black Lives Matter, and everyday sexism.

Beresford (2016) suggests the weakening and reduction in public services and state spending, prioritised the market and been based on increasingly expecting to pay for services and support, and based on business management models. These have become more divisive pressures rather than unifying people under consumerist ideology. New alliances, new social movements co-creation, participation, and partnership have gone some way to enlarging the notion of care and the communities involved in its provision and consumption of care goods and services.

The Current Socio-economic System

The socio-economic system of 'soft', surveillance, spectacular, zombie and neo-liberal capitalism remains fundamentally unaltered. Surveillance capitalism (Zubboff 2019), zombie capitalism (Harman 2010), spectacular capitalism (Debord 1964), and neo-liberal capitalism (Harvey 1989) have had the effect of revaluing 'care', prioritising market interests and reconfiguring the landscape of health and social care.

'Soft' capitalism (Thrift 1995) is concerned with looser organisational forms which are more able to 'go with the flow' which are now more open to a world which is now figured as complex and ambiguous, and the production of subjects who can fit these forms (Thrift 2005, pp. 32–33). There is a danger that a focus on participation has the illusion of empowerment (the decorated sheds of postmodernism) and leaves the status quo unchallenged and unaffected. Current political organisation appears to have left the 1% unchallenged and focused on the proletariat of 99%. In much the same way as David Harvey (1989) provided a forensic analysis of postmodernism, participation, social work, education and health and social care requires the same analysis. As the mode of production changes to more flexible regimes of accumulation, so the cultural and aesthetic reflection changes. 'If we believe that people in organisations contribute to organisational goals by participating inventively in practices that can never be fully captured by institutional processes then we will minimise prescription, suggesting that too much of it discourages the very inventiveness that makes practices effective' (Wenger 1999, p. 11). Social solidarity provides a counter to individualised and privatised health and social care.

Political Leadership

It is worth reflecting on the context of our leaders. The previous Prime Minister, Boris Johnson, was American born, he is educated at Eton College, and studied classics at Balliol College, Oxford. A central part of the establishment (Jones 2015) and a representative of one nation Toryism. He was political editor for the Telegraph, editor of the Spectator, and published a biography of Winston Churchill comparing him to expensive cheese. The establishment is as irrelevant as it is unjust (Jones 2015, p. 293).

It is contradictory with a growth in destitution amongst many and a concentration of wealth amongst a few. The opportunity for leadership in progressive, democratic and supportive ways is remaining opaque with increasing control and order being brought in under the veneer of health and social care. The Government response has been 'troubled', with a lack of leadership and 'mixed messages' on the best course of action for individuals, groups and communities. Dorling (2018, p. 4) suggests the UK's government is an 'unusually shambolic administration, motivated by 'big money'' with ever-present injustices across housing, education and health'. The need for a critical health and social care is more necessary now than ever as is a levelling of the 'existential threat' of continuing care in health and social care. The impact of the neo-liberal agenda has continuing and long-lasting consequences for women and marginalised groups.

Ethics

Lipsky's (2010) central argument is that street-level problems for social work and nurses lie in the structure, system and organisation of work. The social and cultural contexts can permeate and pervade services which provide assistance, help and support. The impact this has is wider ranging across health and social care and can mitigate against the most progressive social policies. Tronto (1993) presents the key outlines of attentiveness, responsibility, competence and responsiveness as the basis for an ethics of care. Grint (2010) refers to the 'cuckoo clock syndrome' where we repeatedly pattern and configure the world in certain, repeated and fixed ways. Moral panics, service failings and catastrophic errors in system-wide failures are responded to with increasing regulation, standards, checking and performance reviews. Perceptively, Tronto (1993) locates ethics in social and cultural practices not rules. Lipsky (2010, p. vx) calls for a response that would 'secure or restore the human interactions in services that require discretionary intervention or involvement'.

Future solidarities between individuals, groups and organisations and new allegiances and alliances of value-based health and social care offers hope for the future. These require a re-orientation of values; efficiency, prediction, control and impact have given way to human values of 'kindness' and looking after each other. There are new alliances, different ways of working and a more caring attitude. The ethical sensibility is re-oriented away from market-driven mechanisms to be with other people and communities.

The outbreak of a pandemic has caused a significant re-ordering of health and social care services. The stress and strain on stretched services experienced a fatal and critical incident through an unprecedented global health crisis in living memory. The moral panic exacerbated by social media lead to widespread anxiety and concern over health and social care services. Schools, universities and workplaces were on 'lockdown' with remote working, social distancing and increased use of digital media part of the suppression and delay of the spread of the virus. The cultural depiction of series on Netflix of 'Preppers' and 'Zombie Apocalypse' has provided fertile ground for a concern over pandemics. A new etiquette has emerged; the digital practices that we now seem accustomed to have been positively responded to. Change in the world of work and services, flexible working, not having physical locations, remote, distant and blended working have become commonplace. The learning of new information technology systems has been exponential with 'knowledge workers' having to learn how to coordinate meetings, deliver teaching, write research bids on virtual platforms like Zoom, Skype, Skype for Business, MS Teams. This paradoxically has brought the outside inside and people have a more intimate connection with established groups and setting up new groups. Virtual 'meals out' with friends and family plus an Internet interface, pub quizzes hosted remotely, online training, have all reconfigured the way of interacting with individuals, groups and communities. It has been interesting to see the range of diverse living arrangements from virtual meetings to see people's spare rooms, offices and the everyday interruptions. Having to tidy rooms or play with backdrops have all become commonplace.

The hidden costs of the pandemic are still to be revealed. The longer-term consequence of people's health is still to be known and Professor Chris Whitty, the UK Chief medical advisor, referred frequently to the 'indirect costs' of the pandemic during the pandemic's daily briefings from Downing Street. These costs are people not getting the care they need from the NHS as resources are diverted to tackling the front-line of the pandemic, the 'gigantic' backlog of 'routine' treatments, and the 'knock on effects' of treatments not being performed or delivered during the pandemic. Disease and illness have been recast as a perfect storm for mental health and well-being is gathering. Who would have thought that monitoring and keeping and eye on rising death tolls would be a commonplace feature of new reporting? 'Normal' health needs such as heart attacks and strokes sway a marked reduction in people presenting with these symptoms at the NHS during the pandemic outbreak. The full impact of the pandemic could take years to unravel. It is an opportunity to sharpen our skills, protect against despondency and work at resilience. These changes in times have led to significant changes for health and social care.

The pandemic created opportunity to break 'business as usual' and create a whole new set of responses to the challenge created to something more agentic and self-determined. Who would not have desired for time off, more time to do those self-maintaining projects or periods of reflection from a different vantage point. They have also widened and deepened in the breadth and scope how far these relationships reach, but also intensified and deepened, becoming richer and fuller. The amount, range and depth of relationships, whether weak or strong, and new solidarities are developing. New community and actions are taking place such as collective clapping, collective choruses, solidifying solidarities and taking care of communities for greater togetherness. Interestingly, these are beyond politics and political parties, based on a humanism of mutual aid. Relationships although conducted at a distance have taken on an intimacy through video calling for a potential culture of attention. The value and importance of protective, enabling and facilitative relationships for children, adults, vulnerable individuals and groups and health and social care staff has been apparent, particularly in global pandemics. We are becoming more 'response-able' rather than the responsible and enable to find our new obsessions. Energy for mobilising protest and challenging local authorities have been diverted to initiating action, self-organisation, and delivering food, service and social care.

New challenges have emerged, such as advocacy for children and young people to prevent becoming a lost generation. Young people are suffering from detrimental impacts from lower incomes, and access to the labour market educational loss. Mental health, safeguarding, LGBT youth, policing are identified gaps in provision of services for children and young people. Child poverty is an ongoing issue and disproportionately effecting specific groups. Widening educational attainment gaps are disproportionally experienced by different groups, inequalities in home learning environments, access to information technology, negative impact in widening gap. It will take 560 years to level the attainment gap in education (Equality and Human Rights Commission 2020). Adverse experiences can be mitigated by protective factors poverty, discrimination, community disruption, lack of mobility, lack of opportunity, multiple disadvantages, poor housing, violence. This exacerbates inequalities and existing disadvantages for the most at risk. Intergenerational cycle of disadvantage is transmitted for a generation. The shadow pandemic of the effects of pandemics. Diversion of health services to adult care from children's health.

Mutual Aid as a collective working together is part of human development and for human communities to survive. The replacing of competition with co-operation (with a sprinkling of universal love) from a stronger basis for future society. It extends public provision, solidarity and charity to work out collective solutions to human and environmental need against a system that has created these problems. Non-hierarchical, non-bureaucratic, member-led and participatory approaches, against wealth, power and privilege.

The shift in health and social care has led to a 'heightened epistemic reflexivity'. Greater phenomenological understanding focusing on the lived experience of people, more narrative focus hearing the stories of people, grounded theory with less prescriptive protocols and allowing the data to speak, greater understanding of ethnographic accounts of the culture in which people find themselves in, through the systems of power, prestige, privilege and authority of marginalisation groups. The valuing of oral histories as the biographical gathering of personal recollection of events and increased reflexivity (of radical doubt) and reflection (of taking stock) are part of the process with more symmetrical power relations. There is clear evidence of a growth in socially extended and heightened epistemologies, allowing disparate voices to speak and be heard, greater forms of participation from 'care' experienced groups, and changes to policy, services and practice. Greater democracy and horizontal power relationships have started the process of power-sharing. There is a greater focus on practice-based work and the experience of being in receipt of services.

Care

Valuing care and care work does not simply mean attributing care work more monetary value. The political economy of care awaits sustained examination. To really achieve change, we must go so much further. As the world becomes seemingly more uncaring, the calls for people to be more compassionate and empathetic towards one another—in short, to care more—become ever more vocal. The prioritisation of 'being kind' has prompted a move in the right direction. Dowling (2021) in *The Care Crisis* challenges the idea that people ever stopped caring, but also that the deep and multi-faceted crises of our time will be solved by simply (re)instilling the virtues of empathy. There is no easy fix. Dowling (2021) charts the multi-faceted nature of care in the modern world, from the mantras of self-care and what they tell us about our anxieties, to the state of the social care system. She examines the relations of power that play profitability and care off in against one another in a myriad of ways, exposing the devastating impact of financialisation and austerity. *The Care Crisis* enquires into the ways in which the continued offloading of the cost of care onto the shoulders of underpaid and unpaid realms of society, untangling how this offloading combines with commodification, marketisation and financialisation to produce the mess we are living in. *The Care Crisis* charts the current experiments in short-term fixes to the care crisis that are taking place within Britain, with austerity as the backdrop. It maps the economy of abandonment, raising the question: to whom care is afforded? What would it mean to seriously value care? Even the previous Prime Minster states that the response to Covid was driven by capitalism and greed. Care is in crisis in its inability to access care to live well, and magnified inequality.

Restructuring the welfare state and everyday experiences of individual's life is caused by globalisation and finalisation and reproductive deal moving from post-war settlement. Rising care needs, increased exclusions and exploitations, greater female labour market creating domestic 'second shift' from primary paid work to informal care duties, primacy of wage work and wage stagnation, austerity measures and welfare state retrenchment, privatisation and commodification of care, politics of personal responsibility, reducing care provision with rising needs makes for a heady mix.

Dowling (2021) develops a short-term care fix, offloading into the home, devaluing care work, new ideologies of caring to instrumentalise, redrawing the boundaries of care and 'labour of love'. The way of compassion, sense of responsibility, to be kind, is drawn into care provision. This creates a double bind and uses ideologically controlled mechanisms to promote market and technological solutions to care, with an unassailable valuation of 'care'. During the pandemic, the 'clap for heroes' mobilised common-sense ideological constructions of carers as heroes, devaluated nurses as trained professionals doing a paid job framing them as 'caring angels', ignored unpaid carers, and smoothed over the cracks in a care system from an exhaustion care resources.

Social and preventative strategies and social determinants of health needed for a public mental health and a community psychology to ensure a more collective dimension to bio-psycho-social models and different models of how to address peoples' distress. This demands critical engagement with dominant perceptions, narratives and discourses to address the lack of community work in health and social care, local provision of safe spaces and a falling between local authorities and national health services.

For Practitioners

Harvey (1989) stated that capitalism has been transformed from its rigid and centralised post-war form to a flexible (for the capitalists at least) and global form. The need for safe working and an end to gender violence, the promotion of disability and human rights, the challenge to discrimination and oppression, mean we stare at disbelief that these are recurrent themes. This is not a way for women and children to live their lives, Black Lives Matter has reinvigorated the discussion on race and ethnicity and discrimination and oppression that are propagated in contemporary society. We have been here before and upsettingly are still here. There is little evidence that we have moved to a Utopian situation or even a modest resolution for equal rights.

'Clean self-care' has become a toxic mantra in a form of self-care solutionism that carries with it, neo-liberal market solutions, individualised and privatised forms of care. Thus, self-care is not simply privilege and self-indulgence, especially to those who have less social privilege and whose self-esteem is constantly undermined by society. Self-care actually has more radical roots in approaches that seek to protect the welfare of those on whom a disproportionate burden of care is placed, have to care for others or for whom society does not care adequately (Dowling 2021). There are difficult questions for the future discomfort and challenge that people will encounter as we are 'positioned' in power relations.

So, What is the Future?

The very notion of 'care' within health and social care, would benefit from a revision. The infrastructure of the common good and growth in co-production would enable a wider understanding of care. Not located, individualised and privatised but an enlargement of care beyond the family. Progressive taxation and reconfiguring care provision would help. Education holds a force for good and offers the possibility of critical education for critical practice (Brookfield 1991, 1994, 1995, Giroux 2021, 2010, 1992). Giroux (2021) provides some guidance. Education and critical pedagogy are needed now more than ever to combat injustices in our society caused by fake news, toxic masculinity, racism, consumerism and white nationalism. In a UK context British exceptionalism in its various forms pave a way to entrenched privilege rather than a world set on the correct course. Giroux (2021) argues that pedagogy has the power to create narratives of desire, values, identity, and agency at time when these narratives are being manipulated to promote right-wing populism and emerging global fascist politics. The notion of the plague is not only a medical, health and social care crisis but also a crisis of politics, ethics, education, and democracy. Covering a range of topics beginning with historical perspectives on fascism and moving on to issues of social atomisation, depoliticisation, neo-liberal pedagogy, the scourge of staggering inequality, populism, and pandemic pedagogy. Giroux (2021) concludes with a call for educators to make education central to politics, develop a discourse of critique and possibility, reclaim the vision of a radical democracy, and embrace their role as powerful agents of change.

The Health and Social Care Act 2022 awaits full implementation and evaluation but leaves unanswered workforce development and funding. The future of Health and Social Care is pressing, growing need that will continue.

This book has charted the challenges ahead but with vision, application and a critical appreciation of how to provide high-quality, caring, compassionate, kindly and empathic care, individuals and groups are set to make the future.

The second decade of the 21st century saw unprecedented challenges to health and social care. The outbreak of pandemics was the ultimate stress test for people and processes providing care. It called for a revaluing of what is important, what is vital, what is expendable and what factors impede or block 'good health and well-being' and what enables good health. Alternative models of social care should be driven by the values of inclusion, inter-professionalism and internationalisation, professionalism, participation, and partnership. Prevention, community connections, independent lives, choice and control. Our world is increasingly a world of science and technology, the future will depend on the nature of the good life, how we live it, what we aspire to and what resources we have to mobilise, and the implications for ethics and values. They are qualitative and philosophical problems that energise policymakers, politicians, stakeholders, patients and their carers.

References

Bell, D., 2018. A pedagogical response to decoloniality: decolonial atmospheres and rising subjectivity. *American Journal of Community Psychology* [online], 62 (3–4), 250–260. DOI: 10.1002/ajcp.12292

Bergström, G., Lennart Bodin, L., Hagberg, J., Lindh, T., Aronsson, G., and Josephson, M., 2009. Does sickness presenteeism have an impact on future general health? *International Archives of Occupational and Environmental Health* [online], 82 (10), 1179–1190. DOI: 10.1007/s00420-009-0433-6

Beresford, P., 2016. *All Our Welfare: Towards Participatory Social Policy*. Bristol: Policy Press.

Brookfield, S., 1991. On ideology, pillage, language and risk: critical thinking and the tensions of critical practice. *Studies in Continuing Education*, 13 (1), 1–14.

Brookfield, S., 1994. Tales from the dark side: a phenomenography of adult critical reflection. *International Journal of Lifelong Education*, 13 (3), 203–216.

Brookfield, S., 1995. *Becoming a critically reflective teacher*. San Francisco: Jossey-Bass.

Cesaire, A., 2000. *Discourse on colonialism*. New York, NY: Monthly Review Press.

Debord, G., 1964. *Society of the spectacle*. London: Red and Black.

Dorling, D., 2018. *Peak inequality: Britain's ticking timebomb*. Bristol: Policy Press.

Dowling, E., 2021. *The care crisis*. London: Verso.

Equality and Human Rights Commission, 2020. *Risking a lost generation*. London: EHRC.

Fanon, F., 1963. *The wretched of the earth*. New York: Grove.

Fanon, F., 1965. *A dying colonialism*. New York: Monthly Review.

Fanon, F., 1967. *Black skins, white masks*. New York, NY: Grove.

Giroux, H., 2021. *Race, politics and pandemic pedagogy*. London: Bloomsbury.

Giroux, H., 2010. *The mouse that roared*. Lanham, Maryland: Rowman and Littlefield.

Giroux, H., 1992. *Border-crossings: cultural workers and the politics of education*. London: Routledge.

Grint, K., 2010. The cuckoo clock syndrome: addicted to command, allergic to leadership. *European Management Journal* [online], 28 (4), 306–313. DOI: 10.1016/j.emj.2010.05.002

Harman, C., 2010. *Zombie capitalism: global crises and the relevance of Marx*. Chicago: Haymarket Books.

Harvey, D., 1989. *The condition of postmodernity: an enquiry into the origins of cultural change*. Cambridge: Basil Blackwell.

Jones, O., 2015. *The establishment: and how they get away with it*. London: Penguin.

Lipsky, M., 2010. *Street level bureaucracy: dilemmas of the individual in public services*. New York, NY: Russel Sage Foundation.

Mignolo, W., 2003. *The darker side of the renaissance: literacy, territoriality, and colonization*. 2nd ed. Ann Arbor: The University of Michigan Press.

Ross, K., 1996. *Fast care, clean bodies: decolonization and re-ordering of French culture*. Cambridge, Massachusetts: MIT Press.

Thrift, N., 1995. *Soft capitalism*. London: Routledge.

Thrift, N., 2005. *Knowing capitalism*. London: Routledge.

Tronto, J.C., 1993. *Moral boundaries: a political argument for an ethics of care*. New York, NY: Routledge.

Wenger, E., 1999. *Communities of practice: learning, meaning and identity*. Cambridge: Cambridge University Press.

Zubboff, S., 2019. *The age of surveillance capitalism: the fight for a human future at the new frontiers of power*. London: Profile Books.

20 Glossary

*Adam Barnard, Verusca Calabria, and
Louise Griffiths*

This chapter is a collection of annotated key terms that will aid your understanding in your health and social care journey. They are an amalgam of research terms, key concepts, legislation and key concept in health and social care.

A priori A term indicating an idea is derived from theory rather than practice.

Able-bodiedism the assumption that the bodily characteristics of non-disabled people are superior to those of disabled people, who should accept an inferior status as a result' (Pierson and Thompson 2010: 1).

Acceptance Perceiving and dealing with users as they really are, including strengths and weaknesses and retaining dignity and worth of individuals.

Accountability where social workers give an explanation and justification of their actions to somebody else who might reasonably expect to be given such an explanation' (Shardlow 1995: 67).

Accretion measure A type of unobtrusive measure that arises from the deposit of material (e.g. graffiti or litter) that can be analysed as having a significance (Gray 2004).

Action research Research that involves close collaboration between researchers and practitioners, and which usually aims to achieve measurable, practical benefits for the company, organisation or community (Gray 2004).

Advocacy speaking up of being helped to speak up'. In health and social care advocacy involves making sure the views and wishes of service users are heard and understood' (Pierson and Thompson 2010: 20).

Analysis of variance (ANOVA) A statistical test used to determine whether there are differences between two or amongst three or more groups on one or more variables. ANOVA is determined using the F-test.

Analytical survey A survey design that uses a quasi-experimental approach that attempts to measure the impact of independent variables on dependent variables, while controlling for extraneous variables.

Anonymity An assurance that data will not be traceable to participants in a research project.

Areas of acceptance or rejection For a one-tailed hypothesis test, the area of rejection is either the upper or lower tail of the distribution. For a two-tailed test both tails are used. (not in text).

Arnstein's ladder a way of mapping out the different degrees of participation by local residents and users in the services or community projects that affect them' (Pierson and Thompson 2010: 34).

Association The tendency of two events to occur together. When applied to variables it is more usual to refer to this as a correlation.

Audit trail The presentation of material gathered within a naturalistic enquiry that allows other researchers to trace the original researcher's analysis and conclusions.

Autobiography The form of biographical writing is the narrative account of a person's life that he or she has personally written or otherwise recorded (Cresswell 2007: 233).

Axial coding A type of coding that treats a category as an axis around which the researcher delineates relationships and specifies the dimensions of the category.

Axiological What is the role of values?' (Cresswell 2007: 17).

Bauman, Zygmunt (1025–2017) Contemporary writer on postmodern ethics.

Bentham, Jeremy (1748–1832) British philosopher who argued for the Principle of Utility by which he meant that an action should be judged according to the results it achieved. Founder of Utilitarianism.

Bereavement and grief the loss of a close relative or friend and the feelings associated with such loss' (Pierson and Thompson 2010: 52).

Bias In general, any influence that distorts the results of a study. In statistics, a case of systematic error in a statistical result. Unconscious bias is the assumptions and unacknowledged influence that people exert.

Care Quality Commission the regulatory agency for health and adult social care in the UK' (Pierson and Thompson 2010: 64).

Case study A research design focusing on one person or sample. Case studies provide limited information on a single issue, person or organisation. There are dangers in generalising from such limited samples, but results may be indicative of trends.

Categorical data Data that include both nominal and ordinal data.

Cell Area containing values in a table of data.

Census The measurement of a complete population rather than a sample – particularly useful when researching organizations.

Chi-square distribution Statistical test used with nominal data to determine if patterns or characteristics are common across populations.

Chi-square test How well observed data fit an expected or theoretical distribution.

Chronology This is a common approach for undertaking a narrative form of writing in which the author presents the life in stages or steps according to the age of the individual (Cresswell 2007: 233).

Closed question A question where the possible answers are predetermined.

Cluster sampling A sampling strategy involving successive sampling of units or clusters, progressing from larger units to smaller ones.

Clusters of meanings This is the third step in phenomenological data analysis, in which the researcher clusters the statements into themes of meaning units, removing overlapping and repetitive statements (Cresswell 2007: 235).

Coding The process of transforming raw data into a standardized format for data analysis. In quantitative research this means attaching numerical values to categories; in qualitative research it means identifying recurrent words, concepts or themes.

Coding frame A template of key coding instructions for each variable in a study (e.g. Agree = 1).

Confidence interval   This identifies a range of values that includes the true population value of a particular characteristic at a specified probability level (usually 95 per cent).

Confidentiality   a system of rules and norms applied to information given by clients to social workers: it is expected that social workers will not divulge this information to others except in certain specified circumstances' (Shardlow 1995: 67).

Confounding variable   A variable, other than the variable(s) under investigation, which may distort the results of experimental research, and so has to be controlled for.

Consequentialism   The theory or perspective that is interested in the outcomes, consequences, results or effects of action.

Constant comparison method   A method of qualitative analysis that generates successively more abstract concepts and theories through the inductive process of comparing data with data, data with categories, categories with categories and categories with concepts.

Construct or Construction   The particular way in which an individual expresses meaning about a concept.

Construct validity   The extent to which an instrument measures a theoretical concept (construct) under investigation.

Constructivism   A perspective that assumes that people construct the realities in which they participate.

Content analysis   The examination of qualitative data by either qualitative or quantitative methods by systematically identifying special characteristics (classes or categories).

Content validity   An estimate of the extent to which a research tool takes items from the subject domain being addressed, including not only cognitive topics but also behaviours.

Contingency table   A display of frequencies for two or more variables.

Control group   As part of an experimental design, a group not given the intervention so that the effects of the intervention on the experimental group can be compared with it.

Convenience sampling   A non-probability sampling strategy that uses the most conveniently accessible people to participate in the study.

Conversational analysis   The formal analysis of everyday conversations, often based upon transcribed tape recordings.

Co-production   A slippery concept, that can be too broad, too narrow or indistinct. A project or intervention that involves stakeholders in a meaningful way and produces positive outcomes for those involved in the project. Organisations, communities, individuals and groups should have shared and agreed agendas and principles that guide the research, service or intervention (SCIE https://www.scie.org.uk/publications/guides/guide51/what-is-coproduction/).

Core category   The central category that is used in grounded theory to integrate all the categories identified.

Correlation   The extent of an association between and among interdependent variables such that when one variable changes, so does the other. Variables that are independent are not correlated.

Correlation coefficient (r)   A measure of the linear relationship between two numerical values made on the same set of variables. It ranges from –1 (a perfectly negative relationship) to +1 (a perfectly positive relationship), with 0 meaning no relationship. Linear relationships can be measured by Pearson's product moment correlation; changes in one variable causing changes in another in a fixed direction can be measured by Kendall's coefficient of rank correlation or Spearman's rank correlation coefficient.

Covert participant Someone who participates in the activities of a research study without revealing his or her identity as a researcher.

Credibility Seen by some supporters of qualitative approaches as more important than validity or reliability. Established through building confidence in the accuracy of data gathering and interpretation.

Criterion-related validity Assessed through comparing the scores on an instrument with one or more external criteria such as a well-established existing test.

Critical inquiry A process which questions currently held values and challenges conventional social structures.

Cross-sectional study A study in which data are collected at one time only, usually for a large number of cases.

Data Findings and results which, if meaningful, become information.

Data saturation The point at which data collection can cease, because data have become repetitive with the emergence of no new themes or ideas.

Deduction Drawing logical conclusions through the process of reasoning, working from the general to the specific.

Deductive approach Experimental approach that uses a priori questions or hypotheses that the research will test.

Degrees of freedom (df) The number of components in results that are free to vary. Measured by the number of categories minus 1.

Dementia a progressive and irreversible decline in intellectual abilities, usually of gradual onset, affecting all areas of the brain' (Pierson and Thompson 2010: 158).

Deontology Ethical philosophy concerned with questions of duty.

Dependent variable A variable that forms the focus of research, and depends on another (the independent or explanatory) variable.

Descriptive statistics Statistical methods used to describe data collected from a specific sample (e.g. mean, mode, median, range, standard deviation).

Design An approach to the collection of data that combines a validity of results with an economy of effort. Includes decisions on the case site, sample, data collection and analysis.

Deviation The difference between the value of a variable and the mean of its distribution.

Discourse analysis The study of how both spoken and written language is used in social contexts.

Emic Specific language or cultural distinctions, meaningful to a cultural group (as opposed to etic, ideas meaningful to researchers). An insider's view of reality.

Empirical Research methods in which data are collected.

Empirical data The results of experiments or observations used to check the validity of assertions.

Empowerment More than just 'enabling', it is a commitment to challenging and combating injustice and oppression shown in action and words with a focus on consultation, participation and information.

Epiphanies   These are special events in an individual's life that represent turning points. They vary in their impact from minor epiphanies to major epiphanies and they may be positive or negative (Cresswell 2007: 234).

Episodic records   Archival records that are insufficiently complete to allow for the identification of trends.

Epistemology   A branch of philosophy that considers the criteria for determining what constitutes and what does not constitute valid knowledge. 'What is the relationship between the research and what is being researched?' (Cresswell 2007: 17).

Epoche or bracketing   This is the first step in 'phenomenological reduction' the process of data analysis which the researcher sets side, as far as humanly possible, all preconceived experiences to best understand the experiences of participants in the study.

Essentialism   Is the tendency to treat fluid, changing processes as if they were fixed entities incapable of change. For example, an essentialist view of self-hood would see identity as a fixed and unchangeable rather than as a developing process. Anti postmodern ideas.

Ethics   The study of standards of conduct and values, and in research, how these impact both the researcher and research subjects. Ethics are coherent bodies of ideas that deal with morals (distinguishing between right and wrong). Ethics is concerned with the systematic study of ethical principles that can form 'schools' or traditions, e.g. Marxism.

Ethnography   A qualitative approach that seeks out the perspectives about the culture of individuals, groups or systems occurring in settings or 'fields'. Originally associated with anthropology and sociology (Gray 2009: 683).

Ethnomethodology   A research tradition that argues that people continually redefine themselves through their interactions with others.

Etic   Ideas meaningful to researchers (as opposed to emic, language and cultural distinctions meaningful to a cultural group). An outsider's view of reality.

Evaluation   The systematic collection of data about the characteristics of a programme, product, policy or service. Often performed to identify opportunities for change and improvement.

Expected frequencies   Frequencies that are observed in a contingency table if the null hypothesis is true.

Experimental group   In experimental research, the group of subjects who receive the experimental treatment, in contrast to the control group who do not.

Experimental research   A research methodology based upon cause-and-effect relationships between independent and dependent variables by means of the manipulation of independent variables, control and randomization.

External validity   The extent to which research results can be generalized to the population as a whole.

Extraneous variable   A variable that needs to be controlled for because it has the potential to adversely affect the results of a study.

Face validity   The extent to which a measuring instrument appears to be measuring what it claims to measure.

Field notes   Notes written when conducting interviews or observations in the field. They may include the researcher's personal comments or interpretations.

Fieldwork   The gathering of data at a research site.

Filter question A question designed to exclude some respondents or direct them to later questions in a questionnaire.

Fisher's exact test Used to test the null hypothesis that nominal characteristics are not associated. Usually used when the sample size is too small for the chi-square test.

Focus group A group interview, usually framed around one issue.

Foucault, Michel (1924–1984) Twentieth-century philosopher concerned with webs or matrices of power and knowledge in discourses of language and practices

Frequency count Calculation of frequencies to determine how many items fit into a category (e.g. number of sales per product, members of a team, men and women in the workforce).

Gatekeepers Individuals who have the power or influence to grant or refuse access to a field or research setting.

Generalisability The extent to which the results of a study based upon evidence drawn from a sample can be applied to a population as a whole. Often referred to as external validity.

Goodness-of-fit How well a given set of data fit a distribution. It may be measured by the chi-square statistic.

Grounded theory An inductive approach to the analysis of qualitative data involving open, axial and selective coding.

Health a state of complete physical, mental and social well-being and not merely the absence of disease or infirmity. Health is a resource for everyday life, not the objective of living. Health is a positive concept emphasizing social and personal resources, as well as physical capacities' (World Health Organisation).

Hedonism The theory or perspective that makes happiness the goal of life.

Hermeneutics An approach based on the interpretation of literary texts and human behaviour.

Hermeneutic phenomenology A form of phenomenology in which research is orientated towards interpreting the 'texts' of life (Hermeneutical) and lived experience (phenomenological) (Cresswell 2007: 235).

Heuristic inquiry A process of open-ended inquiry that begins with a question that is usually focused on an issue that has posed a personal problem for the researcher.

Horizontalisation This is the second step in the phenomenological data analysis, in which the researchers lists every significant statement relevant to the topic and gives it equal value.

Hypothesis A statement that should be capable of measurement about the relation between two or more variables. Testing hypotheses, and especially the null hypothesis, is part of inferential statistics.

Ideographic An approach that emphasizes that explanation of human behaviour is only possible through gaining access to participants' subjective interpretations or culture.

Independent variable Used to explain or predict a result or outcome on the dependent variable.

Induction The development of theory or inferences from observed or empirical reality. It is associated with naturalism and the 'grounded theory' approach to theory formation. It is the opposite of deduction.

Inductive approach The establishment of facts on which theories or concepts are later built, moving from specifics to generalizations.

Inference An assertion made on the basis of something else observed.

Inferential statistics Used to draw inferences from a sample being studied to a larger population that the sample is drawn from.

Informed consent The obtaining of voluntary participation in a research project based on a full understanding of the likely benefits and risks.

Instrument A tool such as a questionnaire, survey or observation schedule used to gather data as part of a research project.

Inter-judge reliability The extent to which two or more observers agree on what they have seen.

Internal validity The extent to which changes in the dependent variable can be attributed to the independent variable, rather than to an extraneous variable.

Interpretivism Interpretations of the world are culturally derived and historically situated. Interpretivist approaches include symbolic interactionism, phenomenology, hermeneutics and naturalistic inquiry.

Intersectionality The interconnected relationship of social divisions such as class, gender, 'race' and ethnicity, disability, geography and interdependent overlapping discrimination, oppression, advantage and disadvantage experienced by individuals and groups.

Interval scale A quantifiable, continuous scale that has an arbitrary zero point (e.g., the Fahrenheit and Celsius temperature scales). Unlike ratio scales (where a score of 120 represents a figure twice as large as a score of 60), an IQ score of 120 (interval data) is not twice as large as one of 60.

Intervening variable A hypothetical internal state that is used to explain relationships between observed variables.

Kant, Immanuel (1724–1804) Eighteenth-century German Protestant philosopher who was concerned with questions of duty.

Leading question A question that suggests a possible answer, and hence promotes bias.

Likert scale A scale in which items represent different sub-concepts of the measured object and responses are presented to indicate different degrees of agreement or disagreement with the item.

Linearity An assumption that the relationship between variables is linear.

Literature review The selection of documents (published and unpublished) on a topic, that contain information, ideas and evidence, and the evaluation of these documents in relation to a particular piece of research.

Lived experience This term is used in phenomenological studies to emphasise the importance of individual experiences or people as conscious human beings (Cresswell 2007: 236).

Longitudinal study A research study that examines phenomena over a relatively long period of time.

Lyotard, Jean-François (1924–1996) Twentieth-century French philosopher who suggests we no longer believe 'grand narratives' and are involved in language games.

Manipulation Intentionally changing the value of an independent variable.

Mann-Whitney U test See Wilcoxon signed-rank test.

Maturation A threat to internal validity caused by changes in the value of the dependent variable that occurs without any intervention by the researcher.

Mean The arithmetic average of observations. A measure of central tendency for interval or ratio data.

Measure of central tendency Used in descriptive statistics, comprising measures of the mean, median and mode.

Measures of dispersion Descriptive statistics that describe the spread of numerical data. They include measures of the range, standard deviation and percentiles.

Median A measure of central tendency where 50 per cent of observations are above it and 50 per cent below.

Method The systematic approach towards the collection of data so that information can be obtained.

Methodology or methodological The analysis of, and the broad philosophical and theoretical justification for, a particular method used in research, for example, action research. 'What is the process of research?' (Creswell 2007: 17).

Mill, John Stuart (1806–1873) Nineteenth-century British liberal philosopher who advocated Utilitarianism and distinguished between higher and lower pleasures.

Mixed methods Refers to an emergent methodology of research that advances the systematic integration, or 'mixing', of quantitative and qualitative data within a single investigation or sustained program of inquiry.

Mode A measure of central tendency comprising the value of the observation that occurs most frequently.

Mortality A threat to the validity of the research caused by subjects prematurely withdrawing from the study.

Narrative research This is an approach to qualitative research that is both a product and a method. It is a study of stories or narrative or descriptions of a series of events that accounts for human experience (Creswell 2007: 234).

Narratives The use of oral or life histories to capture personal lived experiences.

Naturalistic paradigm A paradigm that assumes that there are multiple interpretations of reality and that the goal of researchers is to work with people to understand how they construct their own reality within a social context.

Nietzsche, Fredrich (1844–1889) Nineteenth-century German philosopher who proclaims, 'God is Dead' and that the world is without fixed values or standards. We need to create our own ethics.

Nominal scale Describes characteristics that have no numerical value (e.g. the name of organizations, products, departments, etc.). Sometimes referred to as a categorical scale.

Nomothetic Approaches that seek to construct a deductively tested set of general theories that explain and predict human behaviour. It is the opposite of ideographic.

Non-judgementalism Not judging a person but evaluative judgements of behaviour characterised by open-mindedness and not assigning guilt or innocence.

Non-parametric tests Tests that do not make any assumption that the population is normally distributed (sometimes called distribution-free tests). These include all tests involving the ranking of data, including Kendall's rank correlation and Spearman's rho.

Non-probability sampling   Techniques used to draw a sample in such a way that the findings will require judgement and interpretation before being applied to a population. Often necessary in practice.

Non-stereotyping   Not giving negative attributes to individuals or groups, working without preconceptions and not forming mental representations of groups and individuals.

Normal distribution   Based on the assumption that the distribution of a population will be a smooth, bell-shaped curve that is symmetric around the mean and where the mean, median and mode are equal. Symbolized by the Greek letter mu (m).

Null hypothesis (H0)   A statement of the relationship between two variables which argues that no difference exists in the means, scores or other numerical values obtained for the two groups. These differences are statistically significant when the null hypothesis is rejected – suggesting that a difference does, in fact, exist.

Observed frequencies   Frequency scores actually obtained through research – in contrast to expected frequencies (see above).

One-sample t-test   See paired t-test.

One-tailed test   The area of a normal distribution curve showing the region of rejection for the null hypothesis where the direction predicted by the hypothesis is known.

One-way ANOVA   Used to test for differences for studies with one dependent variable with ratio or interval data. This test uses the F-statistic.

Ontology   The study of the essence of phenomena and the nature of their existence. 'What is the nature of reality' (Cresswell 2007: 17).

Open question   A question without fixed categories of answers.

Operational definition   A concise statement that assigns meaning to a construct or variable by specifying the activities necessary to measure it.

Oral history   is the recording of people's memories and past life experiences in the form of an audio or video recording.

Ordinal scale   An ordering or ranking of values with no implication that the differences between the values are equal. Examples include: Strongly agree, Agree, Disagree and Strongly disagree; Frequently, Often, Sometimes, Never.

Outliers   An observation that is numerically distant from the rest of the data.

Paired sample   Two samples in which each member is paired with a member in the other sample (e.g. comparing the output of two groups of assembly-line workers). The paired t-test is used to measure whether any differences on the random variable (e.g. output) are significant.

Paired t-test or a one-sample t-test   Compares the difference or changes in ratio or interval variables that is observed for two paired or matched groups. It can also be used for before and after measures on the same group.

Paradigm   A perspective or world view based upon sets of values and philosophical assumptions, from which distinctive conceptualizations and explanations of phenomena are proposed. Basic belief system based on ontological, epistemological and methodological assumptions.

Parameter   A limit or boundary which defines the scope of a particular process or activity.

Parametric test   Tests that assume that the data for a population are normally distributed. Examples include t-tests and the F-test. To be used for interval and ratio numerical data, but not ordinal data.

Participant observation Qualitative research, when a researcher both collects data and becomes involved in the site of the study.

Participatory action research A research tradition in which people themselves act as participants to investigate their own reality.

Pearson product-moment A statistical formula for calculating the correlation coefficient between two variables. Assumes that both variables are interval and that the relationship between them is linear.

Percentile A number that indicates the percentage of a distribution that is above or below that number. A statement that a person scored on the 75th percentile indicates that 75 per cent of the others scored the same or below this. (not in text)

Phenomenology The search for how participants experience and give meaning to an event, concept or phenomenon.

Pilot survey A small-scale survey carried out before a large-scale one to evaluate processes and research tools such as questionnaires.

Plausibility An assessment of whether any truth claim is likely to be true, given the present state of knowledge. Associated with postmodern critiques.

Population The totality of people, organizations, objects or occurrences from which a sample is drawn.

Positivism A philosophical assumption that the purpose of theory is application, that the truth can be distinguished from untruth, and that the truth can be determined by either deduction or by empirical support.

Postal survey A survey in which survey instruments such as questionnaires are distributed by post.

Postmodernism A movement, from the liberal arts, that is characterized by relativism, juxtaposition, pastiche and cut up elements. The artistic work of Cindy Sherman is emblematic of postmodern aesthetics. A set of theories that argue that objective truth is unobtainable. All we have is 'truth claims' that are partial, partisan and incomplete.

Post-positivist Sometimes referred to as anti-positivist, a research tradition that rejects the belief that human behaviour can be investigated through the use of the methods of scientific inquiry.

Post-test A test that occurs after a treatment has been administered in an experimental study.

Predictive validity The extent to which scores on an instrument can predict a subject's future behaviour in relation to the test's content (e.g. do scores on an engineering aptitude test predict the ability to perform engineering tasks?)

Pre-test A test that occurs before a treatment has been administered in an experimental study.

Probability sampling Techniques used to ensure that a sample is representative of the population, so that findings can be generalized to that population.

Probe An interviewing technique in which the interviewer seeks clarification and elaboration of a respondent's answers. Can also mean to thoroughly investigate and analyse deeper.

Progressive-regressive method This is an approach to writing a narrative in which the researcher begins with a key event in the subject's life and then works forward and backwards from that event (Cresswell 2007: 234).

Proposition A formal statement that relates two or more concepts.

Purposive sampling   A non-probability sampling strategy in which participants are selected on the basis that they are considered to be typical of a wider population.

p-value   The probability value that helps to determine the significance of a statistical test. A small p-value (typically ≤ 0.05) indicates strong evidence against the null hypothesis.

Qualitative methods   Techniques by which qualitative data are collected and analysed.

Quantitative methods   The systematic and mathematical techniques used to collect and analyse quantitative data.

Quasi-experimental design   Approach using elements of experimental design such as the use of a control group, but without the ability to randomly select the sample.

Quota sampling   A non-probability sampling strategy in which various strata are identified by the researcher who ensures that these strata are proportionately represented within the sample to improve its representativeness.

Random probability sampling   The method of drawing a proportion of a population such that all possible samples have the same probability of being selected.

Range   The difference between the largest observation and the smallest in a sample of a set of variables. Can also mean a set of different things within a similar type for example a range of settings.

Rank   The position of a member of a set in an order.

Ratio scales   A measurement in which equal differences between points correspond to equal differences on the scale. Used for characteristics where there is an absolute zero point that does have some meaning, that is, an absence of the construct being measured (in contrast to interval scales where the zero is arbitrary) – for example, zero length on a ruler.

Reactivity   The potential for the behaviour of research subjects to change due to the presence of the researcher.

Realism   A research philosophy that presumes that a knowable, objective reality exists.

Reflexivity   The monitoring by a researcher of her or his impact on the research situation being investigated. A stance associated with postmodernism and anti-realism.

Relativism   The idea that there are no objective standards of ethics, truth or knowledge.

Reliability   The degree to which an instrument will produce similar results at a different period.

Representative sample   A sample in which individuals are included in proportion to the number of those in the population who are like them.

Research design   A strategic plan for a research project, setting out the broad structures and features of the research.

Research methodology   Approaches to systematic inquiry developed within a particular paradigm with associated epistemological assumptions (e.g. experimental research, survey research, grounded theory, action research).

Research question   A specific formulation of the issues that a research project will address, often describing general relationships between and among variables that are to be tested.

Restorying   This is an approach in narrative analysis in which the researchers retell the stories of individual experience, and the new story typically has a beginning, middle and ending (Cresswell 2007: 234).

Rhetoric What is the language of the research?' (Cresswell 2007: 17).

r-square The square of the correlation between the response values and the predicted response values.

Sample A set of objects, occurrences or individuals selected from a parent population for a research study.

Sampling error The fluctuations in the value of a statistic from different samples drawn from the same population.

Sampling frame A complete list of the people or entities in the entire population to be addressed by a research study, from which a random sample will be drawn. (not in text)

Secondary data analysis A reworking of data that have already been analysed to present interpretations, conclusions or knowledge additional to, or different from, those originally presented.

Significance level The probability of rejecting a true null hypothesis. This should be chosen before a test is performed and is called the alpha value (a). Alpha values are usually kept small (0.05, 0.01 or 0.001), because it is important not to reject the null hypothesis when it is true (a Type I error), that is, there is no difference between the means of the groups being measured.

Skewed distribution An asymmetrical distribution, positively skewed meaning the larger frequencies being concentrated towards the lower end of the variable, and negatively skewed, towards the higher end. (not in text)

Snowball sampling A non-probability sampling strategy through which the first group of participants is used to nominate the next cohort of participants.

Spearman's rank-order Used to describe the relationship between two ordinal correlation (Spearman's) characteristics or one ordinal and one ratio/interval (rho) characteristic. Represented by the symbol rs.

Standard deviation A measure of the spread of data about the mean (average), symbolized by the Greek letter sigma (s), or the square root of the variance.

Standard distribution The distribution that occurs when a normal random variable has a mean of zero and a standard deviation of one.

Statistical inference A procedure using the laws of probability to generalize the findings from a sample to an entire population from which the sample was drawn.

Statistical significance See Significance level.

Statistical validity The extent to which a study has made use of the appropriate design and statistical methods.

Stratified random sampling Drawing a sample from a specified stratum – for example, from a company's rural, out-of-town and town centre stores.

Subject error A measure of the scores achieved on a test that is taken at two different time periods.

Subjects A term most frequently used in positivist research to describe those who participate in a research study.

Survey An investigation into one or more variables in a population that may involve the collection of both qualitative and quantitative data.

Symbolic interactionism A school of sociology in which people are seen as developing a sense of identity through their interactions and communication with others.

t-test A test used on the means of small samples to measure whether the samples have both been drawn from the same parent population.

Teleology   The tendency to ascribe purpose and intentionality to a phenomenon inappropriately. For example, to argue that the 'purpose' of unemployment is to discipline the workforce (to make sure they 'tow the lines') is to fall foul of teleology. This argument implies that unemployment is deliberately designed for a particular purpose. It, therefore, confuses a historical outcome or effect (the existence of unemployment) with an assumed cause ('they' made it that way).

Theoretical sampling   The selection of participants within a naturalistic inquiry, based on emerging findings during the progress of the study to ensure that key variables are adequately represented.

Theoretical sensitivity   Often used in grounded theory, involves maintaining an awareness of the subtleties of meaning in data.

Thick description   A detailed account of life 'inside' a field of study. Associated with humanistic ethnography but rejected by postmodern ethnography as just selective or partial descriptions.

Time sampling   An observational method in which data are collected at periodic intervals.

Time series   A set of measures on a single variable collected over time.

Traces   An unobtrusive measure in which physical evidence is collected to provide evidence about social behaviour.

Triangulation   The use of a variety of methods or data sources to examine a specific phenomenon either simultaneously or sequentially in order to improve the reliability of data.

Two-tailed test   The two areas of a normal distribution curve showing the regions of rejection for the null hypothesis where the direction predicted by the hypothesis is not known (hence the need for two tails).

Type I error   An error that occurs when the null hypothesis is rejected when it is true and a researcher concludes that a statistically significant relationship exists when it does not.

Type II error   An error that occurs when the null hypothesis is accepted when it is false and a researcher concludes that no significant relationship exists when it does. (not in text)

Unit of analysis   The set of objects (individuals, organisations or events) on which the research is focused.

Unobtrusive measures   A non-reactive method of data collection using sources such as archives, documents or the Web.

Utilitarianism   The ethical philosophy that argues actions are right in proportion to how much they promote happiness.

Validity   The degree to which data in a research study are accurate and credible.

Values   The things we attach value to, for example principles or ethics. Values are often to be fund in formal 'set of values', such as religious or political values. However, we also have personal values that are broader than organized and systematic ethical beliefs. They are more personal in nature, include moral worth and value, and what we choose to see as ethically relevant or worthy. Values are 'a set of fundamental moral/ethical principles to which social workers are/should be committed' (Banks 1995: 4).

Variable   A characteristic that is measurable, such as income, attitude, colour, etc.

Variance   The differences measured in repeated trials of a procedure. The standard deviation squared – a measure of dispersion.

Verification Drawing the implications from a set of empirical conclusions to theory.

Wellbeing World Health Organisation (WHO) defines health as 'a state of complete physical, mental and social wellbeing and not merely the absence of disease or infirmity' (WHO, 1948) .... 'Wellbeing' refers to a positive rather than neutral state, framing health as a positive aspiration. Mental health wellbeing, stay connected, stay physical active, learn new skills,b give to others, pay attention to the present moment (mindfulness) (NHS https://www.nhs.uk/conditions/stress-anxiety-depression/improve-mental-wellbeing/) WHO (World Health Organisation).

Wilcoxon signed-rank test A non-parametric test for comparing ordinal data from two dependent samples or interval/ratio data that is not normally distributed.

Health and Social Care Timeline

Adam Barnard, Verusca Calabria, Louise Griffiths, and Bailey Foster

Table 21.1 Time Line in Health and Social Care

Date	Health	Social care	Political administrations	Key concepts
1834	Poor Law			
1853	Vaccination Act			
			Sir Winston Churchill, Conservative, 1951–1955	
1913	Mental Deficiency Act			
1933		Children and Young Persons Act Person posing a risk to children, Schedule 1 Offender.		
1946	National Insurance Act National Health Services Act			
1948	The National Health Service launched 'the greatest gift a national can ever give itself'.	National Assistance Act set out the basis for an insurance-based system for health services and unemployment support. The Act established the framework for the establishment of the welfare state, which separated local responsibilities for welfare from national responsibility for social security. This created the National Health Service (NHS), as well as social care	Sir Anthony Eden, Conservative, 1955–1957	Post-war Settlement

(*Continued*)

Table 21.1 (Continued)

Date	Health	Social care	Political administrations	Key concepts
1958		Mental Health Act aimed to establish community-based services for people with mental health needs and to close down long-stay hospital provision	Harold Macmillan Conservative 1957–1963	
1961	Suicide Act			
1967	Abortion Act		Sir Alec Douglas-Home, Conservative, 1963–1964	
1968	**Health Services and Public Health**	Publication of Seebohm report, Local Authority and Allied Personal Social Services, which recommended the establishment of a family service and 'one door to knock upon'.	Harold Wilson Labour 1964–1970 **Theft Act 1968**	
1969	**Divorce Reform Act**			
1970		Local Authority and Social Services Act addressed the establishment of integrated local authority personal social services departments in England **Equal Pay Act**	Edward Heath Conservative 1970–1974	
1974	Regional, area and district health boards replace regional hospital boards, taking over public health, ambulance and other services from local authorities.		Harold Wilson Labour 1974–1976	
1975		White Paper, Better Services for the Mentally Ill, sought the expansion of local authority social services, with specialist mental health services provided through local general hospitals		
1976	**Race Relations Act**		James Callahan Labour 1976–1979	

(Continued)

Table 21.1 (Continued)

Date	Health	Social care	Political administrations	Key concepts
1978		Consultative document, A Happier Old Age, published with the intention of setting the agenda for a wide-ranging debate 'to develop a long-term strategy to ensure the well-being and dignity of all elderly people'		
1979			Margaret Thatcher Conservative 1979–1990.	
1980	**Housing Act**			
1981	Reorganisation of NHS	White Paper, Growing Older, emphasised that, in future, 'care in the community must increasingly mean care by the community' and the role of public services should be 'helping people to care for themselves and their families'		Anti-discriminatory Practice
1982			Criminal Justice Act	
1983	**Mental Health Act**	Establishment of Care in the Community initiative to support the resettlement of people from long-stay hospitals		
1984	**Police and Criminal Evidence Act**			
1988		Publication of Residential Care: A positive choice, a report of the independent review of residential care chaired by Gillian Wagner. The review had been commissioned in 1985 and set out to promote a change in the perception of residential care and its place within 'the spectrum of social care'		
1989	*Working for Patients* creates an 'internal market' with self-governing NHS Trusts and G.P. fund holding. Implemented in 1991. Children Act	Publication of the White Paper Caring for People: Community care in the next decade and beyond		

(*Continued*)

Table 21.1 (Continued)

Date	Health	Social care	Political administrations	Key concepts
1990	**NHS and Community Care Act**	**Social care** departments were given the responsibility for **community care** for older people. These services would be geared to what the older person needed rather than what was available.	John Major Conservative	
1995		**The Carers (Recognition and Services) Act** introduced the right for carers providing regular and substantial amounts of care to request an assessment of their needs when the person they are caring for is being assessed for community care services **Disability Discrimination Act.**		
1996	**Education Act**	**The Community Care (Direct Payments) Act** introduced powers for certain categories of people to be able to receive a cash payment in lieu of services that they could use to arrange their own support		
1997	Labour wins power. Pledged to 'abolish' NHS markets. Does abolish fundholding but retains purchaser-provider split.		**Tony Blair** Labour 1997–2007	
1998	**Human Rights Act**	Publication of White Paper, Modernising Social Services: Promoting independence, improving protection, raising standards Data Protection Act		
1999		Publication of With Respect to Old Age: Long term care – rights and responsibilities. Report of the Royal Commission on Long Term Care	Youth Justice and Criminal Evidence Act 1999 Crime and Disorder Act	

(Continued)

Table 21.1 (Continued)

Date	Health	Social care	Political administrations	Key concepts
2000	NHS plan – focus to improve access primary care and hospitals, with target to drive down waiting times. Carers and Disabled Children Act.	The Carers and Disabled Children Act extended carers' rights to an assessment and introduced powers for services to be provided to carers in their own right including direct payments Children (Leaving) Care Act Leaving care (services), pathway plan.		
2001	**Health and Social Care Act**	The National Service Framework for Older People set out standards to improve the quality of support in health and social care. Four themes informed the NSF: respecting the individual; developing intermediate care; providing evidence-based specialist care, and promoting healthy, active lives		Participatory action
2002	**Patient (Assisted Dying) Bill** – did not progress **Homelessness Act**			
2003	Assisted Dying for the Terminally Ill Bill – did not progress	Direct Payments Guidance: Community care, services for carers and children's services (direct payments) extended the scope of direct payments, making it a duty (and not merely a power) for direct payments to be offered to eligible people The Community Care (Delayed Discharges etc) Act introduced new duties for councils with social services responsibilities and the NHS to communicate about the discharge of patients from hospitals	Sex Offences Act 2003 Criminal Justice Act Electronic tagging, hate crime, multi-agency public protection arrangements, parole, pre-sentence report	

(*Continued*)

Table 21.1 (Continued)

Date	Health	Social care	Political administrations	Key concepts
2004	First foundation trust created. Practice-based commissioning announced. Pilots of 'choice' of hospital for routine treatments announced.	The Carers (Equal Opportunities) Act meant that carers' assessments had to take account of carers' lives in terms of employment, life-long learning and leisure activities. Carers had to be informed of their rights and local authorities could enlist the support of other agencies in supporting carers		
2005	Basic ideas for NHS reform. Delegation of budgets to G.P.s, need for independent providers to have a 'right to supply' NHS with a new 'pro-competitive' economic regulator, drawing on lessons from private utility providers.	Publication of a Green Paper, Independence, Well-being and Choice: Our vision for the future of social care for adults in England, focusing on 'choice, excellence and quality' within the context of promoting independence		
2006	**Equality Act Safeguarding Vulnerable Groups Act**	Publication of a White Paper, Our Health, Our Care, Our Say: A new direction for community services, presenting key policy reforms for health and social care focused on better prevention; more choice; tackling inequalities, and support for people with long-term needs		
2007	**Mental Health Act**		Gordon Brown Labour 2007–2010	
2008	**Care Standards Act Health and Social Care Act**	Children and Young Person's Act Independent reviewing officer, kinships care.		

(Continued)

Table 21.1 (Continued)

Date	Health	Social care	Political administrations	Key concepts
2010	NHS White paper – *Liberating the NHS*. **Education Act**	The Equality Act 2010 established equality duties for all public sector bodies which aim to integrate consideration of the advancement of equality into the day-to-day business of all bodies subject to the duty.	Crime and Security Act David Cameron Conservative, 2010–	
2011			Police and Social Responsibility Act 2011	
2012	NHS Green paper – Health and Social Care Act. **Health and Social Care Act**	The Social Value Act 2012 requires public sector commissioners – including local authorities and health sector bodies – to consider economic, social and environmental well-being in procurement of services or contracts.		
2013	Health and Social Care Act 2013	Introduced the first legal duties about health inequalities. 100 billion pounds of NHS budget 65 billion to Clinical Commissioning Groups (CCGs) of G.lPs, Nursing, the public, hospital doctors, to choose and buy (commission) services for their population from a competitive market place (mental health services, hospitals, community health services, private, voluntary sectors) monitored by Care Quality Commission. CCGs are supported by commissioning support units (collecting and analysing data, supporting commissioning, contract negotiations, contract management) and clinical senates. Around 200 CCGs overseen by 'small and live' NHS England to commission regional,	Theresa May Conservative	

(Continued)

Table 21.1 (Continued)

Date	Health	Social care	Political administrations	Key concepts
		specialist services. Local Government, Public Health England, Health and Well-being boards. Social Care is part of this process. Health Watch. www.kingsfund.org.uk		
2014	Assisted Dying Bill – did not progress			
2015	Assisted Dying (No 2) Bill – did not progress **Modern Slavery Act**		Criminal Justice and Courts Act 2015	
2016	Assisted Dying Bill – did not progress			
2018		The 70th anniversary of adult social care		
2020			Boris Johnson Conservative	The Great Pandemic of Covid
2021	White Paper *Integration and innovation: working together to improve health and social care for all* (Department of Health and Social Care, 2021)			

Index

Entries in *italics* refer to figures; entries in **bold** refer to tables.

Printed in the United States
by Baker & Taylor Publisher Services